Black...

C...e Essenti...

Emergency Medicine

Blackwell's Primary Care Essentials Series

Other books in Blackwell's Primary Care Essentials Series:

Blackwell's Primary Care Essentials: Cardiology
John Sutherland

Blackwell's Primary Care Essentials: Gastrointestinal and Liver Disease
David W. Hay

Blackwell's Primary Care Essentials: Geriatrics, Second Edition
Karen Gershman and Dennis M. McCullough

Blackwell's Primary Care Essentials: Sports Medicine
Thomas M. Howard and Janus D. Butcher

Blackwell's Primary Care Essentials: Travel Medicine
Robert P. Smith and Stephen D. Sears

Blackwell's Primary Care Essentials: Urology
Pamela Ellsworth and Stephen N. Rous

Coming Soon:

Blackwell's Primary Care Essentials: Dermatology, Second Edition
Stanford I. Lamberg

Blackwell's Primary Care Essentials: Psychiatry, Second Edition
David P. Moore

*Blackwell's Primary Care Essentials: The Complete Guide,
    Fourth Edition*
Daniel K. Onion

Blackwell's Primary Care Essentials: Emergency Medicine

Steven E. Diaz, MD

Attending, Emergency Medicine
Maine General Medical Center
Waterville, Maine

Series Editor

Daniel K. Onion, MD, MPH, FACP
Professor of Community and Family Medicine
Dartmouth Medical School
Director of Maine-Dartmouth Family Practice Residency Program
Augusta, Maine

**Blackwell
Science**

Library of Congress Cataloging-in-Publication Data

Diaz, Steven E.
    Blackwell's primary care essentials. Emergency medicine / by Steven E. Diaz.
        p. ;   cm. — (Blackwell's primary care essentials series)
    ISBN 0-86542-579-5 (pbk.)
    1. Emergency medicine.   2. Primary care (Medicine)
    [DNLM: 1. Emergencies—Handbooks. 2. Evidence-Based Medicine—Handbooks. 3. Primary Health Care—Handbooks.   WB 39 D542b 2002]   I. Title: Primary care essentials. Emergency medicine.   II. Title: Emergency medicine.   III. Title.   IV. Series.
    RC86.7.D547 2002
    616.02′5—dc21
                                                    2001002323

Acquisitions: Nancy Anastasi Duffy
Development: Julia Casson
Production: Andover Publishing Services
Manufacturing: Lisa Flanagan
Marketing Manager: Toni Fournier
Cover design by Leslie Haimes
Typeset by Graphicraft Limited, Hong Kong
Printed and bound by Edwards Brothers

Printed in the United States of America
01 02 03 04 5 4 3 2 1

The Blackwell Science logo is a trade mark of Blackwell Science Ltd., registered at the United Kingdom Trade Marks Registry

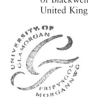

Contents

Preface   xiii
Medical Abbreviations   xv
Journal Abbreviations   xxv

1. ALLERGY   1

    1.1 Anaphylaxis   1
    1.2 Angioedema   2
    1.3 Envenomations   3
    1.4 Urticaria   5

2. CARDIOVASCULAR   7

    2.1 Acute Coronary Syndromes   7
    2.2 Atrial Fibrillation and Flutter   15
    2.3 Congestive Heart Failure   18
    2.4 Heart Block and Bradycardia   21
    2.5 Hypertensive Emergencies   22
    2.6 Infectious Endocarditis   25
    2.7 Myocarditis/Cardiomyopathy   26
    2.8 Pericarditis   28
    2.9 Paroxysmal Supraventricular Tachycardia 30
    2.10 Shock   31
    2.11 Thoracic Aortic Aneurysm/Dissection   33
    2.12 Ventricular Arrhythmias   35

3. DENTAL CONDITIONS   39

   3.1 Infection   39
   3.2 Oral Lacerations   40
   3.3 Trauma   41

4. ENDOCRINOLOGY   43

   4.1 Acute Adrenal Insufficiency   43
   4.2 Diabetic Ketoacidosis   44
   4.3 Hyperosmolar States   46
   4.4 Hypoglycemia   47
   4.5 Myxedema Coma   49
   4.6 Thyroid Storm   50

5. ENVIRONMENTAL   52

   5.1 Altitude (AMS, HAPE, HACE)   52
   5.2 Electrical Injury   55
   5.3 Frostbite   56
   5.4 Heat-Related Illnesses   57
   5.5 Hypothermia   59
   5.6 Lightning   61
   5.7 Near-Drowning   62

6. GASTROENTEROLOGY   64

   6.1 Diverticulitis   64
   6.2 Esophageal Foreign Bodies   65
   6.3 Esophageal Rupture   66
   6.4 Esophageal Varices   67
   6.5 Food-borne Illnesses   68
   6.6 Gallbladder Disease   70
   6.7 Hepatitis   72
   6.8 Infectious Diarrhea   76
   6.9 Lower GI Bleed   78
   6.10 Pancreatitis   79

6.11 Peptic Ulcer Disease/Gastritis   82
6.12 Proctitis   85
6.13 Upper GI Hemorrhage   85

7. GENERAL SURGERY   87

7.1 Abdominal Aortic Aneurysm   87
7.2 Appendicitis   88
7.3 Bowel Obstruction   89
7.4 Incarcerated Hernia (Abdominal)   90
7.5 Ischemic Bowel   92
7.6 Perforated Viscus   93
7.7 Perirectal Abscess   95
7.8 Pilonidal Cyst Abscess   96
7.9 Thrombosed Hemorrhoids   97

8. GYNECOLOGY   99

8.1 Bartholin's Cyst Abscess   99
8.2 Ovarian Cyst Rupture   100
8.3 Ovarian Torsion   101
8.4 Pelvic Inflammatory Disease   102
8.5 Sexual Assault   103
8.6 Sexually Transmitted Diseases   105
8.7 Vaginitis   110

9. HEMATOLOGY/ONCOLOGY   113

9.1 Acute Leukemia   113
9.2 Primary CNS and Spinal Cord Neoplasms   114
9.3 DIC Management   116
9.4 Febrile Neutropenic Patient   117
9.5 Hemophilia and Replacement Factor Guidelines   118
9.6 Sickle Cell Crisis   120
9.7 Transfusion Guidelines   122
9.8 Venous Thrombosis   124

10. INFECTIOUS DISEASE 127

   10.1 Fournier Gangrene 127
   10.2 HIV 128
   10.3 Lyme Disease 134
   10.4 Meningitis 136
   10.5 Periorbital Cellulitis 139
   10.6 Peritonitis (Bacterial) 140
   10.7 Rabies 142
   10.8 Sepsis 143
   10.9 Syphilis (Lues) 144
   10.10 Tetanus 147

11. METABOLIC 149

   11.1 Acidosis 149
   11.2 Calcium Disorders 150
   11.3 Magnesium Disorders 152
   11.4 Phosphorous Disorders 153
   11.5 Potassium Disorders 154
   11.6 Sodium Disorders 156

12. NEPHROLOGY 159

   12.1 Acute Renal Failure 159
   12.2 Dialysis Patient Issues 160
   12.3 Renal Calculi 161
   12.4 Urinary Retention 163
   12.5 Urinary Tract Infection 164

13. NEUROLOGY/NEUROSURGERY 168

   13.1 Acute Serotonin Syndrome 168
   13.2 Acute Stroke Syndrome 169
   13.3 Bells Palsy 176
   13.4 Increased Intracerebral Pressure 177
   13.5 Encephalitis 178

13.6   Epidural Abscess   181
13.7   Head Trauma   182
13.8   Low Back Pain   185
13.9   Migraine Headache   187
13.10 Neuroleptic Malignant Syndrome (NMS)   189
13.11 Grand Mal Seizure/Status Epilepticus   191
13.12 Spinal Cord Injury   194

14. OBSTETRICS   196

14.1 Abdominal Trauma/Uterine Rupture   196
14.2 Ectopic Pregnancy   197
14.3 Perimortem Delivery   199
14.4 Placental Abruption   200
14.5 Placenta Previa   200
14.6 Precipitous Delivery   201
14.7 Abnormal Presentations   202
14.8 Preeclampsia and Eclampsia (Toxemia)   206

15. OPHTHALMOLOGY   208

15.1 Acute Glaucoma (Angle Closure)   208
15.2 Conjunctivitis   209
15.3 Corneal Abrasion/Foreign Body   210
15.4 Herpetic Keratitis   211
15.5 Iritis   212
15.6 Ruptured Globe   213
15.7 Sudden Vision Loss (Traumatic)   214

16. ORTHOPEDICS   215

16.1 Bursitis/Tendonitis   215
16.2 Dislocations   216
16.3 Fracture Management   219
16.4 Gout/Pseudogout   229
16.5 Septic Arthritis   231

17. OTOLARYNGOLOGY 233

17.1 Barotrauma 233
17.2 Epiglottitis 234
17.3 Epistaxis 235
17.4 Foreign Bodies (Nasal, Aural, Pharyngeal) 237
17.5 Otitis Externa 238
17.6 Otitis Media 240
17.7 Parotitis/Parotid Duct Stone 242
17.8 Peritonsillar Abscess (Quinsy) 243
17.9 Streptococcal Pharyngitis 245
17.10 Retropharyngeal Abscess 246
17.11 Sinusitis 248
17.12 Vertigo 249

18. PEDIATRICS/PEDIATRIC SURGERY 251

18.1 Bronchiolitis/RSV 251
18.2 Cervical Adenitis/Cat-Scratch Disease 252
18.3 Child Abuse 253
18.4 Croup 254
18.5 Hirschsprung's Disease 255
18.6 Hypercyanotic Episode of Tetralogy of Fallot 256
18.7 Intussusception 257
18.8 Kawasaki Disease 258
18.9 Pyloric Stenosis 259
18.10 SIDS 260

19. PLASTIC SURGERY 262

19.1 Bites (Human and Animal) 262
19.2 Topical and Local Anesthesia 264
19.3 Wound Management 267

20. PROCEDURES   270

20.1 Airway Management   270
20.2 Conscious Sedation   274
20.3 Intraosseus Technique   276
20.4 Pediatric Bladder Catheterization   276
20.5 Ventricular Shunt Management   276

21. PSYCHIATRIC/SUBSTANCE ABUSE   278

21.1 Chemical and Physical Restraint   278
21.2 Delirium   279
21.3 Intoxication   280
21.4 Medical Screening Exam   282

22. PULMONARY   284

22.1 Aspirated Foreign Body   284
22.2 Asthma   285
22.3 Community-Acquired Pneumonia   287
22.4 COPD   289
22.5 Massive Hemoptysis   291
22.6 Pneumothorax   292
22.7 Pulmonary Embolus   293

23. RHEUMATOLOGY   296

23.1 Acute Rheumatic Fever (ARF)   296
23.2 Behçet's Syndrome   297
23.3 Temporal Arteritis   298

24. TOOLS   300

24.1 ACLS Guidelines   300
24.2 Apgar Scores   300
24.3 Glasgow Coma Scale   301

25. TOXICOLOGY   303

    25.1   Acetaminophen   303
    25.2   Antidepressants   305
    25.3   Aspirin   307
    25.4   Benzodiazepines   309
    25.5   Carbon Monoxide   310
    25.6   Cyanide   310
    25.7   Digitalis   312
    25.8   Ethylene Glycol   313
    25.9   Iron   314
    25.10 Isoniazid   315
    25.11 Lead   316
    25.12 Theophylline   317

26. TRAUMA   319

    26.1 Burns   319
    26.2 C-Spine   322
    26.3 Compartment Syndrome   325
    26.4 Pressure Injection Injuries   326

27. UROLOGY   327

    27.1 Epididymitis   327
    27.2 Priapism   328
    27.3 Testicular Torsion   329
    27.4 Urethritis (Males)   330

INDEX   333

Preface

The most difficult aspect of medicine is blending the art and science, and knowing the difference. Clinical medicine is undergoing large transformations in the 21st century, and the buzz word is "evidence-based."

The crux of this book is to provide information in a concise yet complete manner, taking advantage of the available data in the journals that should direct the way that we practice. Unfortunately, evidence-based medicine has many different connotations. Although my application of evidence-based emergency medicine is not unique, I should explain what it means to me.

The availability of data is overwhelming, and as of yet, we cannot rely on journal publications to be entirely correct. Critically evaluating data is a skill that must be practiced continuously in order to maintain expertise, and often times historical data has never been subject to an appropriate challenge.

In medicine, the scientific grounds that determine diagnostic or therapeutic standards may be weak in methods or statistics. Yet many times this is all that we have to offer patients. We cannot afford to disregard information based on anecdotal evidence, case reports, or even flawed studies, since it is possible that the conclusions may be correct even though the scientific support is weak.

Additionally, there are studies that are well done, but where the authors may be challenged on having reached the correct conclusion. And finally, there are the studies that are well designed *and* that have strongly supported conclusions.

When we evaluate patients, we are relying on pattern recognition to suggest potential disease processes, and this listing gives us our differential diagnoses. Based on what we have been taught and what we have researched, we then give weight to the different possibilities based on history, physical exam, and laboratory data.

As we offer therapies, we again offer interventions that we were taught and that we have researched. After time, our interventions also begin to resemble standard patterns.

Dan Onion asked me to join his collection of authors and develop this "Emergency Medicine" text. My approach was to blend historical teaching in diagnostics and therapeutics with data available in the medical journals. This is what I consider to be evidence-based, in that it is inherent that some supporting evidence is weaker than others. The key is to know where you stand when you are hypothesizing about a disease process or offering some intervention.

As mentioned above, some authors may be challenged on having reached the correct conclusions. Where a citation abstract appears to offer conclusions contrary to the text, there I believe that the study supports my conclusion. Controversies in medicine will have both "pro" and "con" articles cited.

This book is geared towards medical students, residents, and physicians practicing in primary care. It is intended to help teach and sharpen the information that comes at a rapid pace during the formative years. For those in practice, it may provide information and a framework with which to practice emergency medicine. As well, I would like to see my colleagues become more comfortable with dissecting and interpreting journal articles, and I hope that they will find this publication useful.

I had tremendous help from Lawrence Kassman, MD, my mentor, colleague, and boss, who reviewed and improved this writing. Any errors, though, are solely my own.

Steven E. Diaz, MD

Medical Abbreviations

A_2	Aortic (first) component of S_2	ALS	Amyotrophic lateral sclerosis
ab	Antibodies	ALL	Acute lymphocytic leukemia
ABGs	Arterial blood gases		
ABX	Antibiotics	ALT	SGPT; alanine transferase
ac	Before meals		
ACE	Angiotensin converting enzyme	AMI	Anterior myocardial infarction
ACEI	ACE inhibitor	AML	Acute myelogenous leukemia
Ach	Acetylcholine		
ACLS	Advanced cardiac life support	ANA	Antinuclear antibody
		ANCA	Antineutrophil cytoplasmic autoantibodies
ACTH	Adrenocorticotropic hormone		
AD	Right ear	AODM	Adult onset diabetes mellitus
ADH	Antidiuretic hormone		
ADHD	Attention deficit hyperactivity disorder	AP	Anterior-posterior
		AR	Aldose reductase
ADLs	Activities of daily living	ARA	Angiotensin receptor antagonist
AF	Atrial fibrillation	ARDS	Adult respiratory distress syndrome
AFB	Acid-fast bacillus		
Afib	Atrial fibrillation	AS	Aortic stenosis, or left ear
AFP	Alpha fetoprotein		
Aflut	Atrial flutter	ASA	Aspirin
ag	Antigen	ASCVD	Arteriosclerotic cardiovascular disease
AGN	Acute glomerular nephritis		
		ASD	Atrial septal defect
AI	Aortic insufficiency	ASHD	Arteriosclerotic heart disease
aka	Also known as		
Al	Aluminum	ASLO	Antistreptolysin O titer
ALA	α levulinic acid		

ASO	Antistreptolysin O titer	CAD	Coronary artery disease
AST	SGOT; aspartate transferase	cAMP	Cyclic AMP
asx	Asymptomatic	CAPD	Continuous ambulatory peritoneal dialysis
atm	Atmospheres		
ATN	Acute tubular necrosis		
AU	Both ears	cath	Catheterization
AV	Arteriovenous; or atrial-ventricular	CBC	Complete blood count
AVM	Ateriovenous malformation	CEA	Carcinoembryonic antigen
AVN	Avascular necrosis	cf	Compare
		CF	Complement fixation antibodies
Ba	Barium		
bact	Bacteriology	CHD	Congenital heart disease
BAL	British anti-Lewisite		
BCG	Bacille Calmette-Guérin	CHF	Congestive heart failure
BCLS	Basic cardiac life support	CI	Cardiac index
		Cl	Chloride
BCP	Birth control pill	CLL	Chronic lymphocytic leukemia
bid	twice a day		
BiPAP	Bi-level positive airway pressure	CML	Chronic myelocytic leukemia
biw	twice a week	CMP	Comprehensive metabolic profile
BJ	Bence Jones		
BM	Basement membrane	cmplc	Complications
		CMV	Cytomegalovirus
BP	Blood pressure	CN	Cranial nerve; or cyanide
BPH	Benign prostatic hypertrophy		
		CNS	Central nervous system
BS	Blood sugar		
BSE	Breast self-exam	CO	Cardiac output
BSOO	Bilateral salpingo-oophorectomy	c/o	Complaining of
		col	Colonies
BUN	Blood urea nitrogen	COPD	Chronic obstructive lung disease
bx	Biopsy		
		CP	Cerebral palsy
Ca	Calcium, or cancer depending on context	CPAP	Continuous positive airway pressure
CABG	Coronary artery bypass graft	CPC	Clinical/pathologic conference

CPK	Creatine phophokinase	DPI	Dry powder inhaler
CPR	Cardiopulmonary resuscitation	DPT	Diphtheria, pertussus, tetanus vaccine
cps	Cycles per second	DS	Double strength
CRH	Corticotropin releasing hormone	dT	Diphtheria tetanus adult vaccine
CRP	C reactive protein	DTRs	Deep tendon reflexes
crs	Course	DTs	Delerium tremens
c + s	Culture and sensitivity	DU	Duodenal ulcer
C/S	Cesarian section	DVT	Deep venous thrombosis
CSF	Cerebrospinal fluid	dx	Diagnosis or diagnostic
CT	Computerized tomography		
Cu	Copper	EACA	ε-aminocaproic acid
CVA	Cerebrovascular accident	EBV	Ebstein-Barr virus
		ECM	Erythema chronicum marginatum
CVP	Central venous pressure	EF	Ejection fraction
		EGD	Esophagogastroduo-denoscopy
d	Day(s)		
dB	Decibel	ELISA	Enzyme-linked immunosorbent assay
DBCT	Double blind controlled trial	EM	Electron microscopy
DES	Diethylstilbesterol	EMG	Electromyogram
DI	Diabetes insipidus	EMT	Emergency Medical Technician
dias	Diastolic		
DIC	Disseminated intra-vascular coagulation	Endo	Endoscopy
		Epidem	Epidemiology
dig	Digoxin	ER	Estrogen receptors; or emergency room
dip	Distal interphalangeal joint	ERCP	Endoscopic retrograde cholangio-pancreatography
DJD	Degenerative joint disease		
DKA	Diabetic ketoacidosis	ERT	Estrogen replacement therapy
DMSA	Dimercaptosuccinic acid	ESR	Erythrocyte sedimentation rate
DNA	Deoxyribonucleic acid	et	Endotracheal
d/o	Disorder	ETOH	Ethanol
DOE	Dyspnea on exertion	ETT	Exercise tolerance test
DPG	Diphosphoglycerate		

F	Female; or Fahrenheit	HBIG	Hepatitis B immune globulin
FA	Fluorescent antibody, or folic acid	HCG	Human chorionic gonadotropin
FBS	Fasting blood sugar	HCl	Hydrochloric acid
Fe	Iron	HCO_3	Bicarbonate
FFA	Free fatty acids	hct	Hematocrit
fl	Femtoliter	HDL	High density lipoprotein
FMF	Familial Mediterrranean fever	H & E	Hematoxylin and eosin
freq	Frequency	hep	Hepatitis
FSH	Follicle stimulating hormone	H. flu	Hemophilus influenza
		Hg	Mercury
FTA	Fluorescent treponemal antibody	hgb	Hemoglobin
FTT	Failure to thrive	$HgbA_1C$	Hemoglobin A_1C level
f/u	Follow up	HGH	Human growth hormone
FUO	Fever of unknown origin	5-HIAA	5-Hydroxy indole acedic acid
FVC	Forced vital capacity	Hib	Hemophilus influenza B vaccine
fx	Fracture		
		his	Histidine
g	Gauge	HIV	Human immunodeficiency virus
GABA	γ-Aminobutyric acid		
gc	Gonorrhea		
GE	Gastroesophageal		
GFR	Glomerular filtration rate	HLA	Human leukocyte antigens
GHRH	Growth hormone releasing hormone	HMG-COA	Hydroxymethylglutaryl-coenzyme A
gi	Gastrointestinal	h/o	History of
glu	glucose	H + P	History and physical
glut	Glutamine	hpf	High power field
gm	Gram	HPV	Human papilloma virus
GN	Glomerulonephritis		
GnRH	Gonadotropin releasing hormone	hr	Hour(s)
GTT	Glucose tolerance test	HRIG	Human rabies immune globulin
gtts	Drops	hs	At bedtime
gu	Genitourinary	HSP	Henoch-Schönlein purpura
GVHD	Graft vs. host disease		

HSV	Herpes simplex virus	IUD	Intrauterine device
HT	Hypertension	IUGR	Intrauterine growth
5HT	5-Hydroxytryptophan		retardation
HUS	Hemolytic uremic	IVC	Inferior vena cava
	syndrome	IVP	Intravenous pyleogram
HVA	Homovanillic acid	IWMI	Inferior wall
hx	History		myocardial infarction
I or I_2	Iodine	J	Joule
IBD	Inflammatory bowel	JODM	Juvenile onset diabetes
	disease		mellitus
ICU	Intensive care unit	JRA	Juvenile rheumatoid
I + D	Incision and drainage		arthritis
IDDM	Insulin dependent	JVD	Jugular venous
	diabetes melitus		distension
IEP	Immunoelectrophoresis	JVP	Jugular venous
IF	Intrinsic factor		pressure/pulse
IFA	Immunofluorescent		
	antibody	K	Potassium
IgA	Immunoglobulin A	kg	Kilogram
IgE	Immunoglobulin E	KOH	Potassium hydroxide
IgG	Immunoglobulin G	KS	Kaposi's sarcoma
IgM	Immunoglobulin M	KUB	Abdominal X-ray
IHSS	Idiopathic hyper-		("kidneys, ureters,
	trophicsubaortic		bladder")
	stenosis		
im	Intramuscular	L	Liter; or left
incr	Increased	LA	Left atrium; or
INH	Isoniazid		long acting if after a
INR	International		drug
	normalized ratio	LAP	Leukocyte alkaline
IP	Interphalangeal		phosphatase
IPG	Impedance	LBBB	Left bundle branch
	plethysmography		block
IPPB	Intermittent positive	LDH	Lactate dehydrogenase
	pressure breathing	LDL	Low density
IPPD	Intermediate purified		lipoproteins
	protein derivative	LES	Lower esophageal
ITP	Idiopathic thrombo-		sphincter
	cytopenic purpura	LFTs	Liver function tests
IU	International units	LH	Luteinizing hormone

LMW	Low molecular weight	MRFIT	Multiple risk factor intervention trial
LP	Lumbar puncture	MRI	Magnetic resonance imaging
LS	Lumbosacral		
LV	Left ventricle	MRSA	Methicillin resistant staph aureus
LVH	Left ventricular hypertrophy	MS	Multiple sclerosis; or mitral stenosis
lytes	Electrolytes		
		mtx	Methotrexate
m	Meter(s)	Multip	Multiparous pt
M	Male	μ	Micron
MAI	Mycobacterium avium intracellulare	μgm	Microgram
MAO	Monamine oxidase	Na	Sodium
mcp	Metacarpal-phalangeal joint(s)	NCI	National Cancer Institute
MD	Muscular dystrophy; or physician	neb	nebulizer
		neg	negative
MDI	Metered dose inhaler	NG	Nasogastric
meds	Medications	NH₃	Ammonia
MEN	Multiple endocrine neoplasias	NICU	Newborn intensive care unit
mEq	Millieqivalent	NIDDM	Noninsulin-dependent diabetes mellitus
mets	Metastases		
METS	Metabolic equivalents	nl	Normal
mg	Milligram	nL	Nanoliter
Mg	Magnesium	nm	Nanometer
MHC	Major histocompatibility locus	NNH	Number needed to harm
MI	Myocardial infarction; or mitral insufficiency	NNT	Number needed to treat
MIC	Minimum inhibitory concentration	NPH	Normal pressure hydrocephalus
min	Minute	npo	Nothing by mouth
MMR	Measles, mumps, rubella	NS	Normal saline
		NSAID	Nonsteroidal anti-inflammatory drug
mOsm	Milliosmole/s		
mp	Metocarpal phalangeal	NSR	Normal sinus rythmn
6MP	6-mercaptopurine	NST	Nonstress test
MR	Mitral regurgitation	Nullip	Nulliparous pt
MRA	Magnetic resonance angiography	NV + D	Nausea, vomiting and diarrhea

O₂	Oxygen	PCTA	Percutaneous transluminal angioplasty
OB	Obstetrics		
OCD	Obsessive compulsive disorder	PCR	Polymerase chain reaction
OD	Overdose; or right eye		
OGTT	Oral glucose tolerance test	PCWP	Pulmonary capillary wedge pressure
OH	Hydroxy-	PDA	Patent ductus arteriosus
OM	Otitis media		
op	Operative, or outpatient	PEG	Percutaneous endoscopic gastrostomy
O + P	Ova and parasites		
OPV	Oral polio vaccine	PEP	Protein electrophoresis
OS	Left eye	PFTs	Pulmonary function tests
osm	Osmoles		
OTC	Over the counter	PG	Prostaglandin
OU	Both eyes	phos	Phosphatase
oz	Ounce	PI	Pulmonic insufficiency
		PID	Pelvic inflammatory disease
P	Pulse		
P₂	Pulmonary (2nd) component of S₂	PIH	Pregnancy induced hypertension
PA	Pernicious anemia; or pulmonary artery	pip	Proximal interphalangeal joint
PABA	Paraminobenzoic acid	PMI	Point of maximal impulse of heart
PAC	Premature atrial contraction	PMNLs	Polymorphonuclear leukocytes
PAF	Paroxysmal atrial fibrillation	PMR	Polymyalgia rheumatica
PAN	Polyarteritis nodosa		
Pap	Papanicolaou	PND	Paroxysmal nocturnal dyspnea
PAP	Pulmonary artery pressure	PNH	Paroxysmal hemoglobinuria
par	Parenteral		
PAS	p-Amino salicylic acid	po	By mouth
PAT	Paroxysmal atrial tachycardia	PO₄	Phosphate
		polys	Polymorphonuclear leukocytes
Pathophys	Pathophysiology		
Pb	Lead	pos	Positive
PBG	Porphobilinogen	ppd	Pack per day
PCP	Pneumocystis pneumonia	PPD	Tuberculin skin test
		PPG	Protoporphyrinogen

pr	By rectum	RDS	Respiratory distress syndrome
pRBBB	Partial right bundle branch block	re	About
pre-op	Pre-operative	REM	Rapid eye movement
prep	Preparation	RES	Reticuloendothelial system
primip	Primiparous pt	retic	Reticulocyte/s
prn	As needed	Rh	Rhesus factor
PROM	Premature rupture of membranes	RHD	Rheumatic heart disease
PS	Pulmonic stenosis	RIA	Radioimmunoassay
PSA	Prostate specific antigen	RIBA	Radio-immuno blot assay
PSVT	Paroxysmal supraventricular tachycardia	RMSF	Rocky mountain spotted fever
PT	Protime	ROM	Range of motion
pt(s)	Patient(s)	ROS	Review of systems
PTH	Parathormone	RNP	Ribonucleoprotein
PTT	Partial thromboplastin time	R/O	Rule out
		RSI	Rapid sequence intubation
PUD	Peptic ulcer disease	RSV	Respiratory syncytial virus
PVC	Premature ventricular tachycardia	RTA	Renal tubular acidosis
q	Every	rv	Review
qd	Daily	RV	Right ventricle
qid	4 times a day	RVH	Right ventricular hypertrophy
qod	Every other day	rx	Treatment
qow	Every other week		
qt	Quart	S_1	First heart sound
		S_2	Second heart sound
R	Right, or respirations	S_3	Third heart sound, gallop
RA	Rheumatoid arthritis		
RAIU	Radioactive iodine uptake	S_4	Fourth heart sound, gallop
RAST	Radioallergosorbent test	SAB	Spontaneous abortion
RBBB	Right bundle branch block	SAH	Subarachnoid hemorrhage
rbc	Red blood cell	Sb	Antimony
RCT	Randomized controlled trial	SBE	Subacute bacterial endocarditis

sc	Subcutaneous	T°	Fever/temperature
SD	Standard deviation	T_3	Triiodothyronine
sens	Sensitivity	T_4	Thyroxin
SER	Smooth endoplasmic reticulum	TA	Temporal arteritis
		T + A	Tonsillectomy and adenoidectomy
serol	Serology(ies)		
SGA	Small for gestational age	tab	Tablet
		TAH	Total abdominal hysterectomy
si	Signs		
SI	Sacroiliac	tbc	Tuberculosis
SIADH	Syndrome of inappropriate ADH	TCAs	Tricyclic antidepressants
SIDS	Sudden infant death syndrome	TBG	Thyroid binding globulin
sl	Sublingual	tcn	Tetracycline
SLE	Systemic lupus erythematosis	Td	Tetanus/diphtheria, adult type
SNF	Skilled nursing facility	TEE	Transesophageal echocardiogram
soln	Solution		
s/p	Status post	TENS	Transcutaneious electrical nerve stimulation
specif	Specificity		
SPEP	Serum protein electrophoresis		
		Tfx	Transfusion
SR	Slow release	THC	Tetrahydro-cannabinol
SRS	Slow reacting substance		
		TI	Tricuspid insufficiency
SS	Sickle cell disease	TIA	Transient ischemic attack
SSKI	Saturated solution of potassium iodide		
		TIBC	Total iron binding capacity
SSRI	Selective serotonin reuptake inhibitor	tid	3 times a day
SSS	Sick sinus syndrome	TIPS	Transjugular intrahepatic porto-systemic shunt
Staph	Staphylococcus		
STD	Sexually transmitted disease		
		tiw	Three times a week
STS	Serologic test for syphilis	TM	Tympanic membrane
		Tm	Trimethoprim
SVC	Superior vena cava	Tm/S	Trimethoprim/sulfa
SVT	Supraventricular tachycardia	TNF	Tumor necrosis factor
		TNG	Nitroglycerine
sx	Symptom(s)	TPA	Tissue plasminogen activator
sys	Systolic		

TPN	Total parental nutrition	VIP	Vasoactive intestinal peptide
TRH	Thyroid releasing hormone	vit	Vitamin
TS	Tricuspid stenosis	VLDL	Very low density lipoprotein
TSH	Thyroid stimulating hormone	VMA	Vanillymandelic acid
TTP	Thrombotic thrombocytopenic purpura	vol	Volume
		V/Q	Ventilation/perfusion
		VSD	Ventricular septal defect
TURP	Transurethral resection of prostate	VT	Ventricular tachycardia
U	Units	Vtach	Ventricular tachycardia
UA	Urinanalysis	V-ZIG	Varicella-zoster immune globulin
UBO	Unidentified bright object		
UGI	Upper gastrointestinal	W/s	Watt/seconds
UGIS	Upper GI series	w/u	Work up
URI	Upper respiratory illness	wbc	White blood cells or white blood count
US	Ultrasound	wgt	Weight
USPTF	US preventive task force	wk	Week(s)
		WNL	Within normal limits
UTI	Urinary tract infection	WPW	Wolff-Parkinson-White Syndrome (short PR interval)
UV	Ultraviolet		
UVA	Ultraviolet A		
UVB	Ultraviolet B	yr	Year(s)
vag	vaginally	ZE	Zollinger-Ellison syndrome
val	Valine		
VCUG	Vesico-urethrogram	Zn	Zinc
VDRL	Serologic test for syphilis ("Venereal Disease Research Lab")	>	More than
		>>	Much more than
		<	Less than
		<<	Much less than
VF	Ventricular fibrillation	→	Leads to (eg, in a chemical reaction)
Vfib	Ventricular fibrillation		

Journal Abbreviations

The journal abbreviations from the National Library of Medicine were used throughout the book. Some common examples are the following:

Acad Emerg Med	Academic Emergency Medicine
Ann Allergy	Annals of Allergy
Ann Emerg Med	Annals of Emergency Medicine
Am Family Physician	American Family Physician
Ann Intern Med	Annals of Internal Medicine
Arch Intern Med	Archives of Internal Medicine
Arch Surg	Archives of Surgery
BMJ	British Medical Journal
Clin Obstet Gynecol	Clinical Obstetrics and Gynecology
Crit Care Med	Critical Care Medicine
Emerg Med Clin N Am	Emergency Medicine Clinics of North America
Eur Heart J	European Heart Journal
Eur J Cardiol	European Journal of Medicine
JAMA	Journal of the American Medical Association
J Am Coll Cardiol	Journal of the American College of Cardiology
J Emerg Med	Journal of Emergency Medicine
J Trauma	Journal of Trauma
Med Clin N Am	Medical Clinics of North America
Med Lett Drugs Ther	The Medical Letter on Drugs and Therapeutics
NEJM	New England Journal of Medicine

Notice

The indications and dosages of all drugs in this book have been recommended in the medical literature and conform to the practices of the general community. The medications described do not necessarily have specific approval by the Food and Drug Administration for use in the diseases and dosages for which they are recommended. The package insert for each drug should be consulted for use and dosage as approved by the FDA. Because standards for usage change, it is advisable to keep abreast of revised recommendations, particularly those concerning new drugs.

1 Allergy

1.1 ANAPHYLAXIS

Med Clin North Am 1992:841; Ann Allergy 1992:87

Cause: Aspiration, ingestion, and/or parenteral use of drugs or other haptens including foreign antigens (insect stings), desensitization shots, semen, or polysaccharides

Epidem: True anaphylaxis not common

Pathophys: Respiratory distress due to both upper tract edema and lower tract bronchospasm, consider leukotrienes, also known as slow-reacting substance. Histamine release causes hypotension. Diarrhea and GI symptoms due to serotonin. Some reactions not IgE mediated

Sx: Dizziness, dyspnea, pruritus, nausea, vomiting, diarrhea

Si: Diffuse erythema (lobster red skin), tachypnea, decreased breath sounds, hypotension, altered mental status

Crs: Onset in 1/2–3 minutes, death usually in 15–120 minutes; recurs in 28% if rechallenged

Cmplc: Respiratory or vascular collapse, death

Lab: Check for other reasons for respiratory and/or vascular collapse, and monitor vital functions: CBC with diff, ABG, serum tryptase level (Lik Sprava 1992:76)—increases and helps distinguish from other forms of shock, EKG, pan culture, metabolic profile, CXR, ETOH, urine toxic screen, O_2 sat

Prehospital Rx: Epinephrine as below (Ann Emerg Med 1995:785)

ED Rx:
- Secure airway
- IV access (Crit Care Clin 1993:313)
- Trendelenburg if hypotensive, short term (J Trauma 1986:718) with potentially minimal effects (Ann Emerg Med 1985:641; Crit Care Med 1979:218)

- Epinephrine 0.5–1.0 mg IV or IM; peds dose 0.01 cc/kg of 1:1000; not SC (J Allergy Clin Immunol 1998:33)
- Diphenhydramine 25–50 mg IV (peds 1 mg/kg) (J Appl Physiol 1988:210; J Allergy Clin Immunol 1990:684)
- Methylprednisolone 125 mg IV (peds 2 mg/kg) (Ann Allergy 1989:201)
- O_2
- Nebulizers (beta agonists, ipratropium)
- Selective H_2 blockers controversial but may dose cimetidine 300 mg IV (Ann Allergy 1987:447)
- Aminophylline controversial (9 mg/kg load, 0.7 mg/kg/hr) (Br J Pharmacol 1980:467)

1.2 ANGIOEDEMA

J Am Acad Dermatol 1991:146; Pediatr Rev 1992:387

Cause: Genetic, autosomal dominant type (Clin Immunol Immunopathol 1991:S78); medications (e.g., ACE inhibitors), foods (e.g., beer), environmental challenges, bacteria (e.g., hep C, not *Helicobacter pylori*), drugs of abuse (e.g., cocaine)

Epidem: Most Western races

Pathophys: Deficiency of inhibitor of complement C'1a esterase, which also inactivates clotting factors XII and XI; the latter build up and release kallikreins/kinins, causing pain, shock, etc. (Blood 1991:2660)

Sx: Frequently precipitated by trauma, psychological stress; pharyngitis; abdominal pain

Si: Edema of skin, upper GI tract, and respiratory tracts; recurrent, acute, nonpitting, nonpruritic, circumscribed, transient; involves localized areas; edema of uvula (Quincke's edema (Arch Otolaryngol Head Neck Surg 1991:100))

Crs: Onset not until 20–50 years of age

Cmplc: Laryngeal edema causing asphyxia (26% of patients die this way); R/O the following:
- Acquired angioedema—common, benign—Rx with prednisone plus hydroxyzine
- "Pseudo-angioedema" associated with lymphoma and colon CA

- Uvular edema of Franklin's disease (N Engl J Med 1993:1389)—a B-cell lymphoma with uvular edema as a prominent symptom
- ACE inhibitor angioedema (Immunopharmacology 1999:21)

Lab: Assess for other reasons and severity of airway compromise—CBC with diff, ABG, carbon monoxide level, urine tox screen

ED Rx:
- See 1.1
- C′1a inhibitor forms vapor-heated pooled plasma concentrate

1.3 ENVENOMATIONS

Crit Care Clin 1999:353, ix; Pediatr Rev 1999:147, quiz 151)

Cause: Bites from spiders and reptiles, or scorpion stings

Epidem: Annual number of significant spider envenomations in the U.S. is not well known but about 50 species in the U.S. are considered dangerous. Approximately 8,000 envenomous snakebites occur per year in the U.S. with about 19 species being responsible. Scorpion stings are also difficult to track, but only *Centruroides exilicauda* produces a significant systemic envenomation response. *C. exilicauda* is also known as the black scorpion

Pathophys: Local or systemic reactions may occur. The venom may carry a variety of proteins that may cause local tissue destruction due to proteases, phosphatases, lipase, and complement system inhibitors, such as seen in the *Loxosceles reclusa*, or brown recluse spider. Neurotoxic proteins may also play a factor, such as in the black widow spider venom. Other venoms may carry a combination of local tissue destructors and neuroproteins, such as seen in rattlesnake venom. The black scorpion venom carries proteins that activate sodium channels—the resultant neurologic sequela is that of firing of sympathetic, parasympathetic, and somatic efferent nerves. Others such as scorpions may carry proteins which disrupt K^+ channels (Methods Enzymol 1999:624)

Sx: Pain, edema, and erythema. Possibly systemic reaction, including blurry vision, difficulty breathing, difficulty swallowing, dizziness, muscle fatigue or stiffness

Si: Puncture wound, ulceration, local tissue necrosis, muscular rigidity, ptosis, respiratory distress, drooling, nausea, vomiting, hypotension, tachycardia

Crs: Variable course depending on type of envenomation, dose and depth of wound
- Spider and snakebites generally respond to general supportive measures, with severe respiratory and neurologic problems weaning after 2–3 days, and hematologic complications taking longer to resolve
- Scorpion stings initiate neurologic compromise that should respond to airway management and antivenin—scorpion sting antivenin pro (Toxicon 1999:1627) and con (J Toxicol Clin Toxicol 1999:51)

Cmplc: Shock, airway edema, coagulopathy (coagulopathy not seen in scorpion stings)

Lab:
- CBC with diff, metabolic profile, PT/PTT, ABG, CPK, U/A
- R/O other causes of airway compromise and shock: ETOH, urine toxic screen, EKG, consider lateral neck X-ray, consider head CT (consideration of CNS insult with neurogenic pulmonary edema); if coagulopathy suspected: d-dimer, fibrin split products, fibrinogen

ED Rx:
- Airway and shock management, with specific antivenin therapy if indicated
- Consider pretreatment with IV methylprednisolone and/or diphenhydramine for antivenin pretreatment, or IV midazolam for muscle fasciculations (Ann Emerg Med 1999:620)
- State Poison Control for specific guidelines; Jeffrey Bernstein in Tampa, FL, at 1-813-251-6911 or 1-813-253-4444 for clinical questions; Wyeth Labs at 1-800-934-5556 for questions regarding use and availability of antivenin
- Local measures for wound cleaning; perhaps constriction band between bite and torso although not proven effective; specific antivenin measures such as suction, incision, ice, or electric therapy have not been shown to be effective

1.4 URTICARIA

Clin Exp Allergy 1999:31; Clin Exp Dermatol 1999:424

Cause: 80% idiopathic, and as under **Pathophys**.

Epidem: 25% of adult population has had chronic urticaria (including mild form)

Pathophys: Direct histamine release by opiates, NSAIDs, IVP dye, thiamine, curare, dextrans, and some antibiotics; ubiquitous involvement of cytokines (J Allergy Clin Immunol 1999:307)

Immunologic

- C′ activation by cryoglobulins (IgG or cold agglutinins produced by tumors, multiple myeloma, SLE, arteritis, etc.) or by B1C globulin damage (snake venom, DIC). Angioneurotic edema is C′ mediated but not urticaria
- Antibodies vs. mast cells or, in chronic urticaria, their IgE receptors
- Mast cells as "innocent bystanders," e.g., SLE, serum sickness, antigens in all lesions, leukemias, and other malignancies, drugs, parasites, hepatitis B, perhaps mononucleosis plus ampicillin; nearly all recurrent erythema multiforme and most primary episodes are due to herpes simplex, but a few of the latter are due to mycoplasma and drugs
- Mast cell fixed antibody (IgE), e.g., to fish, bee sting, PCN
- Type IV (DHS) immune reaction leads to vasculitis

Physical/"Neurogenic"

- Cold urticaria (test with ice cube); perhaps IgE attaches to a cold-dependent skin antigen and releases platelet-activating factor (N Engl J Med 1985:405)
- Local heat urticaria
- Systemic heat urticaria, cholinergic, seen when core body temperature is elevated; starts around hair follicles; seen in runners, tennis players, etc.
- Light/solar
- Stress
- Dermatographia

Associated Diseases

- Urticaria pigmentosa occasionally and anaphylaxis

Sx: Itching, mucosal swelling (with all but physical types), and abdominal pain

Si: Target skin lesion of erythema multiforme, raised urticarial lesions; bilateral symmetry always suggests drug-induced first

Crs: Most lesions last <24 hours except in vasculitis, immunologic and physical types

Cmplc: Epidermal detachment of mucous membranes, locally in Stevens-Johnson syndrome with 5% mortality, or extensively in toxic epidermal necrolysis with 30% mortality

Lab: Consider R/O of toxic shock and vasculitis: CBC with diff, liver profile, metabolic profile, ESR, U/A; skin biopsy at time of urticaria to also R/O vasculitis

ED Rx: Avoid ACE inhibitors and NSAIDs; 2% ephedrine spray for angioedema; H_1 receptor antagonist antihistamines like loratadine 10 mg po qd (Drugs 1999:31); H_2 blockers like cimetidine with equivocal efficacy (J Allergy Clin Immunol 1995:685)
- Acute Rx: see 1.1
- Chronic: hydroxyzine 25 mg po tid-qid, cetirizine 10 mg po qd (Ann Pharmacother 1996:1075), or terfenadine 60 mg po bid (Ann Allergy 1989:616)
- Cold urticaria: cyproheptadine best (Arch Dermatol 1977:1375); doxepin 10–25 mg po bid (J Am Acad Dermatol 1984:483)
- Heat (cholinergic) type: hydroxyzine
- Vasculitis: steroids
- Mast cell types: ketotifen 2 mg po bid stabilizes mast cells (Ann Allergy 1989:322); acyclovir for, at least, recurrent erythema multiforme

2 Cardiovascular

2.1 ACUTE CORONARY SYNDROMES

Int J Cardiol 1995:S3; J Thromb Thrombolysis 1999:113

Events that have sudden onset and could lead to significant morbidity or mortality if not recognized, such as myocardial infarction, myocardial stunning, coronary artery vasospasm, or unstable angina

Cause: Atherosclerosis (85%) including spasm with superimposed thrombus in 90% of these, emboli (15%), and now occasionally cocaine-induced spasm when used as anesthesia or as a recreational drug

Epidem:

Increased Incidence with History of the Following:

- Carbon monoxide acute exposures (e.g., firefighters) and chronic carbon disulfide exposures (e.g., disulfiram use, rayon manufacturing) (Arch Environ Health 1989:361; N Engl J Med 1989:1426)
- Cholesterol elevations of total and/or LDL (Jama 1998:445). Consider with cholecystitis history, presence of an arcus senilis (Am Heart J 1965:838; Br Heart J 1970:449)
- Lack of hormone replacement in women who would benefit, less of an association with oral contraceptives (Can J Cardiol 1999:419)
- Cocaine use or withdrawal (J Am Coll Cardiol 1990:74)
- Coffee data equivocal (J Epidemiol Community Health 1999:481)
- Exercise test showing ischemia—limited in asymptomatic individuals (Aviat Space Environ Med 1982:379); most sensitive is MIBI-SPECT with dobutamine infusion and most specific is stress echocardiography (Heart 1998:370)
- Family history of MIs prematurely (age <55 years males, <65 years females) (Prev Med 1980:773; Am J Cardiol 1988:708; Br Heart J 1982:78; N Engl J Med 1994:1041)

- Homocysteine levels >15 μM/L correlate with worse prognosis; data equivocal (Semin Interv Cardiol 1999:121; Circulation 1998:204)
- Hypertension (Am Heart J 1988:1713)
- Diabetes mellitus (Am Heart J 1988:1713)
- Sedentary work or lifestyle (Scand J Work Environ Health 1979:100)
- Sexual activity can induce myocardial ischemia, silent or symptomatic (Am J Cardiol 1995:835)
- Smoking increases risk 3 times, but risk decreases to normal over 2 years after cessation; increases risk 5 times if >1 ppd, 2 times if 1–4 cigarettes per day in women; also passive smoking (N Engl J Med 1999:920). Smokers usually have thrombogenic MI rather than diffuse vessel disease, and the mortality/morbidity benefits seen from smoking are due to lack of other risk factors and relative youth of this population—NOT a protective effect of smoking (J Cardiovasc Risk 1999:307)
- Stress, day-to-day but not type A nor distressed personality; possibly hostility (Psychol Rep 1999:505)
- Viral URI in past 2 weeks, or chronic *Chlamydia pneumoniae* infections—pro (Ann Intern Med 1992:273; J Am Coll Cardiol 1998:827) and con (Clin Cardiol 1999:85). Perhaps chronic *Helicobacter pylori* infection as well (Bmj 1995:711)
- Perioperative without β-blockade

Decreased Incidence with:
- Exercise walking or vigorous exercise 3–4 times a week (N Engl J Med 1999:650)
- Fish intake 1–4 times/month (N Engl J Med 1985:1205)
- Daily ASA 325 mg po qod (N Engl J Med 1989:129)
- ETOH 2–3 drinks qd in men vs. 2–3/week in women (Bmj 1999:1523)
- Better control of hypertension, cholesterol, etc., in U.S. (N Engl J Med 1999:1994; 1999:410)

Pathophys: Platelet aggregations and thrombi on plaque fissures cause thrombosis with or without spasm (Intern Med 2000:333), or paradoxical vasoconstriction with stress because plaque prevents normal endothelial cell induction of coronary dilatation

Sx: Chest pain, substernal, in "distribution of a tree," worse supine; diaphoresis, dyspnea; associated with heavy exertion 5–40 times more frequently depending on conditioning state; atypical presentations in women; CNS Sx are the presenting Sx in 50% of patients over 60 years old

Si: Pericardial rub on day 2+, usually without ST changes; S_4 gallop; fever <103°F (39.4°C); transient S_2 paradoxical split. Rectal exam important for guaiac

Crs:

- 25% are unrecognized and half are asymptomatic—yet prognosis is just as bad (N Engl J Med 1984:1144); 15% in-hospital mortality before thrombolytics, now 7–10%; 10% of survivors get severe pump failure, another 10% get persistent angina, 10% flunk discharge mini-ETT, another 10% flunk maximal ETT at 6-week follow-up; remaining 50% do fine (J Cardiovasc Risk 1999:69)
- Age-adjusted survival for women may be worse when compared to men, but studies have yet to prove (Am J Cardiol 2000:147)—treatment should be gender-blind
- Cardiac arrest survival is 3.5% in out-of-hospital CPR, 8.8% if VF/VT; more survivors if bystander CPR initiated (Ann Emerg Med 1999:44)
- In elderly, aggressive invasive study and Rx do not improve mortality

Cmplc:

- Altered binding proteins change meaning of measured levels of quinidine, cholesterol, etc.
- Aneurysm of left ventricle occurs in 40% of those with anterior MI and 13.5% overall, develops in first 48 hours, leads to emboli, CHF, and PVCs, 75% 5-year mortality (Eur Heart J 1990:441)
- Anxiety neurosis, impotence
- Arrhythmias (Physiol Rev 1999:917; Eur Heart J 1999:748); Afib is a risk factor for worse outcome (J Am Coll Cardiol 1997:406)
- CHF
- Dressler syndrome (Cardiol Clin 1990:601), which may be on a continuum of pericarditis of AMI; this may lead to pericardial tamponade from inflammation (R/O RV infarct) since both functionally and acutely constrict pericardial space by fluid or dilated RV
- Heart block occurs in 5% of inferior MIs, 3% of anterior MIs, and in 100% with anterior MI + RBBB causing a 75% mortality (Chest 1976:599; Am J Cardiol 1992:1135)
- Mural thrombi without aneurysm in 11% of acute MIs, 2% of others

CARDIOVASCULAR

- Papillary muscle rupture causes CHF with a normal-sized left atrium by TEE; occurs most often with inferior MIs, and surgery
- Rupture of septal wall to create a VSD or rupture into pericardial sac causing tamponade
- Shock
- Nonhemorrhagic stroke, especially if EF <28% post MI, older age, h/o hypertension or other common stroke risk factors—prevent with warfarin anticoagulation (Circulation 1998:757)

Lab:

Chem

Markers (J Am Coll Cardiol 1999:739; Scand J Clin Lab Invest Suppl 1999:103)—these results may alter hospital course, but should not be the determining factors for those who need admission for cardiac evaluation (Heart 1999:614). CPK and troponin may be "erroneously" elevated in those with renal failure (Nephrol Dial Transplant 1999:1489). Serial evaluation in ED may increase yield for those having acute MIs (Acad Emerg Med 1997:869)

CPK and fractions are up in 12 hours, peak at 2 days, and last 4 days; CPK-MB subfractions MB2 and MB1 rise in first 6 hours after onset of pain and have 95% sensitivity and specificity. Total CPK correlates with MI size; may double in MI but still be less than upper limit of normal. MB band is increased also by increased death and regeneration of skeletal muscle and by decreased clearance in myxedema. MM is increased by hypothyroidism, myopathy. BB band is increased by CNS and/or smooth muscle damage

Cardiac troponin I and T levels elevate in 4–6 hours and are specific to myocardium (Am Heart J 1999:1137); they have 95–100% sensitivity, 22–33% specific for infarction but "false positives" really represent ischemia (unstable angina) (Clin Chim Acta 1999:161) with suggestive history—other etiologies are possible such as sepsis, endocrine, cardiomyopathy, renal failure, and other chronic diseases (Am J Emerg Med 1999:225). Higher levels correlate with worse outcomes (Am J Cardiol 1999:1281); also used perioperatively when surgery may increase CPK

Myoglobin peaks early (2 hours) and is sensitive, but not specific (Ann Emerg Med 1987:851)

LDH and fractions: isoenzymes 4 and 5 (rapidly migrating) increased; R/O renal and red cell source

AST (SGOT) up in 24 hours, peaks at 2–4 days, lasts up to 7 days

Acute phase reactants (C-reactive protein, fibrinogen) and troponin T may have prognostic value if they are elevated (N Engl J Med 2000:1139)

Noninvasive Lab

Echo for mitral regurgitation, aneurysm, ejection fraction estimation, and mural thrombi with 77% sensitivity and 93% specificity. Also looking for wall motion abnormalities—cannot tell us onset of wall motion problems

EKG may show ST elevation (50% sensitivity), duration of elevation correlates with extent of injury, height of at least 1 mm in limb leads and 2 mm in precordial leads; sum of elevation correlates directly with severity of injury (and thus prognosis) (Jama 1998:387); T wave inversions (R/O acute cholecystitis). Persistent ST elevation anteriorly has low association with LV aneurysm (Am J Cardiol 1984:84; Eur Heart J 1994:1500). New RBBB indicates occlusion of anterior descending proximal to first septal branch, new complete right or left bundle branch block denotes higher mortality (J Am Coll Cardiol 1998:105). LBBB to be treated as ST elevation even in patient with ASHD, old LBBB, and a history and physical consistent with acute infarct—i.e., thrombolytic candidate per protocol

Serial EKGs in ED less helpful than serial serum markers (Ann Emerg Med 1992:1445)

ETT

May be useful if done from ED in patients who do not have known CAD, an evolving MI, or unstable angina based on EKG and serial markers, yet they are stable and no plausible explanation for their symptoms; heart rate recovery in first minute is predictive (N Engl J Med 1999:1351)

Radiology

Ventriculogram with technetium scan; ejection fraction—if <40%, 1-year mortality climbs steeply from 5%

Other Reasons for Abnormal EKG or Cardiac Injury

CBC with diff, metabolic profile, CXR, drug reactions (see **Epidemiology**)

Prehospital Rx:
- O_2, IV access
- ASA
- Nitroglycerin and MSO_4

- Prehospital thrombolytics have not been shown to improve outcome and will probably have high skill attrition secondary to paucity of use (Am Heart J 1991:1), but field EKG with telemetry to ED does help (Am Heart J 1992:835)

ED Rx for Acute MI:

(N Engl J Med 1997:847)

Pharmacologic

- O_2
- ASA 81 mg, 2–4 tabs po immediately; no difference in regular vs. prostacyclin-sparing ASA (Eur Heart J 1994:1196)
- Heparin: unfractionated vs. LMWH (J Am Coll Cardiol 2000:1699)
- Thrombolysis with streptokinase, TPA, Retavase, etc.—TPA best (N Engl J Med 1993:673):
  1) Helps all patients including those over 75 years of age
  2) If systolic BP ≥175 or diastolic ≥100, bleeding risk is double
  3) Use if pain is <6 hours duration, or if 6–12 hours and STs still elevated, or LBBB and compelling history
  4) More effective re mortality if used in smokers (Qjm 1999:327)
  5) Potential complications include bleeding, such as intracranial, cardiac rupture (J Am Coll Cardiol 1999:479), or intra-abdominal; intracranial associated with older age and hypertension (Am J Cardiol 1991:166)
  6) Contraindications may include recent stroke, recent major surgery, recent major dental work, trauma, hemoptysis, hematemesis, melena, hematochezia, hematuria, cancer, new headaches, bleeding diathesis, or history of aneurysms
  7) Not for ST depression even if markers positive
- G IIb/IIIa agents (Drugs 1999:609) helpful around time of catheterization (Am J Cardiol 1999:779); but not proven to be helpful otherwise in combination with thrombolytics at this time; ongoing trials to assess whether lower thrombolytic doses could be used if G IIb/IIIa agents given in conjunction (Lancet 2000:337)
- MSO_4 IV to decrease pain
- β-blocker within 24 hours of MI (OK to give in ED and continue indefinitely), helps prevent recurrent MIs and fatal ventricular arrhythmias in all (including the elderly) (Prog Cardiovasc Dis 1993:261), increase survival for 6+ years; one example for loading is metoprolol 5 mg IV over 5 minutes × 3 and then 50–100 mg po
- ACE inhibitors within 24 hours of MI and for 6 weeks, but continue indefinitely if EF <40%; may also help with CHF

emergently as long as no AS with captopril 6.25 mg SL; captopril 50 mg tid increases ETT performance and decreases LV size, especially in anterior MIs; prolong life after MI even if no symptoms

- Nitroglycerin, as patch or IV if volume OK, especially if continued pain, perhaps even if no pain; especially helpful if any element of CHF or if large anterior MI
- MgSO$_4$ perhaps, 8 nM bolus over 5 minutes, then 65 nM over 24 hours; if Mg low, perhaps for all; improves survival in one study from 89% to 92%, but of no help in ISIS-4
- Insulin IV then SC qid for months in all? Diabetics decreased mortality at 1 year; low-dose glucose-insulin-potassium (GIK) is not effective (Cardiology 1966:239; Cardiovasc Drugs Ther 1999:191)

Surgical

- Angioplasty (PCTA) as primary treatment if available (J Invasive Cardiol 1999:61; Circulation 1999:14), after thrombolysis if symptoms or ischemia persist. Preferred if coincident heart failure or cardiogenic shock (J Am Coll Cardiol 1991:1077); thrombolytics of equivocal efficacy (Eur Heart J 1999:128). As acute Rx, 90% successful, 3% require emergency CABG, 5% infarct, 1% mortality
- CABG after angioplasty if low EF (21–49%) and multivessel disease, or if left main disease; can do it 1 month post-MI, although better 6-month survival if done immediately for cardiogenic shock (N Engl J Med 1999:625)
- Atherectomy not as good

RIGHT VENTRICULAR INFARCT

Eur J Cardiol 1976:411

Epidem: Seen with inferior wall MI (IWMI) and increases the mortality from 6% to 30% (N Engl J Med 1993:981); mitral regurgitation, when severe, is associated with a 50% 1-year mortality despite all interventions; increased risk also seems to be age related (Circulation 1998:1714)

Pathophys: Right ventricular infarct syndrome—acute inferior MI, Kussmaul's sign (paradoxical increases in jugulovenous pulsation with inspiration), high CVP with low PA pressure and low PCWP so all nearly equal (like pericardial tamponade), low cardiac output; occurs in 50% of IW MI patients but clinically significant in 30% and nearly 10% of those with CPK levels >2000 IU; reversible with reperfusion Rx

Lab/EKG: ST elevation in RV4; get right-sided EKG in all patients with IWMI

Rx: Consider increasing preload with saline; use dobutamine, nitroprusside, and sequential pacing as needed; avoid nitrates and diuretics; isoproterenol may unload RV but has concerns of increasing mortality. Thrombolytics helpful (Am J Cardiol 1984:951), but not as good as for other regions of the heart unless heart block or hypotension (larger infarct) (J Am Coll Cardiol 1998:876)

UNSTABLE ANGINA/NON-Q-WAVE MI

Circulation 1994:81

Crs: Prognosis is similar for Q-wave and non-Q-wave infarcts although non-Q-wave MIs are followed by more infarcts and angina but are associated with less CHF; is not affected by first-degree heart block, PVCs, Vtach, or RBBB; better prognosis if preinfarction angina preceded

EKG: ST depressions or even no acute changes

Rx: Unstable angina may be amenable to medical therapy, and acutely should use ASA, nitroglycerin drip, and heparin—unfractionated vs. LMWH is an active area of research (Circulation 1999:1593). If ischemia or pain cannot be remedied, this should be treated in a similar fashion to postinfarction angina and coronary angiography is indicated. Whether treatment with primary coronary catheterization with G IIb/IIIa therapy is a better treatment is the question for the TACTICS/TIMI-18 trial (Am J Cardiol 1998:731)

2.2 ATRIAL FIBRILLATION AND FLUTTER

J Cardiovasc Pharmacol Ther 2000:11

Cause: Associated with normal variations; idiopathic, CHF, and rheumatic heart disease; atrial dilatation (e.g., in mitral stenosis or regurgitation); pericarditis, COPD especially with hypoxia and bronchodilators, ASHD; hyperthyroidism especially in the elderly as measured by low TSH, which has a 30% 10-year incidence in contrast to 10% 10-year incidence with normal TSH and with toxic multinodular goiter; alcoholic cardiomyopathy or "holiday heart"; marijuana use (Pediatr Cardiol 2000:284); and Wolff-Parkinson-White (WPW) syndrome (Am J Cardiol 2000:1256)

Atrial flutter and multifocal atrial tachycardia often (60%) from pulmonary disease including pulmonary emboli; theophylline use

Wandering atrial pacemaker (WAP), multifocal atrial tachycardia, and sick sinus syndrome (SSS) are also supraventricular arrhythmias

Epidem: Common; supraventricular prematures are not associated with ASHD or sudden death; 40–65% incidence after cardiac surgery (Ann Thorac Surg 2000:300)

Pathophys: Unknown, hypotheses of conduction problems vs. structural problems as primary insult, probably many variables. Many different frequencies and duration of paroxysmal Afib (Curr Opin Cardiol 2000:54)

Sx: Polyuria, palpitations, and faintness

Si: Tachycardia; irregularly, irregular rhythm with Afib

Crs: Rate control is key to maximize Starling hemodynamics; anticoagulation in chronic/recurrent Afib to prevent thromboembolic sequelae; losing atrial ability to fill the last 10% of ventricular diastolic volume may be an issue with low EF, leading to CHF. Aflutter in neonates is of serious consequence (J Am Coll Cardiol 2000:771)

Cmplc: Chronic Afib, Aflutter, and SSS cause embolic CVA in 20% if recent CHF, HTN, or previous embolus but <1%/year if none of those and no increase in LA size or LV dyskinesis on echo; likewise others find rate only 1.3% after 15 years where no other disease and under 60 years of age; embolic CVA increased 5 times in ASHD type compared to age-matched controls, 17 times in

rheumatic heart disease. In sick sinus syndrome, 16% develop
arterial emboli

Diff Dx: Other SVTs

Lab: CBC with diff, metabolic profile, TSH; consider ETOH, digoxin
level, or theophylline level; experimental—elevated atrial
natriuretic peptide (ANP) (J Am Coll Cardiol 2000:1256)

- EKG:
  1) SSS is diagnosed by SVTs alternating with some heart block, and
     suggested by P <90 after 1–2 mg atropine, or asystole ≥3 seconds
     after carotid sinus massage
  2) MAT, P >100, and >3 different PR intervals and P-wave
     morphologies; looks superficially like Afib but digoxin will not
     help it; WAP is same thing but rate <100
- Holter to find when intermittent; event monitor is even better
- TEE is 99% specific, 100% sensitive for LA thrombus

ED Rx:

Afib

Curr Opin Cardiol 2000:23

- Perioperative prevention post CABG with amiodarone 30 mg/kg po
  (Am J Cardiol 2000:462)
- Rate control: IV verapamil, diltiazem, β-blocker like propranolol or
  esmolol; if time to conversion not a factor, consider digoxin—rate is
  easily overridden by catechol/exercise stimulation; diltiazem does
  not cause significant ionotropic suppression as compared to
  verapamil
- Conversion: especially if LA size is <50 mm, significant CHF or
  ischemia—consider electricity if patient unstable; embolic risk
  postconversion in first 48 hours ≤1% but if >48 hours the risk is
  5–7%, and thus, should anticoagulate first even if TEE is negative,
  whereas others report no emboli if TEE is negative
- Medical conversion with propafenone (Rythmol) 300 mg po
  converts 75% within 8 hours safely, or may use 2 mg/kg IV over
  10 minutes to convert within 30 minutes (Am J Cardiol 1999:345,
  A8); or ibutilide (Corvert) 1 mg IV over 10 minutes, repeat once
  (Clin Cardiol 2000:265); or dofetilide 8 μg/kg 15-minute infusion
  (Am J Cardiol 2000:1031); or perhaps procainamide, amiodarone,
  or clonidine 0.075 mg po repeat in 2 hours by decreasing
  sympathetic tone; digoxin alone is no better than placebo

- Electrical cardioversion with synchronized mode if unstable or eventually if meds fail is OK even if digoxin on board as long as levels therapeutic and not toxic, and K^+ OK
- Maintenance Rx: β-blockers, amiodarone, verapamil, digoxin, sotalol, or dofetilide (Med Lett Drugs Ther 2000;42:41); quinidine po, which holds in NSR but death rate is 3 times placebo; or procainamide
- Anticoagulate chronic or intermittent Afib if clinically able with warfarin to INR >2 but <4—this provides the best risk/benefit balance, which reduces the risk of CVA from 7% to 1–2% at any age especially in SSS variant (Cerebrovasc Dis 2000:39). Annual bleeding risk is approximately 2.5%; no need to anticoagulate chronic Afib if age <60 years, no h/o TIA, no valve disease, normal echo, and no HTN (Lancet 2000:956). Use ASA if cannot use warfarin, might help at least under age 75
- Conduction affected by $MgSO_4$ with delay in RR interval, no change with use of glucose, insulin, or potassium (J Electrocardiol 1998:281)
- AV nodal ablation, area of active research (Pacing Clin Electrophysiol 2000:395) but most are pacemaker dependent afterward (Am Heart J 2000:122); open surgery using the MAZE procedure to let incisions guide impulses from the SA to AV node (Semin Thorac Cardiovasc Surg 2000:2)

Aflutter

Carotid sinus pressure trial, then Rx as Afib

MAT

Rx the primary disease (COPD, sepsis) or theophylline toxicity if appropriate, and may be only treatment necessary; verapamil IV with pretreatment of IV $CaCl_2$ or po for chronic; Mg^+ IV, especially if low serum level; β-blockers if no COPD

SSS

Permanent pacer preferably with atrial pacing to reduce emboli, then medications to control tachycardias

2.3 CONGESTIVE HEART FAILURE

N Engl J Med 1999:577; 1999:759; Med Hypotheses 2000:242

Cause: ASHD, hypertension, dilated cardiomyopathy; occasionally valve disease; and more rarely AV malformations. More uncommonly salt water drowning, Paget's disease, hyperthyroidism, beriberi, severe anemia as with pernicious anemia, multiple myeloma, rarely, peripartum (usually secondary to other complications and then idiopathic (Obstet Gynecol 1986:157)), and NSAID use in the elderly (Arch Intern Med 2000:777)

Epidem: Subclinical coronary disease; associated with hypertension in 40% of men and 60% of women, systolic BP >140; males > females; and inflammation (J Am Coll Cardiol 2000:1628). In U.S., incidence is 400,000/year

Pathophys: Most CHF is due to systolic dysfunction, but a small percentage is due to diastolic dysfunction (e.g., mitral stenosis, constrictive pericarditis, and IHSS, conditions that prevent normal diastolic filling). Hypertrophy in response to load creates dysfunctional myocardial cells. Action of ACE inhibitors, β-blockers, and calcium channel blockers may be to relax hypertrophic myocardium as well as decrease afterload. Inadequate production of endogenous atrial natriuretic peptide, an atrial hormone that promotes diuresis (J Cardiovasc Pharmacol 2000:129). Cardiac asthma is due to bronchial edema and hyperresponsiveness

Sx: Dyspnea on exertion, orthopnea, paroxysmal nocturnal dyspnea, ankle edema, bowel bloating and sense of fullness pc, nocturia

Si: JVD, S_3 gallop, pulse >100, displaced point of maximal impulse, dullness in L 5th intercostal space ≥10.5 cm from sternum. Central apnea in 45%, especially Cheyne-Stokes respirations; Rx with theophylline 250 mg po bid

Crs: 70+% 5-year mortality if due to hypertension, 50% 1-year mortality after starting medications; over age 70, 70% 2-year mortality after pulmonary edema

Cmplc: Sleep apnea (N Engl J Med 1999:949)

Diff Dx: Lymphangitic carcinoma, diffuse pneumonia

Lab:

- EKG—look for underlying rhythm, ischemia, acute injury, pericarditis. QRS dispersion (variability in QRS width as predictor of mortality) (Am J Cardiol 2000:1212)
- CXR—redistribution of blood to apices on upright, perihilar haze, Kerley B lines, increased heart size, pleural effusion R > L
- CBC with diff (assess for anemia and neutrophil percentage >65 post MI associated with risk for CHF (Am Heart J 2000:94)); metabolic profile; consider ABG and/or continuous O_2 saturations; digoxin level if appropriate; cardiac enzymes if severe, hypotensive, or with chest pain; low ESR correlates with acute and severe disease; elevated CRP in some correlates with inflammation of CHF; TSH if not previously tested; lactic acid level if chronic CHF and unable to determine current disease severity (Am J Cardiol 1998:888). Serum interleukin-6 (>10 pg/mL) elevation associated with severe disease (J Heart Lung Transplant 2000:419)

ED Rx:

- O_2, airway—intubate if necessary; consider BiPap in lieu of intubation with settings 10/4 if patient can tolerate (Cmaj 2000:535)
- IV, D_5W
- Nitroglycerin—SL, IV, paste (Circ Res 1976:127; Am J Cardiol 1976:469). Transdermal routes develop tachyphylaxis (Ann Intern Med 1986:295)
- MSO_4 2–5 mg IV, prn
- Foley catheter
- Dobutamine IV (in combination with IV TNG, nitroprusside, or dopamine if hypotensive) if severe for its positive ionotropic properties, better than digoxin or diuretics, no arrhythmias, short half-life; dose at 2.5–15 µg/kg/min (Chest 1980:694)
- Nitroprusside IV for afterload reduction—beware CN build-up; dose at 1–5 µg/kg/min
- Amrinone 40 µg/kg/min for 1 hour, then 10 µg/kg/min for 24 hours at least as efficacious as dobutamine (Am J Cardiol 1981:170); perhaps augmented with use of inhaled nitric oxide (Eur J Emerg Med 1999:161)
- Saterinone (PDE III inhibitor) IV at 0.5–4 µg/kg/min combines actions of dobutamine and nitroprusside (J Cardiovasc Pharmacol 1998:629)

- β-blockers (e.g., metoprolol) if patient can tolerate, especially if rate control is an issue (Jama 2000:1295); (Med Lett Drugs Ther 2000;42:54)
- ACE inhibitor acutely (captopril 6.25–25 mg SL) as long as no AS and not intubated (Int J Cardiol 1990:351). Consider angiotensin II receptor antagonists as well
- Dopamine (with dobutamine) if hypotensive at pressure support doses of 5–20 µg/kg/min, not renal dose. Renal dosing does not help natriuresis (J Am Soc Nephrol 1996:1032)
- Carvedilol (Coreg) combines nonspecific β- and α-blocker effect (J Nucl Cardiol 2000:3); many drug interactions (e.g., with digoxin, cimetidine, SSRIs)
- Dofetilide for CHF and/or Afib conversion, 500-µg dose po for CHF or 250 µg if in Afib (N Engl J Med 1999:857)
- Consider aminophylline 5–10 mg/kg IV load, then 0.3 mg/kg/hour
- Do not use isoproterenol as rescue medication; perhaps some use as prognostic challenge (Am Heart J 1992:989)
- Indications for pacing (Cardiol Clin 2000:55)
- Moxonidine (central acting imidazoline) decreases sympathetic output (J Am Coll Cardiol 2000:398)
- Adrenomedullin infusion is experimental, with pharmacologic ability for vasodilation, diuresis, and natriuresis (Circulation 2000:498)
- Selective adenosine antagonists also experimental, seem to preserve GFR compared to furosemide (J Am Coll Cardiol 2000:56)

Chronic Rx:

Includes some of the above (Med Lett Drugs Ther 1999;41:12)

- Diuretics and digoxin (Eur J Clin Invest 2000:285) do not help emergently, but are for chronic treatment—may begin IV dosing for compromised patient because CHF will decrease po absorption. Furosemide may be used as continuous IV drip (Chest 1992:725); possible paradoxical pump dysfunction 2° to neurohumoral axis activation (Ann Intern Med 1985:1). Spironolactone reduces morbidity/mortality (N Engl J Med 1999:709; Am J Cardiol 2000:1207). Replete thiamine if on long-term furosemide to improve left ventricular function (Am J Med 1995:485)
- Calcium channel blockers for diastolic dysfunction, with even newer agents dangerous if used ubiquitously (Circulation 2000:758)

2.4 HEART BLOCK AND BRADYCARDIA

J Emerg Med 1986:25

Cause: Drug toxicity (especially digoxin), ASHD, myocardial infarction, vasovagal reaction, congenital, granulomatous disease (Eur J Cardiol 1978:349), metastatic calcification. Electrical rhythm without pulses (pulseless electrical activity—PEA) has a myriad of causes including hypothermia, pulmonary embolus, ineffective perfusion volume, cardiac tamponade, pneumothorax with tension physiology, acidosis, hyperkalemia, and drug overdose

Epidem: Rarely associated with HLA-B27 and aortic insufficiency

Pathophys: See 2.1 for ASHD details. Congenital form is associated with maternal autoantibody disease (SLE, Sjogren's, etc.), with anti-SSA (Ro antibodies); parasympathetic and sympathetic function just being elucidated for different etiologies (J Am Coll Cardiol 1988:271)

Sx:
- First degree heart block usually causes no symptoms
- Second degree may cause dizziness or dyspnea
- Third degree may cause syncope, especially on standing

Si:
- First degree heart block has PR >0.22 second
- Second degree has some unconducted P waves: Mobitz type I (Ann Intern Med 1999:58) with prolongation of PR interval until dropped beat; Mobitz type II without PR prolongation
- Third degree has no relationship between Ps and QRSs

Crs: First degree heart block usually benign if not associated with organic disease

Cmplc: R/O Lyme disease if from endemic area, even if no other Sx, with serology; Rx with antibiotics and temporary (not permanent) pacer (Pacing Clin Electrophysiol 1992:252). Low perfusion states can lead to inadequate flow to brain, heart, kidneys, bowel, or any other organ system

Lab: EKG, metabolic profile, digoxin level if appropriate, consider cardiac markers; Holter monitor may still miss a majority of intermittent heart blocks

ED Rx:
    First degree may not need Rx. Second and third degree:
    • Atropine 0.5–1 mg IV (temporary solution) (Resuscitation 1999:47)
    • External pacer until transvenous available; use for 60 minutes is OK
      without increased risk for cardiac damage (J Emerg Med 1989:1).
      External pacer with negative electrode on left anterior chest and
      positive electrode on left upper back (infrascapular); use lowest
      current setting until capture and typical range is from 0–200
      mA—increase slightly postcapture; you also set the rate
      (70–80 bpm). Transvenous is temporary, although in the setting
      of inferior MI a permanent pacemaker is usually not needed
    • Isoproterenol IV (Circulation 1981:427) although controversial—
      effective yet significant side effects in digoxin toxicity, acute MI,
      or those with ASHD
    • Consider aminophylline 100 mg/min IV up to 250 mg, although
      higher doses in chronic therapy (Ann Pharmacother 1998:837)
    • Consider treatment of excessive β-blockade (reverse with glucagon
      1 mg IV (Ann Emerg Med 1997:181)) or calcium channel blockade
      (reverse with calcium chloride 10% 10 cc IV (Am J Emerg Med
      1985:334)) if present

2.5 HYPERTENSIVE EMERGENCIES

Crit Care Clin 1989:477; Clin Cornerstone 1999:41

Cause: Low calcium, and/or potassium intakes? Genetic by defective
    angiotensin gene on chromosome 1; red cell membrane Na^+
    transport correlates with proximal tubule Na^+ resorption; elevated
    insulin levels? Drug use such as cocaine or pseudoephedrine
    (Am J Emerg Med 1986:141)

Epidem: Increased prevalence in blacks (Clin Cardiol 1989:IV13–7)
    (perhaps due to G6PD deficiency) and Hispanic males, especially
    from lower socioeconomic classes (Am J Public Health 1988:636);
    in sleep apnea, especially in older men, is this cause or effect?;
    with >2 drinks of ETOH qd; with insulin resistance

Pathophys: Renally secreted prostaglandins protect; renin-aldosterone-
    angiotensin worsens. Elevated ADH does not increase BP. Calcium
    and sodium intakes modulate BP via parathyroid hormones and
    the renin-angiotensin system. "Salt-sensitive" hypertension

depends on Na⁺ and Cl⁻ together; BP decreases on Na⁺ citrate. Alcohol induces via CRH release. See 14.8 for pregnancy details

Sx: None usually; occasionally causes epistaxis; headache in moderate to severe disease; severe disease may have manifestation of angina, CVA, or other evidence of end-organ dysfunction

Si: Use correct cuff size. Mild HTN if diastolic 90–105 mm Hg and/or systolic 140–160; moderate, diastolic 105–120 and/or systolic >160; severe, diastolic ≥120 and/or systolic ≥210. Systolic false readings increase in elderly due to lead pipe arteries, tell by "Osler's maneuver" (feel artery when occluded above by BP cuff). Controversial significance of "white coat" HTN. Assess for bruits to check for vasculopathology

Crs: In elderly, LVH decreases over 6 months and function improves if Rx with verapamil, atenolol, or thiazides, or better with ACE Inhibitors as first choice, then calcium channel blockers, then β-blockers and diuretics. Treatment of isolated systolic HTN (>160) reduces CVAs by 1/3, stroke mortality by 36%, and cardiac mortality by 25%, as does treatment of systolic and diastolic HTN up to 85 years of age. Isolated moderate systolic HTN still associated with increased cardiovascular risks of 1.5 times

Cmplc:
- Hypertensive crisis: papilledema, obtundation and seizures, renal failure; encephalopathy with stroke; intracranial bleed
- Chronic renal failure
- LVH
- CHF
- Diabetes via hypertension-induced insulin resistance

Diff Dx: Malignant HTN—retinal hemorrhages or papilledema (J Intern Med 1999:513); sleep apnea (present in 30%?), ETOH and other drug/medicine use, primary renal disease, renovascular causes including coarctation of the aorta (check coincident radial and femoral pulses, rarely need to check temporal and radial in proximal type), pheochromocytoma, Cushing's, Conn's, toxemia of pregnancy and BCPs, lead-induced renal disease (most "essential" hypertensives with creatinine >1.5 mg%) (Environ Health Perspect 1988:57), acromegaly

Lab: CBC with diff, metabolic profile, U/A, EKG (3–8% sensitive) or echo (100% sensitive, ? specificity) for LVH

ED Rx:
Drug Saf 1998:99
- HTN crisis—severe numbers with evidence of end-organ disease: nitroprusside drip or propranolol 1–3 mg bolus q 5–10 minutes IV or other β-blocker best; labetalol 20–80 mg over 20 seconds up to 300 mg q 10 minutes IV; diazoxide 50–150 mg IV q 5 minutes with propranolol 3 mg/hour and/or diuretic; hydralazine 10–20 mg IV once, then po nifedipine, clonidine, or captopril
- Nifedipine with substantial complications—not advocated
- In pregnancy, propranolol OK; so are hydralazine, α-methyldopa, clonidine; avoid teratogenic ACE inhibitors
- If able to discharge patient to home, arrange early outpatient medical follow-up (Med Care 1984:755)

Outpatient Treatment
J Hum Hypertens 1999:647; 1999:803
Behavior modification is usually of minimal help
- Increase potassium intake (salt substitute)
- Lose weight
- Regular aerobic exercise (Clin J Sport Med 1999:104)
- Increase fruits, vegetables, and polyunsaturated fats (Clin Cardiol 1999:III6)
- Lessen sodium intake—debatable
- Avoid or stop NSAIDs (Br J Clin Pharmacol 1990:519)
- Perhaps supplemental calcium and magnesium

Drug Regimens
Med Lett Drugs Ther 1999;41:23
- Thiazides, even in diabetics
- β-blockers, all about the same
- ACE inhibitors (Med Lett Drugs Ther 1999;41:105), clearly best in those with NIDDM (preserves renal function in early renal failure). Angiotensin II receptor blockers probably equally good
- Calcium channel blockers, long-acting types only
- Direct vasodilators such as hydralazine or minoxidil, adrenergic inhibitors like clonidine or α-methyldopa, or α-receptor blockers like prazosin
- Endothelin receptor antagonist like bosentan—experimental (N Engl J Med 1998:784)

2.6 INFECTIOUS ENDOCARDITIS

N Engl J Med 1974:832; 1974:1122; Ann Emerg Med 1991:405; Emerg Med Clin North Am 1998:665, ix

Cause: *Streptococcus viridans* (47%); *Staphylococcus aureus* (20%) (usually acute bacterial endocarditis); enterococcus (6%); pneumococcus, nonenterococcal group D strep often misidentified as enterococcus, and rarely anaerobes, fungi, gram negatives, lactobacillus, psittacosis organism, and other unusual organisms like *Bartonella* spp. or *Serratia marcescens* (Ann Intern Med 1976:29)

Epidem: 4000–8000 cases/year in U.S.; 75% in patients with abnormal valves/hearts. Increased in patients with mitral valve prolapse syndrome (yet diagnosis of MVP prior to 1997 was with controversial standards), congenital (VSD, PDA, tetralogy of Fallot), congenital heart disease especially aortic stenosis both repaired and unrepaired (1.5–20% at 30 years) and rheumatic heart disease even when given SBE prophylaxis before dental work and surgical procedures

Pathophys: <5% are right-sided; higher in IV drug users

Sx: Fever, hematuria, and weight loss

Si: Murmur (85% at presentation, 99% eventually; 66% in right-sided type), splenomegaly and/or infarction (25–50%), mucosal petechiae and splinter hemorrhages in nails (29%), clubbing (13%), Roth spots in fundi (2%), Osler's nodes in fingers

Crs: 100% die without Rx; 80% 10-year survival with Rx

Cmplc: CHF (25%) due to chordae rupture and myocarditis; peripheral systemic arterial emboli, mostly with *S. viridans* type; pulmonary emboli (60% in right-sided type); CNS including TIA, CVA, mycotic aneurysm, abscess, encephalopathy, and bacterial as well as aseptic meningitis (Brain 1989:1295); renal failure from diffuse vasculitis, focal "embolic" glomerulonephritis, and renal infarction

Diff Dx: Acute rheumatic fever, collagen vascular disease, anticardiolipin antibody syndrome (Arch Pathol Lab Med 1989:350), acute glomerulonephritis, marantic endocarditis, and rarely atrial myxoma

Lab: CBC with diff, ESR, U/A, CXR, echo (TTE OK in those with native valves if negative (Am J Cardiol 1996:101); otherwise TEE 95% sensitive (J Am Coll Cardiol 1991:391)), 3 10-cc blood cultures unless antibiotics within 2 weeks of presentation—in that case get 5 10-cc blood cultures. Consider RA titer. Biopsy and culture of Osler's nodes (Chest 1987:751)

ED Rx:
- *Therapeutic antibiotics*: empiric treatment consists of ceftriaxone, vancomycin (Int J Antimicrob Agents 1999:191), and gentamicin, antibiotics to be continued 2–6 weeks IV
- *Surgical interventions* rarely needed except for valve ruptures and infections of implanted valves, but over time (10 years) 25% of mitral and 60% of aortic valves need surgery
- *Prevention* in those with valvular disease or previous surgery with pre- and postprocedure doses up to 24–48 h of amoxicillin or alternative antibiotics (Lancet 1966:686; Circulation 1987:376; Med Lett Drugs Ther 1999;41:80)

2.7 MYOCARDITIS/CARDIOMYOPATHY

Emerg Med Clin North Am 1998:665, ix; Circulation 1999:1091; Adv Intern Med 1999:293

Cause:
- Collagen vascular diseases including SLE, polyarteritis nodosa, endocardial fibroelastosis (occasionally seen in children due to a treatable inherited carnitine deficiency), sarcoid, carcinoid (last two may be restrictive and/or congestive)
- Deficiencies like hypophosphatemia from antacid biding, reversible; thiamine (beriberi), selenium, carnitine
- Endocrine: thyrotoxicosis and hypothyroidism; pheochromocytoma; homocystinuria, hypocalcemia
- Giant cell (lymphocytic) myocarditis
- Idiopathic, may be caused by cellular apoptosis (programmed cell death) related to human leukocyte antigen association (J Card Fail 1997:97)
- Infectious from any severe bacteremia, e.g., meningococcus, shigella, diphtheria, mycoplasma; viral including CMV, influenza, echovirus, coxsackie B (Scand J Infect Dis 1970:25), yellow fever, mumps, polio, rubella, HIV; not hep C (Cardiology 1998:75); parasites including toxoplasma, Chagas' disease
- Ischemic

- Neurologic causes including Friedreich's ataxia; dyskalemic myopathies; muscular dystrophies including limb-girdle, Emery-Dreifuss, and myotonic; Refsum's disease
- Peripartum (Obstet Gynecol 1986:157)
- Toxic agents like ETOH (Am Heart J 1976:561), daunorubicin (Daunomycin) and bleomycin, cobalt in beer, arsenic; lead, cocaine, mercury, carbon monoxide, phenothiazines, clozapine (Lancet 1999:1841); most reversible except chemotherapy drugs

Epidem: Idiopathic-type prevalence = 36/100,000: blacks/whites 2.5/1; males/females 25/1

Pathophys: Dilation of both ventricles; mural thrombi

Sx: Dyspnea; muscle weakness in alcoholic type since 83% have skeletal myopathy as well

Si: Afib, other supraventricular arrhythmias; S_3 gallop; CHF signs

Crs: Often chronic and indolent, although may present acutely in infants (Pediatr Emerg Care 1987:110); in alcoholic type, it can rapidly resolve with abstinence; 95% 1-year, 80% 5-year survival. Eosinophilic endocardial fibroelastosis, 4% 3-year mortality. Those with infiltrative types, HIV infection, or doxorubicin-related have worse prognosis (N Engl J Med 2000:1077). Usually good outcome in children (Heart 1999:226)

Cmplc: Systemic emboli from mural thrombi and Afib

Diff Dx: Hypertrophic (IHSS) and restrictive myocardiopathies: amyloid, hemochromatosis, familial, idiopathic, endomyocardial fibrosis, eosinophilic cardiomyopathy, sarcoid, Gaucher's, Fabry's, and Hurler's diseases

Lab:
- CBC with diff, metabolic profile including phosphate level, CXR, EKG—looking for arrhythmia (20% with Afib), cloven T waves, blocks, Q waves, or LVH
- Echo most helpful, EF <45%
- Endocardial biopsy in peripartum and all types to diagnose infiltrative disease; not helpful in dilated types, IHSS, Wilson's disease, etc.; does not correlate well with clinical findings or prognosis once dilated cardiomyopathy has developed (Am Heart J 1989:876)

ED Rx:
- Anticoagulate acutely and chronically; prednisone Rx even when inflammatory by biopsy is no help (Am Heart J 1989:876) or even with immunosuppressive drugs; perhaps human growth hormone 4

IU sc qod or immune globulin 2 g/kg IV (Circulation 1997:2476); transplantation, 75% 5-year survival
- For CHF use vasodilators (see 2.3)
- Indications for pacing (Cardiol Clin 2000:55)

2.8 PERICARDITIS

Emerg Med Clin North Am 1998:665, ix
Cause:
  Arch Intern Med 1979:407; Chest 1999:1564
  - *Acute*: postsurgical or traumatic, uremic, bacterial from a subdiaphragmatic abscess, post-MI, viral especially coxsackie, postsepticemic, mycoplasma, malignancy invading pericardium, actinomycosis, candidal (Ann Thorac Surg 1997:1200). Peds includes Kawasaki disease
  - *Chronic*: tuberculosis, sarcoid, hypothyroidism (Am J Emerg Med 1999:176)
Epidem: Coxsackie viral type probably is the most common cause and occurs in late summer and fall like other enteroviruses
Pathophys: The stiffening causes restriction of ventricular diastolic filling; increased heart rate must compensate for decreased stroke volume; can tolerate 1–3 L if slowly accumulates, only 300–400 cc if rapid accumulation. Paradoxical pulse if constrictive (exaggeration >10 mm Hg of normal drop of systolic BP with inspiration) due to impaired venous return and normal increased pulmonary vascular volume with inspiration
Sx: Dyspnea; chest pain, often pleuritic and better when sitting up
Si: Ascites, poor heart sounds, no PMI, tachycardia; pleural effusions on left more often and larger than on right, unlike CHF. In constrictive pericarditis increased CVP with Kussmaul's sign. Paradoxical pulse >10–20 mm Hg
Crs: Variable secondary to cause and patient's hemodynamic status; those with pericarditis within 1 week of post-MI are likely to have had an anterior MI, less likely to have atrial arrhythmias, but at slightly increased risk for ventricular arrhythmias, CHF, and death (Am Heart J 1974:246)
Cmplc: Cardiac tamponade (Clin Cardiol 1999:446) seen in <1% of thoracic trauma patients who are viable; as complication of

pericarditis presents with hypotension as evidence of shock; co-incident pleural effusions may impact noncritical pericardial effusions and make them symptomatic—drain the pleural effusions (Chest 1999:1820)

Diff Dx: Acute traumatic cardiac tamponade—those intoxicated may be more difficult to diagnose, but fare no worse (J Trauma 1999:346); severe asthma; rapid Y descent and rebound, R/O infiltrating myocardiopathy, e.g., amyloid

Lab:

- CBC with diff, ESR, metabolic profile
- EKG (Chest 1970:460; Am J Cardiol 1970:471) may show Afib or electrical alternans (i.e., alternate QRSs have higher and lower voltages), abnormal P waves, ST elevation, and/or PR elevations in limb and precordial leads, which exclude early repolarization, which usually has precordial lead (STs) or limb (PRs) involvement only and isoelectric V_6 (N Engl J Med 1976:523); Ts invert only after STs back to normal. Consider right-sided EKG looking for RV infarct
- Echo shows pericardial fluid and may show tamponade hemodynamics
- CXR shows large heart—may resemble Erlenmeyer flask or "boot-shaped." Normal CXR does not exclude diagnosis (Nephrol Dial Transplant 2000:719)

ED Rx:

- ASA or other NSAID Rx avoiding indomethacin and/or steroids if ASHD and recent MI
- Pulsed methylprednisolone (30 mg/kg) IV if Kawasaki disease with impending tamponade (Intensive Care Med 1999:1137)
- If constrictive, tap under echo or EKG guidance; pulmonary edema can develop if tap too much too fast, leading to an overload of a deconditioned heart
- Uremic pericarditis: nephrology consult for hemodialysis if patient hemodynamically stable (Am J Kidney Dis 1987:2), pericardiocentesis as above if tamponade
- Cardiac tamponade: pericardiocentesis with 18-gauge spinal needle. If patient responds, emergent pericardial window, reaspirate or place flexible catheter using Seldinger technique if necessary. Anticipate ventricular arrhythmias. Apply aspirated blood to 4 × 4 gauze to determine if it is nonclotting

2.9 PAROXYSMAL SUPRAVENTRICULAR TACHYCARDIA

Cause: Aberrant conduction pathways with different conduction routes within the AV node (AV nodal re-entrant tachycardia—AVNRT) or outside the AV node (AV re-entrant tachycardia or Wolff-Parkinson-White syndrome—AVRT or WPW, respectively), allowing setup of circus movement continuous stimulation when the aberrant or usual pathway conducts retrograde; or ectopic irritable atrial focus (paroxysmal atrial tachycardia—PAT), often associated with digitalis toxicity, especially if manifest with associated block, e.g., 2:1 or 3:1. Different and not as well understood in peds (Br Heart J 1990:317)

Epidem: AVNRT and AVRT of about equal prevalence and represent about 45% of all PSVTs; PAT constitutes 9%, and rare other syndromes like permanent junctional re-entrant tachycardia (PJRT), the last 1%. Common in infancy (Arch Pediatr Adolesc Med 1999:267)

Pathophys: Re-entrant tachycardias occur with increased excitability, decreased refractory period, and increased conduction velocity

Sx: Paroxysmal episodes of palpitations often associated with dizziness, nausea; precipitated by caffeine, alcohol, nicotine, hyperthyroid states, ephedrine in diet supplements, cold/asthma medicines, etc.; relieved by Valsalva maneuver often by patient. Neck pounding in AVNRT types but not accessory pathway (WPW or AVRT) SVT because nearly coincident atrial and ventricular contractions in former cause cannon waves in neck that can be felt

Si: Rapid tachycardia 150–210 beats/minute

Crs: Recurrent from teenage years on

Cmplc: Rare permanent junctional re-entrant tachycardia variant associated with myocardiopathy stays in arrhythmia a long time, reversible if treated. Post-PAT ST depression and T wave inversions may last days or weeks; correlation with CAD without other symptoms is controversial (Am J Cardiol 1999:458, A10)

Diff Dx: Consider Lown-Ganong-Levine syndrome if looks like WPW but no delta waves

Lab: EKG shows SVT with narrow complexes; AVNRT usually has no apparent P waves, AVRT has Ps closer to the last QRS than the next one, and PAT and PJRT have Ps closer to the next QRS and beyond the T wave. PSVT is very regular, even when aberrant and wide, unlike Vtach; QRS aberrancy always <0.14 second whereas Vtach often (>50%) >0.14 second, axis is −30° to +120° unlike the LAD with Vtach 60% of the time

ED Rx:
- Carotid sinus pressure if no bruits
- Adenosine 6–12 mg IV (Br Heart J 1986:291)—peds 0.1–0.3 mg/kg (Circulation 1982:504; Ann Emerg Med 1999:185)—gone in 10 seconds, potentiated by dipyridamole and carbamazepine, inhibited by theophyllines—may induce other more malignant arrhythmias in the post-MI period (Pacing Clin Electrophysiol 2000:140); or verapamil 5–10 mg IV or diltiazem 10–20 mg IV (J Assoc Physicians India 1999:969); or perhaps propranolol 1–5 mg IV or other β-blocker (Br Heart J 1977:834; Ann Clin Res 1979:34)
- Electrical cardioversion with synchronized mode if meds fail or if unstable, OK to do even if digoxin on board as long as levels therapeutic and not toxic, and K⁺ OK; in resistant cases, implanted atrial burst pacers or catheter ablation of atrial slow pathway works 95% of the time (Circulation 1977:727)

For chronic prevention: avoid stimulants; β-blockers; maybe verapamil or digoxin, though both can worsen some

2.10 SHOCK

Resuscitation 1992:55

Cause: Inadequate end-organ perfusion

Epidem: Has not been quantified; covers multiple disciplines

Pathophys: Can be multifactorial, but need to consider if due to heart failure (cardiogenic), hypovolemia (hemorrhage, postsurgical), or loss of vascular tone (septic, anaphylactic, spinal cord)

Sx: Dizziness, dyspnea

Si: Fever in sepsis, hypotension with bradycardia or tachycardia, wheezing is not specific to anaphylaxis, check peripheral limb movement and DTRs to R/O spinal shock, altered consciousness

Crs: Depending upon etiology, cardiogenic and spinal cord shock have worse outcomes

Cmplc: ARDS, ventilator dependent, paralysis

Lab: CBC with diff, metabolic profile, ABG, consider blood cultures and cardiac markers; consider U/A and urine C + S; EKG for acute injury or ischemia; type and crossmatch; stool guaiac. X-ray: CXR to check for sepsis source, tension pneumothorax, pulmonary edema, heart size and morphology, and mediastinum; C-spine evaluation with plain film or CT if neurogenic shock suspected; abdominal CT if AAA or other abdominal source suspected

ED Rx:

- 2 IVs, consider level 1 warmer
- Maintain airway
- Fluid bolus of 20 cc/kg, may repeat once before adding pressors and/or blood products (Jama 1991:1242); type O uncrossmatched blood OK to give emergently (Ann Emerg Med 1986:1282), try to use Rh negative in females of childbearing age; if more than one volume of blood products given, give FFP to replace factors (Am J Surg 1996:399)
- Dopamine (Inotropin) if hypotensive at pressure support doses of 5–20 µg/kg/min, not renal dose. Renal dosing does not help natriuresis (J Am Soc Nephrol 1996:1032)
- Dobutamine (Dobutrex) IV (in combination with IV TNG, nitroprusside, or dopamine if hypotensive and cardiogenic etiology) for its positive ionotropic properties, better than digoxin, or diuretics, no arrhythmias, short half-life; dose at 2.5–15 µg/kg/min (Chest 1980:694)
- Norepinephrine (Levophed), 2–4 µg/min IV (Crit Care Med 1987:687)
- Phenylephrine (Neo-Synephrine), 50–180 µg/min IV, may give 50-µg boluses IV (Crit Care Med 1991:1395)
- Epinephrine, 1–4 µg/min IV (Chest 1990:949)
- Perhaps vasopressin, 40 IU IV (J Trauma 1999:699, discussion 703; Ann Pharmacother 2000:250)
- Isoproterenol (Isuprel), 2–10 µg/min IV (J Oslo City Hosp 1989:23); rarely used
- If suspect adrenal crisis, hydrocortisone 100 mg IV (Mil Med 1996:624)
- Immediate treatment of underlying cause with angioplasty or CABG to be considered if cardiogenic (Ann Intern Med 1999:47)

2.11 THORACIC AORTIC ANEURYSM/DISSECTION

Circulation 1979:1619; J R Coll Surg Edinb 1982:195; Am J Emerg Med 2000:46

Cause:

Aneurysm

Atherosclerotic; connective tissue defect as seen in Marfan syndrome; now rarely due to syphilis

Dissection

N Engl J Med 1987:1060

Elevated pressures in aorta as seen in hypertension or cocaine use (Am J Emerg Med 1997:507). Defect of connective tissue as seen in Marfan syndrome or Ehlers-Danlos syndrome. Traumatic usually at ligamentum arteriosum in chest

Epidem:

Aneurysm

Usually discovered incidentally during "other" evaluation unless medical risk factors prompt serial screening, 1.5 times as common as ruptured abdominal aortic aneurysm. 5% surgical mortality for elective repair and 16% mortality for emergency repair; 21% 5-year survival if no repair (J Thorac Cardiovasc Surg 1985:50). More than half of these will be patients >60 years of age (Ann Chir Gynaecol Fenn 1967:270)

Dissection

Most common acute illness of aorta. If ascending aorta untreated, 50% die within 48 hr and 90% within 12 months (Am J Cardiol 1972:263). Descending aorta with similar medical and surgical outcomes (Circulation 1990:IV39), and surgery if evidence of end-organ ischemia. Increased incidence with advanced age, hypertension, pregnancy, cocaine use, Marfan syndrome, Ehlers-Danlos syndrome, systemic lupus, Turner syndrome, and Noonan syndrome (J Emerg Med 1997:859). Increased risk in those with autosomal dominant polycystic kidney disease (Nephrol Dial Transplant 1997:1711)

Pathophys:

Aneurysm

Dilation of vessel, with increased risk of dissection or aortic insufficiency (Circulation 1975:1202)

Dissection

Medial rupture of vasovasorum causes a dissecting hematoma that ruptures back into lumen, usually, though not always, distally creating a double-barreled lumen. Stanford classification: type A = ascending aorta involved; type B = no involvement of ascending aorta, descending only

Sx (dissection): Pain, thoracic, abdominal or in back; often migrating

Si (dissection): BPs in legs and arms unequal; asymmetric pulses

Crs: Mortality 1%/ hour in type A

Cmplc: Organ ischemia due to vessel occlusion, including distal neurologic deficits (J Thorac Imaging 1994:101)

Diff Dx: Acute coronary syndrome; pulmonary embolus; pneumothorax

Lab:

Ann Emerg Med 1996:278
- Plain X-ray may show aortic knob widening
- Spiral CT of chest with contrast (94% sensitive, 87% specific) (Radiol Clin North Am 1999:575; Clin Radiol 1999:38)
- Do not do echo as first test if clinical suspicion is low: transthoracic echo (57% sensitive, 83% specific), TEE (97% sensitive, 77% specific), and better specificity if combined with CT (Clin Radiol 1992:104) or aortography
- MRI (98% sensitive, 98% specific)
- Aortogram (Chest 1989:124) to define point of origin, aortic insufficiency, and any vessel compromise but MRI + TEE may obviate the need for this

ED Rx for Symptomatic Dissections:
- First, nitroprusside 25–50 μg/min with β-blockers such as Lopressor or esmolol (Dicp 1991:735), or add α-blocking coverage with labetalol. Goal is systolic BP <110 mm Hg
- Second, trimethaphan (Arfonad) 1–2 mg/minute IV
- Surgical for all type A and selected type B

2.12 VENTRICULAR ARRHYTHMIAS

Circulation 2000:1129

Cause:

Ventricular Fibrillation

Annu Rev Physiol 2000:25

Vfib is most likely a terminal rhythm unless noted immediately in hospital setting, and is the end-stage rhythm in many (if not all) terminal conditions. Rare chronic Vfib associated with myocarditis (Jpn Circ J 2000:139). Better outcomes now in those post-MI if definitive intervention available (defibrillation) and treatment of underlying heart disease (Heart 2000:258); out-of-hospital Vfib associated with acute MI usually implicates left coronary artery locus (J Am Coll Cardiol 2000:144)

Ventricular Tachycardia

Vtach may be due to idiopathic reasons, scar from myocardiopathy including alcoholic "holiday heart," MI with re-entry, CHF, metabolic abnormalities, or long Q-T syndrome which may be caused by drugs. Monomorphic is most common, followed in equal frequency by polymorphic VT and torsades de pointes (Acad Emerg Med 1999:609). Mitral prolapse syndrome?

In children and young adults with Vtach, consider IHSS, cardiomyopathies, congenital heart disease such as tetralogy of Fallot and pulmonic stenosis; long QT syndrome, mitral valve prolapse(?), cocaine, Marfan syndrome with aortic dissection, anomalous coronary arteries, Kawasaki's induced coronary aneurysms

Epidem: Vtach and PVCs increased with nicotine (Am J Physiol Heart Circ Physiol 2000:H2124), CO levels >100 ppm, and subtle ST-T wave electrical alternans. The data for caffeine is equivocal. Decreased 50% with weekly fish consumption

Pathophys: Not certain, consider increased sympathetic tone. Vfib is not the asynchronous "Jell-O" as previously thought, but synchronous atrial function is maintained for 8 minutes after disorganization of ventricular activity (Chest 2000:1118)

Metabolic abnormalities may be myriad, but potassium physiology is the most important. Citing disturbances of calcium and magnesium may be due in part to potassium then having a lower threshold to cause arrhythmias (Clin Cardiol 1992:103)

Sx: Syncope that may progress to sudden death

Si: Dizziness, palpitations, unresponsive

Crs:

Sudden Death

47% 2-year mortality after first episode; 86% if no MI, 16% if transmural MI; if asymptomatic, prognosis very good even if complex arrhythmias or VT

PVCs in Asymptomatic Men

Two times the incidence of later MI or other cardiac event

Diff Dx: SVT with aberrancy—no clinical data to differentiate this from VT (Ann Emerg Med 1987:40); digoxin toxicity; mitral valve prolapse(?). "Slow ventricular tachycardia" is a benign regular accelerated idioventricular rhythm <100 beats/minute and asymptomatic, seen often (30%) in inferior MIs; Brugada syndrome, which is idiopathic Vfib with RBBB and elevated ST segments V_1-V_3 on baseline EKG (FEBS Lett 2000:29)

Lab: EKG:

Vfib has an undulating baseline, no other complexes noted

Vtach is unlike SVT with aberrancy due to the following:

- Vtach QRSs are wide (85% >14 seconds—0% false positives, 30% false negatives) with RBBB pattern or >0.16 with LBBB
- Vtach has a left axis deviation
- Vtach is not as regular
- SVT with aberrancy has initial QRS deflection as per normal QRS complexes—may compare if present earlier on strip or from previous EKGs

PVCs differ from supraventricular prematures with aberrancy due to the following:

- PVC QRSs are opposite of the normal beat vector
- T and QRS vectors are in opposite directions
- No atrial depolarization in 70%
- In Afib, if a complex is wide it may be an aberrant conduction rather than a PVC if it follows a previous longer R-R interval

Bidirectional Vtach—Two ventricular foci alternating in bigeminal pattern—is diagnostic of digitalis toxicity

Brugada criteria (98% overall sensitivity) indicating Vtach rather than SVT with aberrancy (Heart 2000:31):

- No precordial RS complex (20% sensitivity), or
- Beginning of R to S nadir >0.10 second (52% sensitivity), or
- AV dissociation present, or

- RBBB pattern + left axis deviation, or R/S <1 in V_6, or positive R forces in V_1 or LBBB pattern + Q in V_6, or in $V_{1\ or\ 2}$ >0.04 second, or beginning of R to S nadir in V_1 or V_2 >0.07, or notching of S down stroke in $V_{1\ or\ 2}$

Prehospital Rx:

Defibrillation by bystanders using automatic external defibrillators saves lives (N Engl J Med 2000;343:1206; 2000;343:1210).

ED Rx:

For Vfib and Unstable Vtach

- Consider precordial thump if defibrillator not available (Am Heart J 1989:248), supposedly delivers approximately 5 kJ of energy to heart
- If field defibrillation unsuccessful, ED Rx considered not worthwhile unless other correctable conditions identified
- Apply O_2 and get IV access
- Bretylium is equivocally effective (Am J Cardiol 1999:115, A9), not available

For Unstable Vtach

- Defibrillation sequence of 200 J, then 300 J, then 360 J in adults. In peds 2 J/kg, then 4 J/kg × 2. If using biphasic, use manufacturer recommended energy equivalents
- Drug Rx:
  1) Lidocaine: 1.0–1.5 mg/kg load with repeat dose in 3–5 minutes if necessary; drip is set at 2–4 mg/min. Peds dose is 1 mg/kg bolus with 20–50 µg/kg/min drip. Data is equivocal (Ann Emerg Med 1981:420)
  2) Procainamide (Clin Cardiol 2000:171): 20–30 mg/min IV until one of the following: arrhythmia suppressed, hypotension, widening of QRS >50%, or maximum dose of 17 mg/kg given. In unstable Vtach or Vfib, OK to give 100 mg IV q 5 minutes; drip rate is 1–4 mg/min. Peds: load 2–6 mg/min over 5 minutes, then drip rate of 20–80 µg/kg/min; max 2 g/24 hours
  3) Amiodarone: 5 mg/kg over 15 minutes IV drip (Am J Cardiol 1983:156) or 150-mg IV bolus, then 0.5–1 mg/min drip
  4) Consider $MgSO_4$ 2 g IV (Chest 1997:1454); especially in those who are known to be hypomagnesemic such as alcoholics, extreme athletes, and those on diuretics or malnourished
  5) Sotalol: 100 mg IV over 5 minutes; may be better than lidocaine
  6) Wide complex without pulses is a form of electromechanical dissociation which has a myriad of causes with either narrow or

wide complexes (hypovolemia; hypoxia; tension pneumothorax; massive MI; massive pulmonary embolus; acidosis; drug overdose such as TCAs, digoxin, β-blockers, Ca-channel blockers; hypothermia; cardiac tamponade), but wide complex may be due to hyperkalemia so consider IV CaCl$_2$ (J Emerg Med 1989:109)

For Vfib

- Defibrillate as above, and one maximum defibrillation after every pharmacologic maneuver. Biphasic waveforms (J Am Coll Cardiol 1989:207; Acad Emerg Med 1999:880; Circulation 2000:2968) appear as effective as monophasic with lower energy levels used
- Drug Rx:
  1) Epinephrine 1 mg of 1:10,000 IV or ET (peds 10 μg/kg which is 0.1 cc/kg of 1:10,000) every 5 minutes or vasopressin 40 IU IV once (Anesth Analg 2000:1067; 2000:627)
  2) Amiodarone as above
  3) Procainamide as above
  4) Magnesium sulfate 2 g IV (J Cardiothorac Vasc Anesth 2000:196), especially if considering torsades de pointes (Herz 1997:51)
  5) Lidocaine as above
  6) Sotalol, verapamil, and flecainide may all be helpful (Circulation 2000:1606); verapamil may convert VF to VT (Circ Res 2000:684)
- IVF should be wide open (LR or NS)
- Consider pacing if able to induce bradycardia with pulses; not routine for refractory Vfib

For Stable Vtach (alert without chest pain, respiratory distress, or hypotension)

- First, try lidocaine and procainamide—procainamide for either a supraventricular or ventricular arrhythmia
- Second, try synchronized cardioversion starting at 100 J, sedate with narcotic and benzodiazepine of choice. Fentanyl avoids hypotension seen with other narcotics (no histamine release), and midazolam (Versed) is of quick onset and short acting

PVCs

- No treatment warranted

3 Dental Conditions

3.1 INFECTION

Compendium 1990:492, 494, 498

Cause: Poor dental hygiene leading to dental and gum disease, or as manifestations of systemic disease as seen in diabetes mellitus, rheumatologic disorders, hematologic diseases, or infectious diseases such as TB

Epidem: Common as first dental visit for many who come to the emergency department, especially children <3.5 years of age (52%) (Pediatr Dent 1997:470). Common pathogens include *Streptococcus pyogenes*, *S. mitis*, *S. salivarius*, *S. faecalis*, *Staphylococcus*, *Escherichia coli*, and *Klebsiella* (Aust Dent J 1978:107)

Pathophys: Breakdown of tooth or gum leading to secondary infectious complication (J Am Dent Assoc 1969:1016)

- Periodontal abscess is an abscess between the tooth and gingiva
- Necrotizing gingivitis is caused by a spirochete very similar to *Treponema pallidum*; it is a fusobacterium

Sx: Halitosis, pain, swelling

Si: Localized edema, erythema, or tenderness; ulcerations; dental caries; lymphadenopathy

Cmplc: Tooth loss; secondary abscess in gingivitis

Lab: None, unless systemic disease sought

ED Rx:

Br Dent J 1989:41

Periodontal Abscess

- Warm rinses
- Antibiotics: penicillin (VK) 500 mg po bid-qid, clindamycin for treatment failures or if PCN allergic—300 mg po qid; perhaps metronidazole for PCN failures (Br J Oral Surg 1977:264)

- I + D if "pointing"—if the abscess has come to a head, perform appropriate block and stab the abscess with a No. 11 blade
- Pain medications, with ibuprofen having physiologic advantage over acetaminophen in dental pain (J Endod 1999:804)
- Dental referral

Necrotizing Gingivitis
- Warm rinses
- Tetracycline 250 mg po qid or PCN or metronidazole 200 mg po tid for 3 days
- Topical lidocaine (2% viscous) may help; avoid overuse or may precipitate lidocaine toxicity
- Dental referral

3.2 ORAL LACERATIONS

Cause: Trauma, usually with tooth or dental hardware as the cutting surface
Epidem: Common
Sx: Cut to inside of lip or mouth
Si: Oral laceration; check for loose tooth or loose dental hardware
Crs: Usually heals quickly
Cmplc: Infection
Lab: None, consider X-ray if looking for foreign body
ED Rx:
- Update tetanus if needed
- Local anesthesia, see 19.2
- Repair with silk, 4-0 or 5-0, after copious irrigation with sterile saline. Place simple sutures loosely and be sure to line up the vermilion border if this has been violated
- May need repair in the OR for children
- Consider 3–5 days of oral antibiotic prophylaxis with penicillin for high-risk wounds; may also elect to leave these open if possible

3.3 TRAUMA

Compendium 1990:526, 528, 530

Epidem: Incomplete tooth fractures more common in older patient population; complete tooth fractures can occur at any age (J Prosthet Dent 1999:226)

Sx/Si:
- Tooth fracture is assigned an Ellis class:
  Class I is a fracture through the enamel
  Class II involves the dentin, as evidenced by air and cold sensitivity
  Class III involves the pulp, evidenced by central blood spot when tooth is gently sponged with gauze
- A subluxed tooth is a loose tooth, with a spectrum of subluxation possible
- An avulsed tooth is a tooth that is missing
- All but Ellis Class I fractures will involve pain

Cmplc: Loss of tooth or secondary infection for all but Ellis Class I

Lab: X-ray if avulsed tooth cannot be located (R/O gingival location) or if tooth fragments suspected in soft tissues; tooth may be in stomach

ED Rx:
Otolaryngol Clin North Am 1972:273
- Ellis Class I: file edges if necessary, elective dental referral
- Ellis Class II: cover the dentin with CaOH and bandage (foil or dry gauze) and avoid hot or cold foods—if minimal dentin showing in adolescents or older patients, may just need dietary changes for a few weeks. Next day dental referral
- Ellis Class III: cover tooth with foil and immediate dental referral—same day, next day at the most. Oral analgesics, nothing on the pulp!
- Subluxed tooth: If minimal, reassurance—if an anterior tooth, explicit instructions to seek dental attention if pain worsening or tooth loosening. Anterior teeth with somewhat tenuous anchoring re neurovascular bundle. Soft diet for 2–3 weeks. If grossly unstable, immediate dental referral for stabilization
- Avulsed tooth (Endod Dent Traumatol 1986:1; Otolaryngol Clin North Am 1991:165; Am J Emerg Med 1990:351): Re-implant

permanent teeth. Gentle rinsing with tap water, avoid touching roots. If unable to re-implant, place in moistened gauze, glass of milk if available, or Hank's solution ideally. Re-implant at ED, and immediate dental referral

Note: Periodontal dressings are widely available for temporary stabilization in the ED

4 Endocrinology

4.1 ACUTE ADRENAL INSUFFICIENCY

Ann Clin Biochem 1999:151

Cause: Primary adrenal insufficiency (Addison's disease) can be atrophic in nature as seen in idiopathic or autoimmune with suppressor T-cell defect, or it can be characterized as destructive as seen in primary or metastatic cancer (Ann Hematol 1999:151); antiphospholipid syndrome (Chest 1998:1136); infection, especially in TB or in peds with sepsis (Arch Dis Child 1999:51), and meningococcemia with Friderichsen-Waterhouse syndrome; in amyloidosis; or in severe hemorrhage with hypotension (Arch Surg 1999:394). Secondary adrenal insufficiency occurs in those who may be panhypopituitary, those on chronic steroids—including the possibility of inhaled beclomethasone (J Allergy Clin Immunol 1999:956), or those who have just come off of corticosteroids and are now under stress; or autoimmune disorders in general (Clin Endocrinol (Oxf) 1998:779). Also seen in HIV in AIDS pts

Epidem: In Addison's disease, peak incidence 20–40 years of age. Associated with HLA-B8 and DR 3/4, and thereby with pernicious anemia, myasthenia gravis, islet cell antibody IDDM, myxedema, vitiligo, alopecia, and primary gonadal failure

Pathophys: 80% of gland must be destroyed to get symptoms. ACTH and MSH similar, hence increased pigmentation; both mineralocorticoid and glucocorticoid deficiencies create the signs and symptoms

Sx: Loss of sense of well-being; nausea, vomiting, and diarrhea; salt craving and weight loss; galactorrhea, rarely; increased pigmentation if chronic

Si: Hypotension; cachexia; hyperpigmentation, vitiligo, longitudinal nail pigment streaks if chronic; diminished axillary and pubic hair;

remember not to rely on abdominal exam for acute abdomen if patient is on exogenous steroids

Crs: 40% of those with Addison's disease will develop other glandular failure (especially thyroid and gonadal)

Diff Dx:

- Hyporeninemic hypoaldosteronism: hyperkalemia and metabolic acidosis due to depressed prostaglandin synthesis
- Adrenoleukodystrophy: in boys, a sex-linked abnormality of fatty acid metabolism

Lab: Chemistry profile with low Na^+, low HCO_3, elevated K^+, order a cortisol level—if less than 15 µgm% then diagnosis most likely; check TSH (J Clin Endocrinol Metab 2000:1388), CBC with diff looking for eosinophilia (Lancet 1999:1675), consider steroid-21-hydroxylase antibody and very long chain fatty acid serum levels looking for elevation for diagnosis of idiopathic (J Clin Endocrinol Metab 1998:3163), consider pan culture and other ID evaluation for hypotension; EKG; graded ACTH stimulation test diagnostic (J Endocrinol Invest 2000:163)

ED Rx:

- IVF with 20-cc/kg bolus
- Hydrocortisone 100 mg IV (and may repeat in 6 hours) (Mil Med 1996:624)
- Methylprednisolone 1–2 mg/kg IV if additional glucocorticoid boost needed (respiratory distress, hypotension)

4.2 DIABETIC KETOACIDOSIS

Acta Paediatr Suppl 1999:14; Emerg Med Clin North Am 1989:859

Cause: IDDM with noncompliance and/or secondary infection most likely

Epidem: ~5% mortality (Med J Aust 1989:439, 441, 444)

Pathophys: Coma from CSF acidosis, hence rarer in metabolic than respiratory acidosis because CO_2 crosses blood-brain barrier easily; HCO_3 Rx may paradoxically induce or worsen coma. Atrial natriuretic peptide suppressed in children to maintain fluid and sodium (J Pediatr 1987:329)

Sx: Malaise, confusion, nausea, vomiting, abdominal pain

Si: Kussmaul's respirations, stupor, coma, hypotension, dehydration

Crs: Onset over 2–3 days

Cmplc: Cerebral edema leading to coma with 90% mortality 6–10 hours after starting treatment—especially in children (N Engl J Med 1967:665). Secondary infection with *Pseudomonas pseudomallei* (melioidosis) ubiquitous in Asia (Arch Intern Med 1972:268)

Diff Dx: Hypoglycemia; infection; drug intoxication; appendicitis; acute renal failure; nonketotic, nonacidotic hyperosmolar coma—seen in the elderly with NIDDM

Lab: Chemistry profile and blood gas, specifically looking for bicarb <10 and pH < 7.2 (Pediatr Emerg Care 1996:347); look for anion gap >15 calculating $Na - (Cl + CO_2)$ = answer (N Engl J Med 1977:814); ABG vs. venous blood gas—venous just as useful (Ann Emerg Med 1998:459); CBC with diff, and >10% bandemia warrants search for secondary infection (Am J Emerg Med 1987:1); U/A; consider pan culture and other ID evaluation if source or febrile; consider serum ketones or acetone level (Diabetes 1986:668); consider measured and/or calculated osmoles—calculated osmoles = glucose/18 + 2 × Na + BUN/2.8

ED Rx:
- IV NS with 1-liter bolus then 1 liter/hr
- Regular insulin 0.33–0.44 U/kg IV push, then 7 U/hr IV continuous until glucose <250 mg%; then 2–6 U/hr IV until glucose <150 mg%; then routine maintenance (Arch Intern Med 1977:1377); check K^+ before infusing insulin unless EKG changes such as wide QRS
- Peds: 0.1–0.2 U/kg IV push, then 0.1–0.2 U/hr
- Fluids: After first liter, NS or change to 1/2 NS if osmoles elevated with 40 mEq KCl/L at 1 L/hr until serum glucose <250 mg%, then change to D5W or D5NS depending on the serum sodium (high sodium, go more hypotonic, and vice versa)
- NGT if vomiting (treatment for gastroparesis)
- HCO_3 IV only if HCO_3 <5 mEq/L or pH < 6.9 (Crit Care Med 1999:2690); gives paradoxical CNS acidosis, and right shift of hemoglobin dissociation curve
- PO_4 Rx rarely needed?; maybe as K_2PO_4 if low (PO_4 <0.1–0.5 mg%) to prevent insulin resistance
- Medical consult for admission

4.3 HYPEROSMOLAR STATES

N Engl J Med 1974:1184; West J Med 1980:16
Cause:
  Diabetes insipidus (Endocrinol Metab Clin North Am 1993:411)
  • Central diabetes insipidus (DI) from idiopathic, sarcoid, eosinophilic granuloma, CNS insult—tumor, trauma, surgery; ETOH ingestion is transient but aggravates all other causes
  • Nephrogenic DI, including drug-induced by lithium, demeclocycline (Declomycin); transient in pregnancy due to increased vasopressinase, renal tubular damage form hypercalcemia, hypokalemia, chronic pyelonephritis, chronic partial obstruction, sickle cell anemia, lead poisoning, renal tubular acidosis
  Dehydration from one of the following:
  • Loop diuretics
  • Inability to drink
  • Betadine Rx of burns
  • Peritoneal or hemodialysis
  • Diminished urine concentration and diminished thirst in elderly, especially with AODM as a comorbid diagnosis, which leads to nonketotic hyperosmolar coma (Drugs 1989:462; Curr Ther Endocrinol Metab 1997:438)
  Perhaps precipitated by glucocorticoids, β-blockers, or diazoxide
Epidem: DI is 3/100,000 (Pediatr Rev 2000:122, quiz 129)
Pathophys: Both types of DI associated with ADH deficiency or resistance (nephrogenic (J Mol Med 1998:326))—normally ADH dilates splanchnic arterioles, increases renin, and stimulates factor VIII clotting factors while causing water resorption in kidney. Dehydration as per etiology
Sx: Confusion
Si: Confusion, stupor, coma, hypotension, dehydration
Crs: Worse prognosis in those who have normal or elevated corrected serum sodium (Ann Intern Med 1989:855); add 1.6 mmol/L to the serum sodium for every 100 mg/dL of serum glucose over 100 mg/dL
Cmplc: Mortality >40% in elderly patients
Lab: CBC with diff, chemistry profile, measured or calculated osmoles (formula above), consider U/A and pan culture to search for ID reasons for hypotension; EKG. X-ray: neuroimaging such as

CT/MRI (J Clin Endocrinol Metab 1999:1954) to evaluate pituitary in central DI, may not be necessary in isolated idiopathic DI or those with growth hormone deficiency only (Lancet 1999:2212)

ED Rx:

- O_2
- IV
- Replace H_2O, but at less than 12 mEq Na change/24 hrs (cerebral edema) or change serum osmolality at less than 2 mOsm/L/hr. Water deficit = 0.6 × (ideal body weight) [1–140/(measured serum sodium)]
- Central DI Rx'ed with desmopressin (vasopressin analog) 5–20 μgm nasal, sc, or IV q 4–20 hours for complete types. Desmopressin is resistant to vasopressinase. Perhaps indapamide 2.5 mg qd (Arch Intern Med 1999:2085). For incomplete type, treat the same way or treat like nephrogenic
- Nephrogenic Rx'ed with thiazides, carbamazepine, or chlorpropamide; amiloride 5–10 mg bid (0.3 mg/kg/day tid in peds) (Arch Dis Child 1999:548)
- NSAIDs (indomethacin) for lithium-induced DI (Ren Fail 1997:183)
- Nonketotic hyperosmolar coma with 0.15 U/kg IV bolus of regular insulin, followed by regular insulin infusion in 1/2 NS at 5–7 units/hour. NS for IV fluid resuscitation, avoid hypokalemia (Diabetes Care 1982:78)

4.4 HYPOGLYCEMIA

Cause:

Exogenous
- Insulin: low plasma C peptide levels; prolonged hypoglycemia with use of β-blockers (Diabetes Care 1984:243)
- Sulfonyureas
- Endotoxic shock (Circ Shock 1982:269)
- Drug list (AIM 1993;118:536)

Fasting
- Pancreatic functioning tumor (Diabetes 1981:377)
- Nonpancreatic functioning tumor (Arch Intern Med 1972:447)
- Liver disease

1) Acquired, especially from CHF
2) Congenital glycogen storage disease or galactosemia
   (J Clin Invest 1998:507)
3) Hepatoma

- ETOH (Endocrinol Metab Clin North Am 1989:75) and/or poor
  nutrition from decreased gluconeogenesis, e.g., in diarrheal disease
  in children
- Endocrine deficiencies, e.g., Addison's, hypopituitarism, decreased
  pancreatic α-cell function
- Normal physiologic responses in women and children

Reactive (Postprandial)

Diabetes 1981:465

Oral GTT no help, get blood glucose prn Sxs; ≤60 mg% is significant

- Rapid gastric emptying
- Fast absorption
- Prediabetes
- Dumping syndrome (Pediatrics 1987:937)
- Leucine sensitivity
- Hereditary fructose intolerance

Sx: Confusion, epinephrine release symptoms—sweaty, pale, nausea

Si: Tachycardia, pallor, diaphoresis, intoxication, coma

Cmplc: CNS insult, coma

Lab: Glucoscan, chemistry profile

ED Rx:

- O_2
- IV access
- 25 g of glucose (50 cc of 50% solution—D50 1 amp) with 100 mg
  of thiamine IV if ETOH related or patient in coma and unknown
  ETOH history. May repeat once. Peds: 2 cc of a 50% solution or
  4 cc of a 25% solution (1 g)/kg IV
- Or may try glucagon 1 mg IV (Diabetes Care 1987:712), IM OK if
  no access
- May give juice or glucose paste if patient alert and able to
  swallow (Diabetes Care 1982:512); rectal glucose not effective
  (Acta Paediatr Scand 1984:560)
- Feed when alert
- Outpatient follow-up if short-lived reason for hypoglycemia and
  patient recovers; otherwise medical admission

4.5 MYXEDEMA COMA

Jama 1974:884; Med Clin North Am 1995:185

Cause: Untreated hypothyroid state, with the hypothyroidism due to any factor such as I_2 deficiency or excess, autoimmune (Ann Intern Med 1985:26), surgical excision, radiation, or iodide after treatment of diffuse toxic goiter (N Engl J Med 1969:816). Less likely from lithium therapy or secondary (pituitary or hypothalamic failure) hypothyroidism

Epidem: Rare, with 50% mortality in elderly even if recognized and treated (J Am Board Fam Pract 1995:376); more common in cold climates

Pathophys: Lack of T3 and T4 has global influence on the body. Autoimmune Hashimoto's has associations with pernicious anemia and insulin-dependent diabetes; phenytoin (Dilantin) and carbamazepine (Tegretol) may precipitate hypothyroidism (Acta Neurol Scand 1980:330)

Sx: Hair loss and coarseness; skin coarseness; fatigue; swollen tongue, constipation, muscle cramps

Si: Hypothermia; goiter; surgical scar on neck; hung-up reflexes (J Psychiatr Res 1967:289) or areflexia; diminished PMI from pericardial effusion; psychosis; respiratory depression; seizures; coma

Crs: Imminent death if not recognized early and treated

Cmplc: Environmental cold, trauma, secondary infection, and drugs as listed above may all be complicating factors. Cardiac arrhythmias may occur with rewarming. Cardiac tamponade (Clin Cardiol 1982:459)

Lab: Chemistry profile, CBC with diff, TSH (N Engl J Med 1971:529), Free T4, EKG, ABG if significant neuro or respiratory compromise, U/A and/or pan culture if considering other reasons for mental status change, CXR—may show Erlenmeyer flask sign as seen in pericardial effusion, consider head CT to R/O intracranial process

ED Rx:
- Coma protocol of O_2, and IV Narcan, dextrose, thiamine if appropriate
- Secure airway if necessary, intubate for hypoxemia
- 500 µg IV of T4 or 40 µg IV of T_3, if possible—give ASAP

- Rewarm gradually
- Medical consult for admission

4.6 THYROID STORM

Jama 1974:592

Cause: Untreated hyperthyroid state, which may have a heightened physiologic response due to cessation of antithyroid meds (Metabolism 1968:893), radiation thyroiditis, infection, trauma, surgery, acidosis, or toxemia of pregnancy

Epidem: Those with previous surgical treatment for hyperthyroidism may relapse (16%) (Br J Surg 1983:408)

Pathophys: Unopposed hyperthyroid state, with T3 and T4 influencing the physiology of the whole body. Autoimmune thyroiditis (Graves' disease) is a classification of many different subtypes (Clin Endocrinol (Oxf) 1992:75); rarely Hashimoto's thyroiditis (Metab Pediatr Ophthalmol 1981:213). Thyroid cancer present in ~6% (World J Surg 1998:473, discussion, 477), more often found in those with solitary adenoma

Sx: Hot and sweaty; smooth skin; diarrhea from steatorrhea, polyphagia of fat, and decreased GI transit time

Si: Fever; muscle wasting; resting tachycardia; temors; hyperactivity; weakness; confusion; psychosis; coma; hepatomegaly

Crs: Death is imminent unless recognized and treated

Complc: Treatment-induced hypothyroidism (Clin Endocrinol (Oxf) 1997:1) or hypocalcemia

Diff Dx: Physical signs of chorea may also be seen in medication reaction, neurologic lesion, or psychiatric disorder (Am J Psychiatry 1979:1208)

Lab: Metabolic profile, CBC with diff, TSH, free T4, free or total T3 (J Am Geriatr Soc 1988:242), consider ID evaluation with U/A and pan culture for fever and mental status changes, EKG, ABG if neuro changes and/or respiratory compromise

ED Rx:
- IVF, have D_5NS ready for bolus with treatment as below
- β-blockade: propranolol 2–10 mg IV—go slow, or esmolol (Brevibloc) 50–200 µg/kg/min; not in heart failure (Br Med J 1977:1505)

- Hydrocortisone 100 mg IV (q 6 hr) and consider dexamethasone to prevent T4 to T3 peripheral conversion
- PTU 1 g po or via NGT
- Iodine as Lugol's solution, 10 gtts po tid (IV sodium iodide?)
- Consider lithium 300 mg po tid instead of SSKI
- Cooling blanket for hyperthermia, cool mist with fan works quicker
- Digitalis if necessary (atrial fibrillation)

ENDOCRINOLOGY

5 Environmental

Some basic environmental facts:
- When we speak of elevation (high altitude), we generally mean >8000 ft above sea level, although high altitude is anything above 5000 ft
- You get colder faster in water
- Hypothermia is also a summertime problem
- Hyperthermia has a myriad of causes besides environmental
- When unable to explain neurologic problems or constitutional symptoms, think CO

5.1 ALTITUDE (AMS, HAPE, HACE)

Am J Emerg Med 1985:217; Emerg Med Clin North Am 1984:503

Cause: Being above altitude (8000–10,000 ft above sea level) with or without appropriate acclimatization. "Climb high, sleep low." (Aviat Space Environ Med 1976:512; N Z Med J 1998:168)

Epidem: Getting to altitude is easier today than in the past; even extreme altitude (18,000 ft above sea level) is attainable at a cost

Pathophys:
- Hypoxia is the problem, with the partial pressure of O_2 decreasing as we attain higher elevations. Initial hyperventilation—due to decreased PaO_2—is blunted by an ensuing respiratory alkalosis. Peripheral vasoconstriction leads to central venous pooling, which causes a diuresis and increasing osmolality. Pulmonary hypertensive tendencies (Adv Exp Med Biol 1999:93) will be exacerbated by altitude due to the global pulmonary hypoxia, and perhaps pulmonary vasoconstrictors such as endothelin-1 (Circulation 1999:2665). Cerebral blood flow will increase in an attempt to increase oxygen flow to the brain, yet this increase in cerebral blood

volume may lead to an increase in intracranial pressure. Perhaps this is due to edema and ischemia (J Appl Physiol 1995:375). Cerebral blood flow is important in high altitude cerebral edema, but probably not the significant physiologic problem in acute mountain sickness (J Appl Physiol 1999:1578)

- Acclimatization may offset some of the problems with attaining altitude, but this is not always certain. Hike high, sleep low—with no more than a 2000–2500-ft increase being allowed in altitude on a single day
- The three major problems with altitude are acute mountain sickness (AMS), high altitude pulmonary edema (HAPE) (Wilderness Environ Med 1999:88), and high altitude cerebral edema (HACE) (Wilderness Environ Med 1999:97)

Sx:
- AMS: Headache, fatigue, nausea, vomiting, anorexia
- HAPE: Same as AMS with cough and dyspnea on exertion
- HACE: Same as AMS and HAPE with change in mental status

Si:
- AMS: Nonspecific
- HAPE: Rales; irregular, nocturnal breathing patterns (Aviat Space Environ Med 1989:786)
- HACE: As with HAPE, as well as stupor, coma, focal cranial nerve deficit

Crs: Rapid physiologic decline in all categories unless rapid diagnosis and Rx

Cmplc: AMS may progress to HAPE or HACE or both, and symptoms may worsen with use of ETOH, respiratory depressants, inadequate fluid intake, and overexertion

Diff Dx: Hypothermia, dehydration, drug side effect or OD (specifically CO poisoning), infection, PE, CVA, diabetic reaction, or simply fatigue or bronchitis

Lab: None for mild episodes. More severe episodes, begin treatment and gather the following: metabolic profile, glucoscan, ABG, CO level, CBC with diff, CXR, EKG, U/A with pan culture if ID evaluation considered, head CT without contrast if CNS insult considered, ETOH or urine toxic screen if drugs of abuse considered

Note: Low resting SaO_2 is a risk factor for developing AMS and HAPE (Aviat Space Environ Med 1998:1182)

ENVIRONMENTAL

Field Rx:
- Descent
- Rest (J Appl Physiol 2000:581) and warm patient
- O_2
- Different scores available for AMS, such as the Lake Louise score (Aviat Space Environ Med 1998:1186)
- Gamow Bag® if necessary and available (Am J Emerg Med 1996:412; Biomed Sci Instrum 1989:79)

ED Rx:

Mild AMS will resolve with some descent (1000 ft), further evaluation per patient symptoms. All other cases should do the following:
- As above
- Good oral hydration, IV access if needed (Aviat Space Environ Med 1999:867)
- Maintain/secure airway; possible use of PEEP valve for prevention (Eur J Appl Physiol 1998:32)
- Acetazolamide (Diamox) 5 mg/kg day divided tid (N Engl J Med 1968:839; 1969:49; Lancet 1981:180; Ann Intern Med 1992:461)
- Dexamethasone 4 mg q 6 h any route (po/IM/IV) (West J Med 1991:289)
- Acetazolamide + dexamethasone better than acetazolamide alone, which is better than dexamethasone alone (Aviat Space Environ Med 1998:883)
- Data on theophylline is equivocal (Eur Respir J 2000:123)
- Potential role of magnesium (orally) (Aviat Space Environ Med 1999:625)
- Perhaps hyperbaric bag in EDs that treat many with altitude illnesses and that are at altitude

HAPE
- MSO_4, 2–3 mg IV, may facilitate splanchnic pooling
- Loop diuretics such as furosemide, 60–80 mg IV, paucity of data
- Nifedipine 10 mg po, data equivocal (Med Sci Sports Exerc 1999:S23)
- Hydralazine 10 mg IV or phentolamine, data equivocal (Int J Sports Med 1992:S68)

HACE
- Consider mannitol and loop diuretics—data equivocal

5.2 ELECTRICAL INJURY

Emerg Med Clin North Am 1992:211; Ann Emerg Med 1993:378;
  J Emerg Med 1999:977; 2000:181; 2000:27

Cause: Children playing around electrical sockets or broken electrical
  cord; nongrounded tools; lack of appropriate barrier secondary to
  material breakdown, sweat, or water

Epidem: 3–5% of burn center admissions, 1000 deaths/yr
  (Ann Emerg Med 1993:378)

Pathophys: More than 1000 volts is significant to humans, with as little
  as 20 mA causing significant morbidity if alternating current.
  Ohm's law: amperage = voltage/resistance. The electrical injury
  can cause conduction problems in nerve or cardiac cells, as well as
  thermal destruction

Sx: Tingling in body part in contact, inability to relax grip, shortness of
  breath, localized pain

Si: Tissue destruction, respiratory distress, arrhythmias, mental status
  changes, paralysis, or sudden death

Crs: Variable

Cmplc: Sudden death from delivery of current on ventricular
  repolarization phase—analogous to R on T phenomenon.
  Children who bite electrical cords may have delayed labial artery
  hemorrhage resulting from sloughing mucosa as underlying tissues
  heal—delay may be as much as 2 weeks

Lab:
  • If localized hand tingling with no other symptoms and no evidence
    of entrance and exit wounds on opposites sides of the body, nothing
    specific
  • All other cases: EKG; CMP, PT/PTT, CPK, U/A and urine for
    myoglobin if suspect significant muscle destruction; check LFTs and
    amylase if intra-abdominal path; head CT if mental status changes

ED Rx:
  • IV access
  • Airway management if facial or neck burns with declining
    respiratory function, or if burns noted in mouth or oropharynx
  • Treat cardiac arrhythmias if lethal pattern. Continuous cardiac
    monitoring is not needed if normal EKG and no acute problems
    (J Emerg Med 2000:181), including loss of consciousness

(Burns 1997:576). Perhaps 24 h observation if exit and entrance wounds through thorax (Br Heart J 1987:279)
- IV fluid for burn resuscitation if significant burns noted during physical or laboratory evaluation (South Med J 1996:869)
- Update tetanus if necessary
- NGT if intra-abdominal process with ileus
- Fracture management as appropriate

5.3 FROSTBITE

J Trauma 2000:171
Cause: Tissue destruction from cold exposure
Epidem: Seen frequently in those with ETOH abuse or psychiatric issues
Pathophys: Peripheral vasoconstriction to maintain core temperature, leaving extremities at risk for cold exposure without rewarming. Local tissue destruction from cell lysis and ice crystal formation. Distal destruction is irreversible with venous and arterial thrombosis, and proximal injury is noted by erythema, with an unknown extent of destruction between these two extremes
Sx/Si:
- First degree: Erythema, edema, border erythema
- Second degree: Partial thickness with blisters and black eschar
- Third degree: Full thickness with subcutaneous involvement, hemorrhagic blisters with skin necrosis
- Fourth degree: Full thickness with subcutaneous involvement as well as tendon, muscle, and/or bone involvement
Cmplc: Refreezing and inadequate treatment leading to extension of tissue destruction is a possible problem. Peripheral vascular disease, diabetes mellitus, dehydration, trauma, and infection all worsen outcome
Lab: As dictated by patients' comorbid diagnoses; consider CBC with diff, ESR, and appropriate X-ray to diagnose osteomyelitis
Field Rx:
- Warm in warm (not hot) water—40°C (104°F)
- Avoid refreezing
- Do not open intact blisters
- Ibuprofen (Ann Emerg Med 1987:1056)
- Topical aloe vera (Postgrad Med 1990:67, 73)

ED Rx:
- Rapid rewarming in water 40°C (104°F) for 10–30 minutes
- Narcotics IV for pain management
- Update tetanus if necessary
- Intra-arterial thrombolysis experimental
- Opening blisters is controversial
- Prophylactic antibiotics are controversial
- Dextran and heparin controversial
- Hyperbaric O_2 controversial
- Pentoxifylline is experimental (Arch Otolaryngol Head Neck Surg 1995:678)

5.4 HEAT-RELATED ILLNESSES

Trans R Soc Trop Med Hyg 1977:402; 1977:412; 1977:419; Lancet 1998:1329; Crit Care Clin 1999:251

Cause: Inability to handle endogenous heat production with exogenous heat augmentation. Anticipatory intervention (Public Health Rev 1985:115; Jama 1996:593) and monitoring weather extremes key in prevention (Jama 1998:1514). Children at risk when left in cars (Pediatrics 1976:101)

Epidem: Heat-related problems increase markedly if environmental T >91°F. Potentially exacerbated by being very young or very old, using drugs of abuse, or being on anticholinergic or neuroleptic medications (see 13.10). Perhaps risk of malignant hyperthermia if episode of heat stroke, or heterozygote status for cystic fibrosis if significant episode of heat exhaustion (J R Army Med Corps 1995:40)

Pathophys: Although dehydration a component of pathophysiology, exact mechanisms for these problems not fully elucidated (Int J Sports Med 1998:S146); perhaps neuro (J Sports Sci 1997:277) or immune dysfunction (Crit Rev Immunol 1999:285)
- Usual cooling methods of conduction, convection, and evaporation are overwhelmed. Evaporation is major cooling mechanism, followed by convection, and finally conduction
- Heat exhaustion is an overheating problem but sweating is still intact, and is considered a diagnosis of exclusion. May be

accompanied by a myriad of minor heat-related problems, e.g., heat cramps, heat syncope, prickly heat
- Heat stroke is the clinical triad of hyperpyrexia (T >105°F), mental status changes, and anhidrosis (anhidrosis is not a hard and fast finding)

Sx: Dizzy, weak, tired, nausea, vomiting, headache

Si: Hypotension (commonly asymptomatic in extreme athletes (Med Sci Sports Exerc 1995:1595)), core temp elevated (may be normal in heat exhaustion), diaphoresis, and anhidrosis in heat stroke (+/−). Mental status change is the *sine qua non* of heat stroke

Crs: Difficult to discern heat exhaustion from early heat stroke

Cmplc: Worse with the very young and very old; associated cardiovascular disease; dehydration; secondary drug use such as sympathomimetics, β-blockers, Ca-channel blockers, MAOIs, or TCAs; high body mass index; inappropriate clothing; and altered skin physiology

Diff Dx: Neuroleptic malignant syndrome (NMS); infection or sepsis; CVA; DKA; thyroid storm; malignant hyperthermia; seizures; drug (ETOH or benzodiazepine) withdrawal; drug abuse such as ETOH, cocaine, amphetamines, LSD, or PCP

Lab: Core temp, CBC with diff, metabolic profile—specifically hyponatremia (Am J Emerg Med 1999:532), Mg, PT/PTT, ABG, TSH, ETOH, salicylate level, U/A, urine toxic screen, urine for myoglobin, pan culture, CXR, head CT with and without contrast to R/O abscess, LP

Field Rx:
- Remove heavy clothing
- Cool thermal windows (neck, axilla, groin); consider sponge bath/cool mist
- IV access, consider fluid bolus
- O_2

ED Rx:
- Cooling methods: thermal windows with cool packs, cool mist with fan blow by, NGT with cool saline, peritoneal lavage, immersion cooling; treat shivering with benzodiazepines or phenothiazines if not contraindicated
- Discontinue cooling when core temp is 104°F

5.5 HYPOTHERMIA

Aviat Space Environ Med 1983:425; Ann Emerg Med 1993:370; Jama 2000:878

Cause: Core temperature less than 35°C (95°F) due to environmental, physiologic, or functional problem

Epidem: Seen all year round, with about 780 deaths/year in U.S. Infants fare better than all others unless coincident septicemia (Intensive Care Med 2000:88). Core temp <26°C associated with 50% mortality (Ann Emerg Med 1982:417). Associated in those with dementia or psychiatric problems if it impairs judgement or protective instincts

Pathophys: Mild hypothermia is 32–35°C (90–95°F). Shivering stops below 32°C. Metabolism slows after an initial and short-lived increase in an attempt to stay warm

Sx: Shivering early, then just cold

Si: Early tachycardia followed by bradycardia, bronchospasm, hypotension, mental status changes, decreased core temperature (use appropriate thermometer)

Crs: Trauma and submersion may be coincident problems that have worse prognosis and longer hospital stays independent of age (Eur J Emerg Med 1995:38). Coincident shock has a multiplicative effect on hemodynamic and coagulation problems (Am Surg 2000:348).

Cmplc: The very young and very old (Clin Geriatr Med 1994:213) are at risk of more sequelae from this problem, perhaps secondary to elevated bacterial lipopolysaccharide concentrations from ischemic gut (Undersea Hyperb Med 2000:1). Data is equivocal for noncardiogenic pulmonary edema (Chest 1993:971)

Diff Dx: Hypothyroidism; hypopituitarism, hypothalamic, or other CNS insult; hypoglycemia; drug abuse such as ETOH, barbiturates, phenothiazines; sepsis; altered skin physiology such as burn victims; chronic disease including metabolic and functional movement problems

Lab: Core temp, CBC with diff, glucoscan, metabolic profile, PT/PTT, amylase, ETOH, U/A, urine for myoglobin, urine toxic screen, consider pan culture for ID evaluation, CXR, head CT, EKG—interval prolongation and Osborne waves (Circulation 1996:372; Acad Emerg Med 1999:1121) may be

ENVIRONMENTAL

present as well as many other potential abnormalities. ABG of equivocal help, with tendency towards acidosis, but perhaps induced alkalosis is preferred (Arch Intern Med 1988:1643), and even if corrected for temperature will give little prognostic information (Arctic Med Res 1995:76)

Field Rx:

Arctic Med Res 1991:28
- Warm patient
- Remove wet clothing and place in dry clothes or sleeping bag as insulator
- IV access
- Check pulses for 1 full minute before considering CPR
- The field treatments of mild hypothermia (T >33°C) with shivering, external heat, and exercise are all about equivalent (J Appl Physiol 1987:2375)
- Inhalation rewarming and peripheral rewarming of no benefit in the field (Ann Emerg Med 1991:896)

ED Rx:

Aviat Space Environ Med 1983:487; Arctic Med Res 1986:16; Ann Emerg Med 1987:1042
- Rewarm
  - Heating blanket, such as a forced air torso blanket (e.g., Bair Hugger) more effective than simple insulating procedures (Aviat Space Environ Med 1994:803; Resuscitation 1999:105; Ann Emerg Med 2000:337)
  - Thermal window warm packs (neck, axilla, groin)
  - Warm inhaled gases (O_2)
  - Warmed IV fluids (e.g., level 1 Warmer)
  - NGT with warm saline lavage
  - Bladder lavage with Foley
  - Two chest tubes on one side (left) with lavage
  - Peritoneal lavage/dialysis (Jama 1978:2289)
  - Thoracotomy with mediastinal lavage
  - Warm water immersion
  - Extracorporeal warming via extracorporeal circuit (Intensive Care Med 1999:520), dialysis, or cardiopulmonary bypass
- No definitive studies exist, thus more invasive methods have not demonstrated higher efficacy. Perhaps cardiopulmonary bypass for the atraumatic cardiac-arrested patient if immediately available (Lancet 1995:493)

- Beware of cardiac arrhythmias; Afib is a stable rhythm in hypothermia
- Treat comorbid problems as they are determined
- Person must be warm to be declared deceased (32°C)
- Vfib refractory to countershock when T <30°C, limit total number to 3 until T >30°C

5.6 LIGHTNING

Emerg Med Clin North Am 1992:211; Ann Emerg Med 1993:378; J Emerg Med 2000:181

Cause: Random strikes, but may be augmented by holding onto metal items and not wearing rubber-soled shoes

Epidem: 150–300 fatalities/yr

Pathophys: Higher energy delivery over a shorter period of time when compared to man-made electrical energy

Sx/Si: Depending on the pathway, any organ system may be affected, with consequent acute injury symptoms for that system; extent of burns, and coincident superior and inferior wounds (one being entrance, and the other exit), should be noted. *Note*: More than one system may be involved, and the hematologic system may be involved as well, and may manifest DIC

Crs: Common to see neurologic and otologic problems after a lightning strike
- Although paralysis may be a factor, a subset of patients have keraunoparalysis which is a lower extremity flaccid paralysis that may resolve over days to hours—acute injury to the spinal cord should still be entertained
- Tympanic membrane rupture is very common as well (>50%)—always check for this if patient unconscious and history unclear; also very common in closed space blast injuries

Cmplc: Mainly from cardiac or neurologic sequelae; may have sudden death or permanent paralysis (Ann Emerg Med 1992:575). A single strike may involve multiple victims (J Trauma 1999:937)

Lab: EKG, CBC with diff, consider metabolic profile if fluid resuscitation or cardiac arrhythmia are problems, CPK, U/A, urine for myoglobin, ABG if respiratory compromise or coma, PT/PTT

ENVIRONMENTAL

if acute neuro or cardiac event suspected, neuroimaging of head or spinal column as appropriate

ED Rx:
- Supportive measures
- Coma protocol if unclear presentation (O_2, naloxone, thiamine, glucoscan)
- Airway
- Treat underlying arrhythmias
- Suspect cardiac involvement if wounds on superior and inferior aspect of body (Crit Care Med 1990:293)
- Warm if hypothermic
- Fluid resuscitation rarely needed secondary to tissue destruction; consider blunt trauma, extrinsic blood loss, or spinal cord shock
- 24-hour cardiac monitoring for all patients is not advocated (J Trauma 1986:166)

5.7 NEAR-DROWNING

Pediatr Clin North Am 1993:321; Ann Emerg Med 1993:366

Cause: Immersion in water with some degree of suffocation. Associated with ETOH and high rates of speed in watercraft

Epidem: Exact numbers unknown, hypothesized that >4000 deaths/yr. Fresh water > salt water—swimming pools. Less alcohol use associated with some decrease in incidence of drowning (Jama 1999:2198)

Pathophys: Hypoxia secondary to aspiration of water or from laryngospasm, leading to neurologic and other end-organ ischemia

Sx: Coughing, shivering, confusion, not responsive

Si: Hypothermia, cold skin, piloerection, tachypnea or apnea, rales, tachycardia or bradycardia, confusion, obtundation, coma

Course: Poor neuro function in ED after warm water drowning is controversial as to whether extended resuscitation has a better prognosis in children—pro (Can Anaesth Soc J 1980:201; Am J Dis Child 1986:571) and con (Pediatrics 1977:364; Am J Dis Child 1981:1006; Pediatr Emerg Care 1997:98)—vs. adults (J Trauma 1982:544); case reports of extended submersion with "good" outcomes in children are in cold water (<20°C) or core temp <32°C (Jama 1980:1233)

Cmplc: Some patients have delayed respiratory insufficiency after appearing stable—aka secondary drowning, which usually manifests in 4–6 hours (Ann Emerg Med 1986:1084); pulmonary edema in salt water drowning (Am Rev Respir Dis 1992:794), fresh water is hypothesized to absorb into the blood stream since it is isotonic (Med J Aust 1966:1282)

Lab: CBC with diff; ABG; metabolic profile; PT/PTT; ETOH; U/A; UTS; EKG; X-ray—C-spine, CXR, head CT if neuro insult

Field Rx:
- Safe removal of patient from water, maintain open airway
- O_2, remove wet clothing, warm patient if necessary
- Rescue breathing, or CPR if needed

ED Rx:
- Airway, O_2; perhaps warm butyl alcohol vapor 7.5% for aspirated sea water near-drownings (Am J Emerg Med 1993:20); Heimlich maneuver probably not helpful (J Emerg Med 1995:397)
- Treat underlying arrhythmias. Role of calcium channel blockers post resuscitation (Am J Emerg Med 1984:148)?
- Warm if hypothermic; perhaps use of cardiopulmonary bypass (Arch Surg 1992:525)
- Fluid resuscitation if necessary
- Pressors if fluid ineffective
- NGT
- Foley catheter
- May discharge children to home if GCS ≥13 and Sao_2 >95% after 4–6 hours of observation (Am J Emerg Med 2000:9)

ENVIRONMENTAL

6 Gastroenterology

6.1 DIVERTICULITIS

Gastroenterol Clin North Am 1988:357; Dis Colon Rectum 2000:289

Cause: Diverticulosis with secondary infection

Epidem: Diverticulosis present in almost all patients age >40 years in U.S. if on a low-bulk diet. Increased risk in alcoholics (Br J Surg 1999:1067)?

Pathophys: Low-residue diet leads to increased intracolonic pressures causing outpocketings

Sx: Left lower quadrant pain, usually, although may be anywhere

Si: Localized abd tenderness (LLQ in 67% <40 years of age); fever; tachycardia (Am J Emerg Med 2000:140)

Crs: Variable, with obesity as risk for accurate diagnosis and surgical treatment, if needed

Cmplc: Perforation, peritonitis, partial obstruction, abscess, fistulas, bleeding from diverticulosis alone

Diff Dx: Intestinal gas; gastroenteritis; abdominal wall muscle strain; colitis; hernia; right-sided angiodysplasia of the colon, often seen in elderly and associated with aortic stenosis

Lab: CBC with diff showing leukocytosis in 91%, consider U/A in atypical cases. X-ray: plain films if looking for free air (Dis Colon Rectum 1970:444); CT delineates site/process

ED Rx:
- Prevent with high-fiber diet
- Antibiotics for acute disease (Bactrim + Flagyl; Cipro + Flagyl; Augmentin)
- Surgical staged colonic resection with temporary colostomy for recurrent disease, perforation, or abscess. Perhaps primary surgical therapy in those <40 years of age (Am J Surg 1997:733, discussion, 735)

6.2 ESOPHAGEAL FOREIGN BODIES

Gastroenterol Clin North Am 1991:691

Cause: Inadvertent ingestion of foreign body or large food bolus

Epidem: 80% peds

Pathophys: Pediatric esophagus with 5 natural narrowings; adults may have rings, webs, dysmotility, or mass lesions

Sx: Foreign body sensation anywhere from oropharynx to epigastrium, inability to swallow saliva

Si: Drooling is almost pathognomonic

Crs: If no foreign body on exam or plain film, no hypersalivation, and no obstruction or foreign body on barium swallow, then expectant management OK (Jacep 1979:101) except as noted under **Cmplc**

Cmplc:
- Button batteries (Ann Otol Rhinol Laryngol 1984:364) and sharp objects may need removal even if they have passed through the esophagus—erosion and laceration are still potential complications. Button batteries are given 48 hours to pass through the pylorus (Jama 1983:2495). Sharp objects past the esophagus may be managed expectantly as long as they are small (relative to patient size) and not causing secondary problems (perforation). All sewing needle ingestions should be referred to a surgeon or gastroenterologist
- Cocaine packet ingestion (patients referred to as mules) may warrant surgery, Golytely®, or expectant passage
- Aspiration
- Tracheal compression in peds (Am J Roentgenol Radium Ther Nucl Med 1974:80)

Lab: CXR to R/O aspiration, and to identify location if radiopaque. Consider lateral neck film or abdominal film if unable to locate object in chest. Barium swallow if still uncertain.

ED Rx: For esophageal foreign bodies without an acute abdomen:
- INT (heplock)
- TNG 0.4 mg SL (N Engl J Med 1973:23)
- If unsuccessful, glucagon 1 mg IV (Jacep 1979:228), or consider pulse doses q 30 minutes of 20–100 µg IV (Gastroenterology 1975:160)

- Perhaps effervescent drink to push bolus forward or facilitate regurgitation (Radiology 1983:299; Ann Emerg Med 1988:693), perhaps with glucagon (Radiology 1986:567)
- If unsuccessful, GI consult for EGD; surgery consult if acute abdomen
- Potential use of radiologists with balloon catheter extraction in selected patients with proximal foreign bodies (AJR Am J Roentgenol 1979:441; Arch Otolaryngol 1983:323), but not first choice (Gastrointest Endosc 1993:626)

6.3 ESOPHAGEAL RUPTURE

Chest Surg Clin N Am 1994:819

Cause: Full thickness esophageal tear, known as Boerhaave's syndrome after the Danish physician who diagnosed this after the grand admiral had vomited portions of a duck. May occur secondary to a weakened esophagus or after violent emesis, but the history is nonspecific most of the time. Ingested sharp or corrosive foreign bodies, or direct penetrating trauma, are also risk factors

Epidem: Uncommon, many diagnoses made postmortem. If diagnosis made promptly, outcome as good as with esophageal perforation secondary to endoscopy (Chest 1987:995)

Pathophys: Cause as above; leakage of enteric contents causes the secondary mediastinitis. One hypothesis is lack of muscularis mucosa at site of rupture (Am J Surg 1989:420)

Sx: History of vomiting; chest pain, abdominal pain, fever, otherwise nonspecific

Si: Rales; subcutaneous emphysema

Crs: Worse with delayed diagnosis; classic triad of vomiting, chest pain, and subcutaneous emphysema is not common (Am Surg 1999:449)

Cmplc: Mediastinitis—mortality >70% with delayed diagnosis

Diff Dx: Stomach rupture (Jama 1982:811); tension pneumothorax; bronchial tear; pulmonary embolus

Lab: Low Sao_2; pleural fluid for food particles if radiographic studies equivocal (Chest 1992:976). X-ray: CXR—pneumothorax, pleural effusion, pneumomediastinum, or subcutaneous emphysema (Am J Gastroenterol 1978:212); Gastrografin swallow (Br J Surg 1985:204) or CT (Arch Intern Med 1988:223) confirmatory

ED Rx:
- Treat/anticipate shock—IV access with fluid resuscitation
- Immediate surgical consult
- Anecdotally, conservative treatment has worked in some patients (Am J Surg 1981:531)

6.4 ESOPHAGEAL VARICES

Gastrointest Endosc Clin N Am 1999:175; Drug Ther Bull 2000:37

Cause: End-stage hepatic failure has many etiologies; one of the four major complications is hemorrhage, and esophageal bleeding is the most life-threatening (common?). Other complications are ascites, renal failure, and encephalopathy

Pathophys: Portal hypertension leading to varices; bleeding from depressed prothrombin and fibrinogen; depressed platelets from bleeding and hypersplenism; perhaps diminished platelet function from increased BUN; increased plasminogen activators due to diminished hepatic filtration

Sx/Si: Hematemesis, melena

Crs: Cause of death in 20% of patients with cirrhosis

Complc: Coagulopathy, encephalopathy

Diff Dx: See 6.13

Lab: Hemoccult emesis and stool, CBC with diff, PT/PTT, type and cross for PRBCs

ED Rx:

Gastrointest Endosc Clin N Am 1999:287
- IV, with fluid resuscitation if necessary to keep sys BP >100 mm Hg
- FFP if coagulopathy
- Somatostatin 250 µg IV bolus, then 250 µg/hr continuous drip (Gastroenterology 1990:1388), or octreotide 25 µg/hr IV drip (Can J Gastroenterol 1997:339)
- Consider nitroglycerin, transdermal (Hepatology 1990:678) or sublingual (Hepatology 1986:406)
- Vasopressin no longer advocated, somatostatin or its analogs (such as terlipressin) with fewer transfusion requirements (Hepatology 1993:61). Terlipressin and nitroglycerin better than balloon tamponade (Hepatology 1990:678)

- Sengstaken-Blakemore tube (Surg Gynecol Obstet 1976:529) with accessory NG tube until endoscopy available if pt hemorrhaging—applying external traction not necessary (Gastroenterology 1978:566); not a substitute nor should it delay endoscopy (Surg Gynecol Obstet 1988:331)
- Endoscopic ligation as good as surgery (50% survival), better than medical treatment (Hepatology 1997:1101) after a bleed but not used prophylactically if pt has never bled, and is better than sclerosis (Surg Gynecol Obstet 1985:438; Endoscopy 1997:241). Sclerotherapy better than medical therapy (Hepatology 1989:274), and better hemorrhage control when combined with octreotide (N Engl J Med 1995:555)
- Perhaps eventual portocaval or splenorenal (Ann Surg 1982:393) surgical shunting

6.5 FOODBORNE ILLNESSES (BACTERIAL GASTROENTERITIS)

Medicine (Baltimore) 1979:95; Arch Dis Child 1984:848

Cause: Inadequately prepared or maintained food, fecal-oral contamination, or water supply (*Campylobacter* (Lancet 1983:287))

Epidem: Most common in U.S. is *Staphylococcus*, *Salmonella* spp., *Clostridium perfringens* (MMWR Morb Mortal Wkly Rep 1994:137, 143), *Shigella*, *Campylobacter* (*jejuni* common, *upsaliensis* rare (Pediatr Infect Dis J 1999:988)), *Escherichia coli*—both invasive (MMWR Morb Mortal Wkly Rep 1991:265) and toxigenic, and *Listeria monocytogenes* (uncommon (N Engl J Med 2000:1236)). Potential current omeprazole use as risk factor for *Campylobacter* infection (Bmj 1996:414)

Pathophys:
- *Staphylococcus* forms a heat-stable toxin, does not stick to bowel wall
- *Salmonella* spp. invade bowel wall
- *Clostridium perfringens* produces a toxin
- *Shigella* demonstrates wall invasion (Infect Dis Clin North Am 2000:41, viii)
- *Campylobacter* invades bowel wall and produces a heat-labile toxin

- Invasive *E. coli* (e.g., 0157:H7) invades colon wall and produces toxin (Infect Dis Clin North Am 2000:41, viii)
- Toxigenic *E. coli* may produce both heat-labile and heat-stable toxins

Sx: Abdominal discomfort, vomiting, diarrhea

Si: Fever in those with *Salmonella*, *Shigella*; less likely or low-grade fever in *Campylobacter* and invasive *E. coli*; no fever in *Staphylococcus*, *Clostridium*, or toxigenic *E. coli*

Crs: Some with persistent problems consistent with irritable bowel syndrome (Bmj 1997:779)

Cmplc:
- Dehydration
- *Shigella* (Clin Diagn Lab Immunol 1996:701) and invasive *E. coli* (Pediatrics 1992:616) may be complicated by the hemolytic-uremic syndrome (HUS)
- *Shigella* may also be complicated by Reiter's syndrome, reactive arthritis, myocarditis (J Pediatr 1993:82), or erythema nodosum (Scott Med J 1984:197)

Diff Dx: Scombroid (N Engl J Med 1991:716; Jama 2000:2927) and ciguatera (J Toxicol Clin Toxicol 1993:1; Med J Aust 2000:176) poisoning if fish eaten; perhaps sorbitol or Olestra (large doses) consumption (Regul Toxicol Pharmacol 2000:59)

Lab: Consider stool culture if bloody diarrhea or if symptoms more than 72 h; perhaps PCR for *Campylobacter* (Epidemiol Infect 1998:547); stool for leukocytes is not sensitive and nonspecific (Diagn Microbiol Infect Dis 1993:313); other laboratory tests rarely alter treatment or disease course (Ann Emerg Med 1989:258; Dig Dis Sci 1996:1749; Acta Paediatr 1999:592)

ED Rx:
- IV hydration if oral rehydration not possible; many oral rehydration solutions available that contain sodium, potassium, chloride, base, and glucose with osmolality 311 mMol/L or less (Nutr Rev 2000:80). OK to IV hydrate children at 20–30 cc/kg over 1–2 hours and then send home if able to take po (Ann Emerg Med 1996:318)
- Antiemetics
- Antidiarrheals—do not worsen clinical picture and prevent ongoing fluid losses, such as bismuth subsalicylate or loperamide (Jama 1986:757)

- Sulfamethoxazole-trimethoprim (Bactrim DS bid) is better than ampicillin 500 mg po qid for 5 days for *Shigella* in areas of ampicillin resistance (Antimicrob Agents Chemother 1980:961)
- Cipro 500 mg po bid for 3–5 days covers all pathogens (Eur J Clin Microbiol 1986:241), including traveler's diarrhea where *E. coli* is prevalent (Ann Intern Med 1991:731); both *Staphylococcus* and *C. perfringens* are self-limited in this setting. This does limit duration and severity of illness (Clin Infect Dis 1996:1019)

6.6 GALLBLADDER DISEASE

Emerg Med Clin North Am 1996:719

Cause: Cholelithiasis may cause lodging of stones in the cystic duct or the common duct, or they may pass to the duodenum. Colic (misnomer) is an obstructed gallbladder, usually due to stones but may be due to a mass lesion. Cholecystitis is inflammation/infection of the gallbladder; acalculous cholecystitis is inflammation without stones. Cholangitis is infection of the biliary system, and may be due to a gallstone lodged in the common duct

Epidem: Cholecystitis is F/M 2:1, with stones present in 10% of adult women in U.S., 70% of Southwestern Native American women. Higher incidence of stones with the following:
- Increasing age
- Multiple pregnancies
- During pregnancy but later reverting to normal
- +/– chronic thiazide treatment
- Hemolytic disease
- Birth control and other estrogen use
- ETOH abuse
- Cirrhosis
- Vagotomy
- TPN—100% have sludge at 6 weeks
- Prolonged starvation/fasting
- Obesity, especially during weight loss
- Ileal disease
- Elevated triglycerides

Pathophys: Stones are usually mucin protein + cholesterol, less often with bilirubin and calcium

Sx: Steady epigastric or right upper quadrant pain (colic is a misnomer in this case) radiates to right scapula, nausea, vomiting—temporary relief after vomiting

Si: Fever, pressure at the right subcostal area inhibits patient from taking deep breath when prompted secondary to pain (Murphy's sign—97% sensitivity (Ann Emerg Med 1996:267))

Crs: Those with stones will have a 10–20% chance of having symptoms over 20–30 years; after first symptoms, 50% will recur over 20 years, with 25–50% getting complications—these are the low numbers and may be higher

Cmplc: Pancreatitis; cholangitis; hydrops, emphysema, or empyema of gallbladder; perforation and peritonitis; gallstone ileus is rare—a small bowel obstruction from a gallstone that has lodged at the ileocecal valve after eroding through the gallbladder into the duodenum; perhaps gallbladder cancer—cause and effect in these cases is uncertain

Diff Dx: Chronic acalculous cholecystitis (seen mainly in white females (Jsls 1999:221)), hepatitis, PUD, pyelonephritis

Lab: CBC with diff, LFTs, amylase, lipase—the elderly may have moderate to severe disease with little supportive serum laboratory data, age ≥65 years (Acad Emerg Med 1997:51); perhaps CRP (Eur J Surg 1992:365); gallbladder U/S (Gastrointest Radiol 1986:334); consider HIDA scan (Radiology 1982:369) if U/S equivocal—no dye in gallbladder is consistent with cholecystitis, no dye into duodenum is consistent with common duct stone. Abdominal X-ray usually not helpful, even for emphysematous cholecystitis (Br J Radiol 1997:986)—U/S better

ED Rx:

- IV access for nausea, vomiting, and pain control—some consider MSO_4 to cause spasm at the sphincter of Oddi but is not supported by good evidence. Perhaps NSAIDs of use, such as diclofenac 75 mg IM (Dig Dis Sci 1989:809)
- Parenteral antibiotics such as ampicillin/sulbactam, cefotetan, cefoperazone, or ceftriaxone (Chemotherapy 1988:30) for acute cholecystitis with fever and/or elevated white count, and surgical consult

- Parenteral antibiotics as above for cholangitis, and GI consult to consider ERCP. Would also get GI consult if concerned about common duct stone for any other reason
- If simple biliary colic, and/or mild cholecystitis (fever <101°F and no abnormal white count), consider outpatient follow-up with explicit instructions for surgical follow-up (1 week), and signs and symptoms to monitor which would necessitate immediate ED follow-up

6.7 HEPATITIS

Am J Clin Pathol 2000:12; hep A (Vaccine 1992:S15); hep B (Vaccine 1998:S11; Microbiol Mol Biol Rev 2000:51); hep C (Cmaj 2000:827; J Clin Gastroenterol 2000:125)

Cause: Inflammation of the liver from infectious, autoimmune, toxin, or metabolic disorder. Common causes are mononucleosis, hepatitis A, hepatitis B, hepatitis C, ETOH, and autoimmune hepatitis (Biomed Pharmacother 1999:255)

Epidem:
- Hepatitis A is usually a fecal-oral passage; higher in parents of day care children and common in developing countries
- Hepatitis B and Hepatitis C are parenteral or via sexual contact
- Hepatitis C is the leading cause of chronic liver disease (J Hepatol 2000:98)
- Other hepatitides are of a more chronic basis and most will be outpt work-up

Pathophys:
- Hepatitis A is an RNA enterovirus, with peak incidence in late summer and early winter
- Hepatitis B is a DNA virus that may incorporate into liver genome, associated with liver carcinoma—perhaps due to secondary carcinogenic exposures (Cancer Surv 1986:765). Hepatitis D (delta particle) (Antivir Ther 1998:37) can only infect in conjunction with hepatitis B
- Hepatitis C is an RNA virus that appears to merit no protective antibody response

Sx:

- Hep A with 15–40-day incubation period. Only 5–15% of children get symptoms, with malaise, anorexia, abdominal pain, nausea, vomiting, diarrhea, light-colored stools, and dark-colored urine being found in symptomatic children and adults
- Hep B has a 60–160-day incubation period, with arthralgias, arthritis, urticaria, and other rashes being common
- Hep C has a 2–20-week incubation period (6–7 weeks being average)
- Chronic hepatitis associated with autoantibodies (Prog Liver Dis 1994:137)

Si:

- Hep A with jaundice, although anicteric form also common and more benign
- Hep B with many cases anicteric
- Hep C with 80% anicteric

Crs:

- Hep A is usually benign, with 15% morbidity and 0.3% mortality; symptoms peak 2 weeks after onset and take about 4 weeks to clear; 6% of patients will relapse in 1–3 months
- Hep B has many possibilities with acute hepatitis, typical or cholangitic, leading to the following:
  - Benign course, recover or relapsing, or chronic persistent—portal—or mild hepatitis, or
  - Acute liver necrosis, all of whom die, or
  - Submassive hepatic necrosis (bridging) of whom 60% die or go on to postnecrotic cirrhosis, the balance of patients recovering completely, or
  - Chronic active hepatitis, usually with a progressive downhill course over 5–10 years, or
  - Asymptomatic carrier state in approx. 90% newborns, 20% school-age children, <1% young healthy adults (WWII vaccine epidemic)
- Hep C also has a variable course; 60–70% of patients still have elevated LFTs 12 months later but overall mortality over decades is not increased. Acute hepatitis, typical or cholangitic, leads to the following:
  - Chronic active hepatitis in most, or
  - Benign course, recover or have relapsing or chronic persistent (mild or "portal") hepatitis, or

– Acute liver necrosis, all of whom die, or
– Submassive hepatic necrosis (bridging) of whom 60% die or go on to postnecrotic cirrhosis, the balance of patients recovering completely

Cmplc:
- Hep A with fulminant hepatitis or relapsing hepatitis
- Hep B with hepatoma; 10% go on to chronic active hepatitis (Ann Intern Med 2000:723); facilitates secondary infection with delta agent (hepatitis D), which is an RNA virus and this leads also to acute hepatitis or a severe chronic active hepatitis; fasting hypoglycemia; serum sickness; polyarteritis (J Clin Invest 1975:930); and nephritis, especially membranous GN
- Hep C with 80% going on to chronic active hepatitis over 10 years, and 20–35% of these people go on to cirrhosis over 20 years; hepatocellular carcinoma over 30 years independent of hep B; and may develop mixed cryoglobulinemia

Diff Dx:
- With fever: mononucleosis, Q fever (Gastroenterology 1982:474), toxoplasmosis, CMV, Fitz-Hugh-Curtis syndrome, psittacosis, hepatitis E and other viral hepatitides
- Without fever: drugs (Baillieres Clin Gastroenterol 1988:385)— ETOH, acetaminophen, NSAIDs, other toxins; chronic autoimmune hepatitis; hemochromatosis; Wilson's disease; α-antitrypsin deficiency; α-methyldopa (Aldomet)-induced hepatitis; oxyphenisatin laxative induction; primary biliary cirrhosis; diabetes; myxedema; hepatitis G and other viral hepatitides; myopathy

Lab: CBC with diff, LFTs, amylase, lipase, PT/PTT if suspect fulminant hepatitis (Vaccine 1992:S21); get CPK, especially if LDH > AST (SGOT) > ALT (SGPT) to R/O myopathy—may also check aldolase

Serologic Markers (see Table 6.1)
- Hep A shows IgM first; this later goes negative as IgG appears and stays positive (J Virol Methods 1980:31)
- Hep B with hep B_SAg first, and then hep B_SAb—if both negative but high suspicion, then retest. A small window exists when both may be negative
- Hep C antibody elevated 4–50 weeks after LFTs abnormal; may check sera for hep C viral RNA via PCR
- Hep E serology accurate (Clin Infect Dis 1995:621)

Table 6.1. Viral Hepatitis (Reprinted with permission from Am J Clin Pathol 2000;113:16)

Type	Clinical Features	Transaminases	Serologic Findings Acute Disease	Immunity
A (RNA)	Acute self-limiting; fecal-oral transmission; no carrier state	Markedly elevated, 3+ to 4+	IgM anti-HAV	IgG anti-HAV
B (DNA)	Acute or chronic; often asymptomatic; 5% infected blood and body fluids	1+ to 3+ (acute); variable; chronic	IgM anti-HBc; HBsAg; HBeAg; HBV DNA	IgG anti-HBs; anti-HBe
C (RNA)	Usually chronic	Mild to moderate elevation, even in acute cases	Total anti-HCV; HCV RNA	Unknown
D (RNA)	Requires HBV coinfection; acute or chronic; rare in United States	Often markedly elevated	IgM anti-HDV; total anti-HDV; may require multiple assays	Unknown
E (RNA)	Epidemic similar to HAV; acute self-limiting; water borne and enteric; transmission in India and Southeast Asia	Variable	Testing not widely available; reference laboratory: CDC	Unknown
G (RNA)	Close homology to HCV; high prevalence (2% of US donors); usually mild disease, if at all; disease spectrum uncertain	Variable	HGV-RNA and EIA (reference laboratory only)	Unknown
Non-A-E, exclude EBV and CMV	Possibly acute or chronic	Variable	None	Unknown

CDC, Centers for Disease Control and Prevention; CMV, cytomegalovirus; EBV, Epstein-Barr virus; EIA, enzyme immunoassay; HAV, hepatitis A virus; anti-HBc, antibody to hepatitis B core; anti-HBe, antibody to hepatitis B e antigen; HBeAg, hepatitis B e antigen; anti-HBs, antibody to hepatitis B surface antigen; HBsAg, hepatitis B surface antigen; HBV, hepatitis B virus; HCV, hepatitis C virus; HDV, hepatitis D virus; HGV, hepatitis G virus.

- X-ray: get U/S of abdomen for imaging study if concerned about anatomic or obstructive problem with liver, especially suspect this if patient elderly. Abdominal CT may further delineate anatomy

ED Rx:
- Hep A exposures should prophylax with 0.02 cc/kg of IgG, max dose 2.0 cc IM. A vaccine does exist (Havrix or Vaqta) for travel or high-risk prophylaxis—booster needs unknown. Vaccine does prevent secondary cases (Lancet 1999:1136)
- Hep B exposures should receive hep B immune globulin (HBIG) if not vaccinated—dose is 0.05 cc/kg × 2 30 days apart within 24–72 hours of exposure. The vaccination series is recommended for everyone not already vaccinated and is 3 injections on day 0, day 30, and day 180. If acute exposure, the vaccine should be given as well. Active disease should be referred to GI for consideration of interferon α-2a or -2b, or possibly lamivudine (3TC) (N Engl J Med 1998:61), but no steroids
- Hep C as with hep B except immune globulin is ineffective, and perhaps use of other nucleoside analogs (N Engl J Med 1998:1493; Lancet 1998:1426). Perhaps vaccine (Proc Natl Acad Sci U S A 2000:297)
- OK to give hep A and hep B vaccines together (Vaccine 2000:1074)
- *Note*: Universal precautions advocated for everyone; wear gloves, wash hands, and get screened if you have a body fluid exposure. If patient has active disease, high-risk behaviors discouraged—IV drugs, sexual promiscuity, blood donation

6.8 INFECTIOUS DIARRHEA (USUALLY NON-FOOD-RELATED)

Cause: Inoculation person-to-person, infected water supplies, or foodborne (see 6.5). Possibly airborne as well (Am J Epidemiol 1988:1261)

Epidem: Common; many outbreaks are episodic, or possibly referable to water supply, day care setting, hospital ward (J Infect Dis 1982:727), or other common variables. United Kingdom evaluating small round structured viruses as predominant factors in outbreaks (J Med Virol 2000:132)

Pathophys: In U.S., acute diarrhea is usually due to a viral agent, with some specific exceptions as noted below. The most common viruses are rotavirus, Norwalk virus, enteric adenovirus, calcivirus, and astrovirus.

- *Clostridium difficile*: seen after antibiotic use, specific risks of advanced age, and/or clindamycin use. Asymptomatic carrier state in peds <1 year of age, even after antibiotic use (Pediatr Infect Dis 1984:433) and increased likelihood with bottle-fed infants (J Clin Microbiol 1983:830)
- *Giardia lamblia*: seen after exposure to untreated fresh water supply, such as mountain lakes or streams
- *Yersinia* colitis: household pets, as well as food- or waterborne exposures, as proposed transmission

Sx: Abdominal discomfort, vomiting, diarrhea. Bloating, gaseous, and profuse and foul-smelling diarrhea in *Giardia*

Si: Fever in rotavirus, *C. difficile*, and *Yersinia*; much less likely in the other types listed above

Crs: Usually self-limited without treatment except in *Giardia*

Diff Dx: See 6.5. Risk factors predispose to other etiologies as listed below:

- Male homosexual: herpes II, gonorrhea, and chlamydial colitis
- Immunocompromised individuals: *Cryptosporidium, Cyclospora cayetanensis, Enterocytozoon bienensis, Isospora belli, Plesiomonas,* and *Aeromonas*
- World travel: *Entamoeba histolytica, Bacillus cereus, Vibrio cholera, V. parahaemolyticus*
- Handlers of seawater: *V. mimicus*
- Radiation enteritis
- Chemotherapeutic induced, specifically fluoropyrimidines and irinotecan (J Pain Symptom Manage 2000:118)

Lab:

- Rotavirus: latex agglutination (fast) and stool ELISA test available —both have sensitivity >90% and specificity ~99% if used in first week of the illness (J Clin Microbiol 1985:846; 1982:562)
- *C. difficile*: stool toxin; perhaps useful in patient with antibiotics within last month, significant diarrhea, abdominal discomfort, or recent hospitalization (and >1 year of age) (Diagn Microbiol Infect Dis 2000:169)

- *Giardia*: stool antigen, 3 O + P samples if antigen test not available
- *Yersinia*: stool culture, antibody titers with 30% false negative

ED Rx:
- Symptomatic treatment with oral or IV rehydration, antiemetics
- Bismuth subsalicylate (Pepto-Bismol) 60 cc in adults or 1.14 cc/kg (100 mg/kg) in children qid helps speed recovery
- Zinc gluconate 20 mg po qd within first 3 days in children in developing countries
- *C. difficile*: metronidazole orally, oral vancomycin if no response or if severe illness; perhaps the probiotic *Lactobacillus GG* (Am J Gastroenterol 2000:S11)
- *Giardia*: metronidazole; furazolidone for children if liquid preferable
- *Yersinia*: consider tetracycline
- Children with mild to moderate diarrhea may fare better with homeopathy (J Altern Complement Med 2000:131), although this group of patients would do OK with WHO ORS and a wide spectrum of individual (different) homeopathic medications

Oral rotavirus tetravalent vaccine at 2, 3, and 4 months of age available (MMWR Morb Mortal Wkly Rep 1999:1)

6.9 LOWER GI BLEED

AJR Am J Roentgenol 1993:703

Cause: Consider upper GI bleed, but lower GI bleed causes include hemorrhoids, diverticulosis, ischemic colitis, AV malformations, polyps, cancer, and Meckel's diverticulum. Rarely TB (Am J Gastroenterol 1999:270)

Epidem: Less common than upper GI bleeds; more common in older age and if male (Am J Gastroenterol 1997:419)

Pathophys: Erosion through mucosa may herald bleeding in ischemic colitis and AV malformations, and the arterial bleeding of diverticulosis is secondary to the diverticula outpouching occurring at the site of weakness from the perforating mucosal vessels. Meckel's diverticulum may have gastric tissue and consequent ulcer formation

Sx: Painless hematochezia usually; may have pain with external hemorrhoids

Si: Bright red blood on rectal exam, obvious hemorrhoids

Crs: Worse prognosis if ongoing bleeding, systolic BP <100 mm Hg, elevated PT (INR >1.2), change in mental status, or other unstable disease process (Crit Care Med 1997:1125)

Cmplc: If significant anemia, secondary cardiac (Chest 1998:1137) or neurologic compromise

Diff Dx: Carcinoma, inflammatory bowel disease, polyps, and infectious (including TB) enteritis may cause lower GI bleeding, but not usually hemorrhage unless some sort of trauma—inadvertent shearing of a polyp, for example—or coagulopathy, such as seen with liver dysfunction or ASA use

Lab: Guaiac stool, CBC with diff, PT/PTT, type and cross, metabolic profile to look for BUN/Cr ratio, EKG to R/O silent ischemia if this is an issue. Consider anoscopy at bedside as diagnostic test. X-ray: barium enema not superior to colonoscopy

ED Rx:
- O_2
- Two large bore IVs, at least one with NS to be compatible with blood
- Blood if no response to fluid resuscitation, tachycardia with no fever or pain in an elderly patient necessitates treatment even with no hypotension or orthostasis
- Nuclear tagged red cell scan (Radiology 1981:465; Ann Surg 1996:29) if pt is stable; consider Meckel scan if previous evaluation has been complete and without source. Only those patients with immediate blush on technitium scan most likely to have useful angiography (Dis Colon Rectum 1997:471)
- Surgical and GI consult for the unstable pt, perhaps urgent angiography (Ann Surg 1989:175; AJR Am J Roentgenol 1992:521) or colonoscopy (Gastrointest Endosc 1995:93)

6.10 PANCREATITIS

Gastroenterol Clin North Am 1999:571, viii

Cause:
- Gallstones in 45–75%; biliary sludge is an ultrasound diagnosis that is underappreciated (N Engl J Med 1992:589)
- ETOH 10–35% responsible from sphincter of Oddi spasm and increased pancreatic secretion via secretin

- Hereditary types I and V hyperlipidemia
- Idiopathic in 10–30%, perhaps association with cystic fibrosis gene (N Engl J Med 1998:653)
- Posterior duodenal ulcer
- Accidental trauma or inadvertent during surgery
- Hyperparathyroidism with calcium stone formation
- Infectious such as mumps, coxsackie, many viruses including HIV, ascariasis (Br J Surg 1992:1335), clonorchiasis
- Cancer of duodenum, pancreas, or ampulla; diabetes seen with pancreatic cancer most likely of recent onset, diabetes not a risk factor for pancreatic cancer (N Engl J Med 1994:81)
- Anatomic variants such as choledochal cysts, duodenal diverticula, or pancreatic divisum
- Pregnancy
- Protein starvation
- Vasculitis, specifically with anticardiolipin antibodies (Am J Emerg Med 1993:230)
- Drugs such as thiazides, steroids, sulfasalazine (Azulfidine) and other sulfas, furosemide, azathioprine
- Post pump after bypass surgery, probably from IV $CaCl_2$ given

Epidem: Male/female: 2:1; incidence approx. 400/million/yr, but in AIDS, 5–20/100/yr

Pathophys: Autodigestion perhaps due to trypsin and lipase, hypocalcemia from calcium soap formation, or perhaps glucagon-induced?

Sx: Epigastric abdominal pain relieved by leaning forward, radiates to back/flank; abdominal distention, nausea, and vomiting

Si: Ileus; guarding; fever, or hypothermia at times; erythema nodosum–like lesions due to focal fat necrosis; Grey-Turner sign is flank ecchymoses with retroperitoneal bleeding, and Cullen's sign is periumbilical ecchymoses from extension of pancreatic enzymes along the falciform or round ligament (Gastrointest Radiol 1989:31)

Crs: 50–80% never recur. Worse prognosis with age >55 years, male gender, and idiopathic or alcoholic pancreatitis (Hepatogastroenterology 1998:1859). Ranson (Am J Gastroenterol 1974:443) and modified Ranson criteria (see Table 6.2): mortality <1% if ≤2 risk factors, 16% if 3–4 risk factors, and 100% if ≥7 risk factors; APACHE III and modified Glasgow Coma score also predictive (Crit Care Med 1999:901)

Table 6.2. Early Objective Prognostic Signs Used to Estimate the Risk of Death or Major Complications from Acute Pancreatitis (Am J Gastroenterol 1982;77:63)

At admission or diagnosis
　Age over 55 yr
　White blood cell count over 16,000/mm^3
　Blood glucose over 200 mg/100 ml
　Serum lactic dehydrogenase over 350 IU/l
　Serum glutamic oxaloacetic transaminase over 250 Sigma Frankel Units %

During initial 48 h
　Hematocrit fall greater than 10 percentage points
　Blood urea nitrogen rise more than 5 mg/100 ml
　Serum calcium level below 8 mg/100 ml
　Arterial pO$_2$ below 60 mm Hg
　Base deficit greater than 4 mEq/l
　Estimated fluid sequestration more than 6000 ml

Cmplc: ARDS; ATN; tetany with hypocalcemia; shock; pancreatic abscess (4%); pancreatic pseudocyst formation (Am J Surg 1996:228), which can result in infection or rupture into peritoneal cavity or spleen or dissection along body planes; GI bleeding and splenomegaly from splenic vein thrombosis rare

Diff Dx: Amylase elevation from 5 sources: pancreas, parotid/salivary glands, small bowel, fallopian tubes, and macroamylasemia—the molecule is too big to filter through kidney

Lab: CBC with diff; metabolic profile including calcium, magnesium, phosphorous; amylase and lipase (J Emerg Med 1999:1027); urine for trypsinogen-2 dipstick, positive is 92% sensitive/specific (N Engl J Med 1997:1788); perhaps phospholipase A$_2$, pancreatitis-associated protein (Ann Med 1998:169), or interleukin-6 (Clin Chem 1999:1762)

　• Amylase serum levels up for 3 days, >225 IU is 95% sensitive and 98% specific; lipase peaks at 4–7 days, correlates with hypertriglyceridemia that follows acute attacks, and is more sensitive (95% vs. 79%) in direct comparison study (Am J Emerg Med 1994:21)

　• Glucose may be elevated from transient glucagon release

　• ALT ≥3 times normal indicates gallstone etiology with 95% certainty

- Isoamylase equally as good as lipase as a confirmation test
- X-ray: G/B U/S to evaluate common duct and cystic duct and to look for stones. Intravenous cholangiography may be better (Jama 1979:342). CT is best for delineating intra-abdominal processes in those with complicated courses (J Gastroenterol Hepatol 1990:103)

ED Rx:
- IV fluid; pt will most likely be volume contracted secondary to plasma loss from third spacing
- Antiemetics and parenteral narcotics for pain management
- NGT if significant ileus or obstruction
- IV H_2 blocker, controversial as far as helping pancreatitis resolve, but helpful for ileus
- Consider IV antibiotics such as ampicillin/sulbactam or imipenem if pt appears septic; this is debatable
- GI consult—consideration of ERCP—this is where the U/S helps

6.11 PEPTIC ULCER DISEASE/GASTRITIS

Dig Dis Sci 1988:129; Am Surg 1990:737; Gut 1993:580

Cause: Due to *Helicobacter pylori* infection; endogenous or NSAID-induced (Gastroenterology 1989:640) increased acid/pepsin secretion, compounded problem with use of corticosteroids (N Engl J Med 1983:21; Br Med J (Clin Res Ed) 1987:1227; Ann Intern Med 1991:735); decreased pancreatic or duodenal HCO_3 secretion; or a decrease in other GI defenses

Epidem:
- Duodenal ulcer 90% associated with chronic *H. pylori* infection that often begins early in life but 28% with NSAIDs if > age 60; occurs in 10% of people, male/female = 4/1 under age 60 years; positive family history in 50% under age 30 years, 20% in those older than 30 years at onset
- Gastric ulcers have an 80% association with chronic *H. pylori* infection (N Engl J Med 1989:1562), found in 3% of people, females > males
- Meckel's diverticulum in <1% of people, usually ulcerates in childhood

Note: Only 15–20% of those chronically infected get duodenal or gastric ulcers

Pathophys:

Increased acid production in the following:

- Zollinger-Ellison syndrome
- Neurogenically increased secretion, e.g., burn or CVA pts
- Nicotine users
- Coffee users, but it's not the caffeine
- TPN pt from the IV amino acids
- Hypersecretors, who can be divided into hypersecretors and hypergastrin responders
- ASA, NSAID, and ETOH users

Diminished pancreatic secretions in the following:

- 10% of those with cystic fibrosis, may be first symptom in heterozygote
- Perhaps with nicotine
- Perhaps with steroids

Impaired GI defenses include the following:

- *H. pylori* infection, which tolerates high-acid environment
- ASA and NSAIDs in elderly, esp. if concomitant steroid use
- ETOH increases permeability of mucosa to H^+ and produces direct mucosal damage
- Smoking inhibits duodenal HCO_3 secretion

Sx: Epigastric pain esp. 1–2 hr pc and 2 am; GI bleeding, occult, melena, or hematemesis

Si: Epigastric tenderness; stool guaiac positive

Crs:

- Duodenal ulcer recurs in 10%, except in smokers, where 72% recur in 1 year; R/O Zollinger-Ellison syndrome if does recur and not a smoker; eradication of *H. pylori* reduces rate of rebleeding (Gastrointest Endosc 1995:1)
- Gastric ulcer recurs in 50%; takes approx. 8 weeks to heal with Rx
- *H. pylori* may be chronic, recurrent, and resistant to multiple treatment attempts, but 96% do not recur after cleared with antibiotic course

Cmplc: Persistent bleeding, perforation, obstruction, pain; possibly adenocarcinoma and non-Hodgkin's gastric lymphoma in pts with *H. pylori*

Diff Dx: Gastroesophageal reflux esophagitis (GERD); gastric carcinoma—document healing; celiac artery compression/obstruction give pc pain—aka abdominal angina

Lab: CBC with diff, LFTs, PT/PTT if bleeding, consider amylase and lipase, consider U/A if considering genitourinary etiology; *H. pylori* antibody titer if considering empiric treatment with proton pump inhibitor, although poor test for screening for ulcer (Aliment Pharmacol Ther 2000:615). X-ray: 3-view abdominal series if suspect perforation to R/O free air

ED Rx:

If actively bleeding, consider immediate endoscopy and possibly IV octreotide. If not actively bleeding, consider the following options:

- GI cocktail:
  - *Silver Slider*—10 cc viscous lidocaine with 20 cc Mylanta
  - *Green Goddess*—10 cc each of viscous lidocaine, Mylanta, and Donnatal
- H_2 blocker of choice: cimetidine (Tagamet) 300–400 mg po bid or 800 mg po qhs, ranitidine (Zantac) 150 mg po bid or 300 mg po qhs, famotidine (Pepcid) 20 mg po bid or 40 mg po qhs, or nizatidine (Axid) 150 mg po bid or 300 mg po qhs
- Proton-pump inhibitor of choice if pt already failed H_2 blocker: lansoprazole (Prevacid) 30 mg po qd, omeprazole (Prilosec) 20 mg po qd or bid (Digestion 1990:64, discussion, 76; Aliment Pharmacol Ther 1989:83), rabeprazole (Aciphex) 20 mg po qd (Med Lett Drugs Ther 1999;41:110), or pantoprazole (Protonix) 40 mg po qd, mainly for GERD (Med Lett Drugs Ther 2000;42:65)
- Antacids work the quickest, such as Maalox or Mylanta (N Engl J Med 1966:921)—avoid those with $CaCO_3$ because of acid rebound seen 1 hour after ingestion
- Black licorice helpful (Scand J Gastroenterol Suppl 1979:117); propantheline (Pro-Banthine) 15 mg ac appears equivocal (Am J Gastroenterol 1967:124)
- Sucralfate (Carafate) 1 gram po qid 1 hour ac (Pharmacotherapy 1982:67) as benign and as good as cimetidine
- Behavioral Rx: stop tobacco, ETOH, NSAIDs, coffee (N Engl J Med 1974:469)
- Outpt referral for consideration of *H. pylori* treatment, radiographic upper GI imaging or endoscopy

6.12 PROCTITIS

Gastroenterol Clin North Am 1987:157; Clin Infect Dis 1999:S84

Cause: Seen in inflammatory bowel disease (ulcerative colitis) and as a sexually transmitted disease (STD). Less common from trauma (Sex Transm Dis 1979:75); iatrogenic from gold (J Rheumatol 1987:142) or radiation therapy (Am J Gastroenterol 1996:1309)

Epidem: Unsure

Pathophys: Seen in ulcerative colitis as an autoimmune phenomenon which is usually refractory to therapy. As an STD, occurs from direct anal intercourse, or as contiguous spread sometimes in *Chlamydia trachomatis* (lymphogranuloma venereum) or *Neisseria gonorrhoeae*. The same organisms implicated in common STDs are seen here—herpes type II, HIV, papillomavirus, and *Treponema pallidum*

Sx: Pain, itching (pruritus ani (Dis Colon Rectum 1994:670)), and discharge

Si: Erythematous mucosa, possible discharge

Cmplc: Ulcerative proctitis may go on to carcinoma or stricture, or be associated with other autoimmune phenomena (see 8.6)

Diff Dx: Perirectal abscess, hemorrhoids, fissure, neoplasm, fistula

Lab: If not consistent with STD, CBC with diff. If STD considered, anoscopy with Gram's stain, culture; serum test for syphilis—e.g., VDRL or RPR; HIV counseling and/or testing

ED Rx:

If ulcerative proctitis, GI consult—timing depends on how symptomatic pt feels. If STD, see 8.6 for females and 27.4 for males. All partners should be evaluated

6.13 UPPER GI HEMORRHAGE

Digestion 1999:47

Cause: Most commonly seen in esophageal varices (see 6.4), Mallory-Weiss tear, peptic ulcer disease (see 6.11), erosive esophagitis and gastritis, and less commonly in arteriovenous malformation, carcinoma, or pure arterial bleed (Dieulafoy's lesion). Those with previous aortic repair are at risk for aortoenteric fistula. Rarely TB (Am J Gastroenterol 1999:270)

Epidem: >60 years of age usually with less ETOH use, and greater likelihood of PUD; less than 60 years of age with more Mallory-Weiss tears and variceal problems (Am J Gastroenterol 1997:42)

Pathophys: Mallory-Weiss tear is a partial-thickness tear at the GE junction usually following vomiting. Erosive esophagitis is a mucosal problem with usually self-limited hemorrhage seen in those who use tobacco, ETOH, and NSAIDs, and may or may not have a coincident hiatal hernia—seems as if a variant of PUD/gastritis

Sx: Hematemesis, melena, abdominal pain

Si: Epigastric tenderness

Crs: Worse prognosis if older, comorbid disease processes, tachycardia or hypotension, or if ongoing bleeding (Scand J Gastroenterol 1995:327)

Cmplc: Secondary to hemorrhage, ischemic/infarcting cardiac (Chest 1998:1137; Mayo Clin Proc 1999: 235) and/or neurologic events

Diff Dx: Upper pharyngeal hemorrhage

Lab: Guaiac positive stools, Hemoccult positive emesis, CBC with diff, PT/PTT, metabolic profile—look for BUN/Cr > 23/1 (Am J Gastroenterol 1997:1796) although not solely discriminatory, type and screen, consider EKG

ED Rx:
- IV, with fluid resuscitation if necessary to keep sys BP >100 mm Hg
- Blood products if fluid bolus ineffective, consider pressors
- FFP if coagulopathy
- Consider somatostatin 250 μg IV bolus, then 250 μg/hr continuous drip (Digestion 1989:190; 1999:1), or octreotide 25 μg/hr IV drip
- H_2 blockers of no help emergently (Scand J Gastroenterol 1984:885)
- Sengstaaken-Blakemore tube with accessory NG tube until endoscopy (Gastrointest Endosc 1999:145) available if pt hemorrhaging
- If due to peptic ulcer disease, proton pump inhibitor to prevent recurrence (Epidemiology 1999:228)
- Nonvariceal bleeding that is not persistent and without significant anemia, no orthostasis or baseline vital sign abnormalities, no liver disease or coagulopathy, and in a nondisabled young patient (<60 years of age) may be considered for outpatient follow-up and treatment (Acad Emerg Med 1999:196)

7 General Surgery

7.1 ABDOMINAL AORTIC ANEURYSM

Cause: Arteriosclerotic disease or genetic cause (Ann Intern Med 1999:637) most likely, such as Marfan syndrome; less likely due to trauma or infection (syphilis, TB (Pediatr Radiol 1999:536))

Epidem: Male:female 10:1

Pathophys: Proposed that degenerative changes in the media of the arterial wall responsible for the aneurysm formation

Sx: Abdominal pain, radiating to or originating in the back, flank, or genital area

Si: Presence of pulsatile mass not as significant as the width—with 5–5.5 cm being significant (Can Fam Physician 1999:2069; J Vasc Surg 1999:191), loss of femoral pulses. Check for bruits

Crs: Spontaneous rupture of this aneurysm increases with size, with aneurysms greater than 5 cm in diameter having a chance of rupture

Cmplc: Vascular collapse resulting in death, this is higher in AAA repairs done emergently after symptoms start (Ann Vasc Surg 1999:613)

Diff Dx: Myocardial infarction, aortitis (J Vasc Surg 1999:189), pneumonia, pancreatitis, nephrolithiasis, bowel obstruction, diverticulitis, sickle cell crisis, mesenteric thrombosis, porphyria, diabetes, cholecystitis, perforated viscus, splenic infarct, incarcerated hernia

Lab: CBC with diff with abnormal platelets (Eur J Vasc Endovasc Surg 1999:434), PT/PTT, type and cross, 10 units PRBCs, U/A may show hematuria. X-ray studies: may be seen on plain abdominal lateral shoot-through; ultrasound for screening (Eur J Vasc Endovasc Surg 1999:472); abdominal CT gives the most information (AJR Am J Roentgenol 2000:181) and may be better than aortography (J Endovasc Surg 1998:222); MRI may have role (Magn Reson Imaging 1990:199)

ED Rx:
- Two large-bore IVs
- Fluid resuscitation if necessary, consider pressors and blood products
- To OR in a timely fashion; resuscitation in OR is considered more appropriate

7.2 APPENDICITIS

Emerg Med Clin North Am 1996:653; Am Fam Physician 1999:2027

Cause: Obstructed appendix from fecolith, lymphoid hyperplasia from viral illness

Epidem: 7% lifetime risk; male to female 1.5 to 1; incidence is 23 cases/10,000 population/year if between second and third decade of life

Pathophys: As above

Sx: Nausea, anorexia; periumbilical pain at first that moves to the RLQ; >36 (Am Surg 1999:453) but <72 hours of duration; sense of constipation and urge to defecate

Si: Fever 37.5–38.5°C; <101°F (Am Surg 1999:453). Right lower quadrant guarding, rebound, and cough tenderness; right-sided rectal tenderness not helpful (World J Surg 1999:133). Iliopsoas, obturator internus, and heel pounding signs may also be positive

Crs: 12–24 hours

Cmplc: Perforation with peritonitis (20–33%—pre CT) (Pediatrics 1979:36); perforation increases prevalence of infertility 5 times

Diff Dx: UTI; urolithiasis; incarcerated inguinal or femoral hernia; intussusception in children <4 years of age; cecal mass (World J Surg 1999:713, discussion, 716) including neoplasm; tuberculosis; schistosomiasis; mesenteric adenitis including *Yersinia* pseudoappendicular syndrome; diverticulitis; epiploic appendagitis; typhlitis, a cecal colitis seen with aggressive chemotherapy for leukemia; strep throat in children

Gynecologic

Ruptured ovarian cyst, ectopic pregnancy, ovarian torsion, tubo-ovarian abscess, PID

Obstetric

Difficult diagnosis during pregnancy, with clinical and serum markers of little help in diagnosis (Acta Obstet Gynecol Scand 1999:758)

Lab: CBC with diff (WBC usually 10K–13K, but not sensitive or specific—perhaps low normal WBC helpful in excluding diagnosis, i.e., <8K (World J Surg 1999:133)); +/– CRP with elevation (large gray zone between 10–50) indicative of acute complicated disease, e.g., abscess or perforation (Br J Surg 1999:501); U/A, hematuria does not necessarily implicate nephrolithiasis with appropriate history for appendicitis; pregnancy test if of childbearing age. X-ray: KUB not helpful, but presence of appendicolith will necessitate surgery, helical CT helpful (N Engl J Med 1998:141) including with gyn diagnoses (Obstet Gynecol 1999:417), +/– Gastrografin enema. U/S not helpful (World J Surg 1999:141). Possible use of a technetium labeled antibody fragment, Sulesomab (91% sensitive, 92% specific (Surgery; 1999:288))

ED Rx: Place IV, pain meds and antiemetics, surgery is curative. Pain meds do not obscure diagnosis (Ann R Coll Surg Engl 1986:209)

7.3 BOWEL OBSTRUCTION

Cause: Inability of intraluminal intestinal contents to be moved forward via peristalsis

Epidem: Complications and death have decreased since 1961 with more timely diagnosis, now being less than 10% if younger than 80 years of age (Ann Surg 2000:529)

Pathophys: May be due to previous surgery with either defect in the mesentery or the development of adhesions causing problems; herniation through the femoral canal, inguinal area, or anterior abdominal wall; inflammatory bowel disease or radiation enteritis with luminal stenosis; volvulus due to medications or loss of ganglion cells (J Surg Res 1996:385); neoplasm; or less likely a foreign body or gallstone ileus or ascaris

Sx: Abdominal pain, nausea, vomiting, bloating, constipation

Si: Diffuse abdominal pain with peritoneal signs, increased or lack of bowel sounds, distended or tympanic abdomen

Crs: May pass spontaneously; others will require surgery

Cmplc: Perforation

Diff Dx: Ileus, Ogilvie's syndrome (Arch Surg 1977:512), partial small bowel obstruction. Peds: intussusception, Hirschsprung's disease, atresia or stenosis

Lab: CBC with diff, metabolic profile to exclude reasons for an ileus, type and cross if surgery considered. X-ray: consider radiographs if at least two of the following (Eur J Surg 1998:777):

- Distended abdomen
- Increased bowel sounds
- History of constipation
- Previous abdominal surgery
- Age >50 yrs
- Vomiting

Abdominal series may disclose no air in the rectum—helpful if X-rays previous to rectal exam, dilated bowel with paucity of bowel gas in distal colon, air/fluid levels on upright film; CT is better (Am J Surg 1999:375), some obstructions have no obvious dilation or air/fluid levels on plain film secondary to the intraluminal regions having no air; small bowel follow-through (SBFT) if CT is not diagnostic—SBFT does not provide treatment (Eur J Surg 2000:39)

ED Rx:

J Pain Symptom Manage 2000:23

- IV access with hydration
- Parenteral antiemetics and narcotics if necessary
- NGT
- Consider dexamethasone 6–16 mg IM for malignant bowel obstruction due to GI or gyn cancer (Cochrane Database Syst Rev 2000)
- Surgical consult

7.4 INCARCERATED HERNIA (ABDOMINAL)

Am J Surg 1967:888; Emerg Med Clin North Am 1996:739

Cause: Outpouching of intra-abdominal contents through wall defect produces a hernia. If complete defect with no covering of contents—including parietal peritoneum—then this is evisceration. Usually due to genetic defect or postsurgical site or augmented by peritoneal dialysis (Surg Gynecol Obstet 1983:541)

Inguinal

Consider femoral hernia in this area as well. A direct inguinal hernia goes through Hesselbach's triangle, which is defined as the area lateral to the lateral border of the rectus abdominis, superior to the inguinal ligament, and medial/inferior to the inferior epigastric artery. An indirect inguinal hernia lies lateral to the inferior epigastric artery and above the inguinal ligament. A femoral hernia lies below the inguinal ligament in the inguinal canal, and this type of hernia is more common in females. An inguinal hernia in pediatrics calls for either laparoscopic or direct inspection of the contralateral side according to some authors

Umbilical

Location as name implies, could be congenital or postsurgical. More common in females and in those who are obese or have ascites or women who are pregnant. Although troublesome in adults, watchful waiting is OK in children. In neonates, consider patent urachus and/or omphalocele

Ventral

May have gastric involvement (Gastrointest Radiol 1984:311). Consider spigelian hernia—this is a potential defect where the inferior border of the posterior rectus sheath (linea semicircularis) and the lateral border of the rectus abdominis muscles intersect. Seen commonly in postoperative sites. In children, consider a diastasis recti—a condition where the linea alba does not form a tough sheath—which is amenable to watchful waiting

Pathophys: Inability to reduce contents back to correct cavity is incarceration, and this may be acute or chronic. Cutting off the blood supply is strangulation. If the hernia sac includes one wall of a hollow viscus so that intraluminal contents can still pass unimpeded, this is called a Richter (sliding) hernia

Sx: Mass felt at site of herniation, pain; nausea and vomiting if incarcerated even with or without obstruction

Si: Palpable mass, may be erythematous if acute incarceration or strangulation, bowel sounds may be present. Increase in intra-abdominal pressure with cough, lifting head from pillow, or Valsalva may make lesion more noticeable and may be diagnostic

Crs: If bowel involved, this may go on to obstruction (Gastrointest Radiol 1984:311)

Cmplc: Perforation possible if bowel involved and if obstructed. Abscess or peritonitis may also ensue. Strangulation induces ischemia, which may cause bowel necrosis

Diff Dx: Testicular problems in males such as torsion, tumor, hydrocele, or epididymitis; lymphadenopathy in the inguinal area

Lab: Clinical diagnosis—CBC with diff may help delineate how ill someone is, as well as give you the H/H for preop. X-ray: Abdominal series may show obstruction. CT can help delineate anatomy if diagnosis is in question (Br J Surg 1999:1243). Perhaps U/S with tangential plain films (Clin Radiol 1991:185) or herniography if site uncertain (Radiographics 1995:315), although CT has largely supplanted this

ED Rx:

If patient has a chronic incarceration and is not ill or obstructed, may elect outpatient surgical follow-up. To avoid activities which increase intra-abdominal pressure. Otherwise:

- IV access
- NGT if obstructed
- Parenteral antiemetics and narcotic analgesia if necessary
- May try gentle reduction if peritonitis not present, advocate the use of IV midazolam if reduction attempted. Gently direct hernia towards defect, and feed contents back into abdominal cavity starting with the contents at the site of the defect
- IV antibiotics if peritonitis or sepsis present, consider ampicillin/sulbactam, imipenem
- Surgical referral

7.5 ISCHEMIC BOWEL

Dis Colon Rectum 1970:275; 1970:283; Radiol Clin North Am 1993:1197

Cause: Atherosclerotic or other arterial or venous disease with low flow states; also consider embolic disease. Rarely post-traumatic (ischemic stenosis) (Arch Surg 1980:1039) or drug-related such as ergotamine (Gastroenterology 1977:1336), oral contraceptives (Gastrointest Radiol 1977:221), or Pitressin (Am J Roentgenol 1976:829)

Epidem: Should increase as population ages

Pathophys: Watershed areas most susceptible if global arteriosclerotic disease of bowel—ileocecal area, splenic flexure of colon, for example. May be seen with occlusion of inferior mesenteric artery. In neonates, systemic hypoxia or incomplete bowel generation may be the nidus for ischemic problems (Perspect Pediatr Pathol 1976:273)

Sx: Crampy abdominal pain, blood in stools

Si: Abdominal exam usually underwhelming (Can J Surg 1974:435); have a high index of suspicion in the elderly

Crs: After initial episode, will develop scarring with consequent lumen narrowing as part of the healing process

Cmplc: Strictures; those with SMA lesions fare poorly

Diff Dx: Lower GI bleed (see 6.9)

Lab: Guaiac positive stool, CBC with diff, PT/PTT, metabolic profile, type and cross; EKG if considering global ischemic disease. X-ray: Consider nuclear red cell tagged scan if unsure of lower GI bleed etiology; abd CT will give most info if considering primary working diagnosis of ischemic bowel (Radiology 1988:149), especially in those with SLE (Radiology 1999:203); barium enema will show "thumbprints"

ED Rx:
- IV access, fluid resuscitation if necessary
- GI consult if stable, possibly considering endoscopy or arteriography/angioplasty (J Vasc Interv Radiol 1995:785)
- Surgery consult as well if patient hemorrhaging or unstable

7.6 PERFORATED VISCUS

Surg Clin North Am 1972:231

Cause: May be seen in peptic ulcer disease, especially at the duodenum; trauma, also in regard to the duodenum and proximal jejunum; inflammatory bowel disease, being more common in ulcerative colitis compared to Crohn's disease; diverticulitis; appendicitis; bowel obstruction from any cause with subsequent perforation—most common at cecum when diameter greater than 10 cm; bowel ischemia; and neoplasm

Epidem: Nontraumatic small bowel perforation with mortality of ~29%, irrespective of timeliness of diagnosis (Am J Surg 1987:355)

Pathophys: Erosion/defect through bowel wall resulting in leakage of intraluminal contents into peritoneal cavity

Sx: Diffuse abdominal pain, nausea, vomiting

Si: Acute abdomen signs with decreased bowel sounds, rebound tenderness, cough tenderness, percussion tenderness

Note: Acute abdomen symptoms and signs may be lacking in those with diabetes and/or being treated with corticosteroids (Ann Surg 1980:581)

Crs: Suspect perforated viscus in those with gunshot wounds to the spine (Spine 1989:808)

Cmplc: Peritonitis, sepsis, abscess formation, multi-organ failure that is not associated with etiology of perforation (Arch Surg 1996:37)

Diff Dx: Gangrenous cholecystitis, abdominal aortic aneurysm, bowel obstruction, ischemic bowel, pancreatitis, nephrolithiasis; more uncommonly—Ogilvie's syndrome, a nonobstructive massive cecal dilatation (Arch Surg 1977:512), sickle cell crisis, porphyria

Lab: CBC with diff, metabolic profile with LFTs, amylase, lipase, U/A. X-ray: Abd series with free air under the diaphragm on upright or along the liver edge on left lateral decubitus—less sensitive in those with atraumatic small bowel perforation (~17%); in those without obvious free air or bowel dilatation, an ileus may be a positive sign in patient with the clinical exam of an acute abdomen (Am J Roentgenol Radium Ther Nucl Med 1973:275); abd CT in stable patient will also disclose free air even if not seen on plain films, and may help define etiology (Gastrointest Radiol 1984:133)—use Gastrografin if giving oral contrast

ED Rx:
- IV fluid
- Parenteral antiemetics or narcotics if needed, consider IV antibiotics such as ampicillin/sulbactam (Unasyn) 1.5–3 g IV or cefoxitin (Mefoxin) 2 g IV preop
- NGT if vomiting
- Surgical consult

7.7 PERIRECTAL ABSCESS

Am J Surg 1973:765; Ann Emerg Med 1995:597

Cause: Infection of anal glands with subsequent loculation forming an abscess

Epidem: Associated with previous abscess, inflammatory bowel disease (Dis Colon Rectum 1990:933), and diabetes mellitus. Association with hemorrhoids may be linked to prior misdiagnosis

Pathophys: Inoculation with cutaneous and enteric organisms, such as *Staphylococcus*, *Streptococcus*, *Eschlrichia coli*, *Bacteroides*, *Peptostreptococcus*, *Clostridium*, and the like (Pediatrics 1980:282)

Sx: Rectal/perirectal pain, purulent drainage

Si: Possible palpable mass, tenderness, erythema, warmth; exquisite pain on rectal exam—clinical exam can diagnosis this abscess ~95% of the time. Anoscopy

Crs: I + D is curative if uncomplicated presentation in a healthy patient

Cmplc: May progress to a secondary cellulitis, fasciitis, or even septicemia. Some may develop fistula-in-ano

Diff Dx: Perianal is most common and easiest to diagnose and treat— if no apparent mass on exam, consider ischiorectal abscess, or an abscess between the internal and external sphincter muscles, or an abscess above the levator ani muscle(s) as the cause. Consider fissure, inflamed hemorrhoids, inflammatory bowel disease, perianal hematoma (Lancet 1982:467), infectious proctitis, uterine pathology, endometriosis, rectal foreign body—po (Dis Colon Rectum 1975:407) or pr source, referred pain from sacral plexus, or neoplasm (Arch Surg 1985:632)

Lab: None for uncomplicated perianal abscess, otherwise CBC with diff (not sensitive nor specific), blood cultures, and specimen culture for fasciitis and/or septicemia. X-ray: CT of pelvis to delineate anatomy if perirectal abscess suspected but cannot define on physical exam; better than U/S

ED Rx:

For perianal abscess:

- Pretreat with antibiotics if patient with congenital heart or valvular disease who would receive pretreatment for dental and/or other invasive procedures

- IV access if narcotics and/or midazolam necessary for conscious sedation, or if IV antibiotics necessary
- Prep the area with Betadine, then drape
- Anesthetize with 1 or 2% lidocaine buffered with bicarb
- Cross-hatch incision over the abscess, trim all edges to keep wound patent—you should end with a hole in the skin tracking directly to the abscess. Either pack or place a drain with 1–2 day follow-up with surgery
- Consider outpatient oral antibiotics for patients who required pretreatment, those with secondary cellulitis, or those with compromised immune function, e.g., diabetes mellitus
- If patient is systemically ill or cannot tolerate procedure in ED, surgical consult

7.8 PILONIDAL CYST ABSCESS

Br J Surg 1990:123; J Wound Care 1998:481

Cause: Congenital predisposition to coccygeal cyst formation from coccygeal sinus blockage; anaerobic bacteria in all cases with mixed aerobic (*E. coli*, group D strep, α-hemolytic strep, *Proteus*) co-infection in ~32%, with *Bacteroides* species, gram-positive anaerobic cocci, and *Fusobacterium* predominating (Am J Dis Child 1980:679)—peds study

Epidem: Although congenital, most come to medical attention in second to fourth decade of life

Pathophys: Cyst formation with secondary infection; ingrown hair etiology?

Sx: Pain in coccyx area, worse with sitting, even worse with driving

Si: Mass at coccyx area that is tender, erythematous, warm, and may have a sinus tract with drainage. Early on, may only be tender

Crs: Repeated infection if not removed, surgical referral for removal once acute episode has waned

Cmplc: Rare cases of CSF involvement with leakage and meningitis (Clin Neurol Neurosurg 1985:131)

Lab: None

ED Rx:

J Emerg Med 1985:295

- IV access if conscious sedation necessary to I + D, consider narcotics and/or midazolam
- Prep area with Betadine, drape, and local anesthesia as per 19.2
- Cross-hatch over abscess, trim edges to prevent closure
- Place drain if deep—may use either Penrose or simply pack with plain Nu-Gauze
- Antibiotics not necessary unless significant secondary cellulitis
- Have wound rechecked in 2 days to ensure healing and remove/change drain/packing
- Surgical referral electively once healed

7.9 THROMBOSED HEMORRHOIDS

Practitioner 1974:221

Cause: External rectal hemorrhoids are equivocally associated with constipation (Am J Gastroenterol 1994:1981), straining at stool, and dehydration, but probably have more to do with increased sphincter tone (Dis Colon Rectum 1998:1534, discussion, 1541) Internal hemorrhoids usually present with bleeding, and are only covered here as advocating surgical referral for persistent bleeding, internal hemorrhoid prolapse through rectum, or incarceration of internal hemorrhoids

Epidem: Common

Pathophys: Some external hemorrhoids thrombose secondary to the stasis that develops in the protruded tissue

Sx: Pain with defecation and sitting, blood in stools, palpable mass

Si: Palpable mass with solid feeling clot in hemorrhoidal tissue

Crs: Behavioral modification usually curative

Cmplc: Recurrent bleeding, incarceration of tissue

Diff Dx: Fissure, cryptitis, rectal foreign body, infectious proctitis, fistula-in-ano, abscess, inflammatory bowel disease, neoplasm

Lab: None if diagnosis obvious on exam, H/H if anemia is a concern. No reason to look for systemic hypercoaguable state (Dis Colon Rectum 1971:331)

ED Rx:

If not thrombosed, then do the following:
- Stool softener, such as Colace
- Suppository with steroid (Med Lett Drugs Ther 1968:105), such as Anusol HC—equivocal data
- Increase bulk in diet
- Drink liberal amount of fluid, i.e., 6–8 8-oz cups of H_2O per day
- Sitz baths

If thrombosed, do the following:
- IV access if patient requires conscious sedation with parenteral narcotics and/or midazolam for incision procedure
- Tape buttocks if necessary for better exposure
- Left lateral decubitus position, prep, drape, and local anesthesia per 19.2
- Incise directly on top of thrombosed hemorrhoid the entire length of the protruded tissue, and express clot with mosquito forceps. Explore the entire length of the hemorrhoid, and if clot not expressed, you may have simply unroofed the mucosa and the hemorrhoid still needs to be lanced (Dis Colon Rectum 1990:249)
- Place pads in area for the expected bleeding
- Follow instructions as above for when thrombosis not present, and pain meds for home as well

8 Gynecology

8.1 BARTHOLIN'S CYST ABSCESS

Br J Clin Pract 1978:101

Epidem: 80% of acute episodes associated with *Neisseria gonorrhoeae*, and may also be associated with *Chlamydia trachomatis*, *Escherichia coli*, or mixed flora. Seen predominantly in Hispanic or black women 20–29 years of age, with multigravid and multiparity as protective (South Med J 1994:26)

Pathophys: Obstruction of Bartholin's duct with abscess formation

Sx: Labial pain and swelling

Si: Usually unilateral lower labial swelling with erythema, warmth, and tenderness

Crs: Recurrence may be treated/prevented with marsupialization of cyst

Cmplc: Work up and treat as with other STDs—8.6

Lab: Gram's stain of abscess contents, GC/Chlamydia from cervix (urine?), test for syphilis (RPR, VDRL, etc.), consider HIV and partner testing

ED Rx:
- IV access if conscious sedation with parenteral narcotics and/or midazolam necessary for procedure
- Lithotomy position, prep with Betadine, then drape
- Anesthetize with 1–2% lidocaine buffered with bicarb
- Incise on mucosal surface, and place gauze packing or Word catheter (South Med J 1968:514)
- To marsupialize, cross-hatch on mucosal surface and carry cross-hatch down to the cyst. The four corners of the incised cyst will be sewn to the superficial mucosal surface, so that the cyst cannot reocclude, and will heal by secondary intention
- Consider silver nitrate for sclerosis (Eur J Obstet Gynecol Reprod Biol 1995:61)
- Sitz baths
- See 8.6 for specific STD treatments

Cause: Rupture of cyst, which may be physiologic, benign, or malignant. Some examples are follicular cysts, mucinous or serous cystadenomas, endometriomas, or cystic teratomas—usually benign

Epidem: 2–5% in prepubertal females (Obstet Gynecol 1993:434)

Pathophys: The size of the unruptured cyst does not correlate with physical symptoms, and a ruptured cyst of any size may cause significant pelvic pain

Sx: Pelvic pain of sudden onset, nausea

Si: Abdominal exam may be nonspecific; pelvic exam may disclose localized tenderness with or without a mass, cervical motion tenderness (chandelier sign) should be lacking, but not 100%

Crs: Most will be self-limited and respond to pain treatment and others will be recurrent. Cysts greater than 5 cm or complex need further evaluation, or if other concerning aspects are noted during a patient's evaluation, e.g., ectopic tooth

Cmplc: Hemoperitoneum (hemorrhage) (Abdom Imaging 1999:304), peritonitis

Diff Dx: Ectopic pregnancy (pseudo-ectopic pregnancy (W V Med J 1989:488)), appendicitis, tubo-ovarian abscess, ovarian torsion, PID, nephrolithiasis, UTI, endometriosis, or mittelschmerz. Endometriosis is difficult to qualify as to whether it is an individual's cause for pelvic pain. It may be found gross or microscopically in either women with chronic pelvic pain or just found incidentally during other procedures without correlation to pain history (Hum Reprod 1996:387)

Lab: Urine pregnancy test—serum quantitative if positive, U/A, CBC with diff if considering infectious etiology, GC/*Chlamydia* for all women of childbearing age and/or if has cervicitis clinically. X-ray: this discussion is for a nonpregnant patient. If unsure of diagnosis or if palpable mass, U/S may show a cyst coincident with pain locale, or free fluid with no other lesions, which may be consistent with a ruptured cyst. U/S may also define simple vs. complex cysts. Hemorrhagic ovarian cyst may be better elucidated with transvaginal ultrasound (Gynecol Endocrinol 1991:123). Right-sided pain may not be easily explained with free fluid but no other lesions noted—this may be consistent with appendicitis as well

ED Rx:

   If pt is pregnant, see 14.2. Otherwise:

   - If pt afebrile, and *left-sided* pain, may elect to treat with NSAIDs and narcotics for breakthrough pain—U/S as outpatient with referral to primary care physician or gynecologist
   - If pain is *right-sided*, must consider appendicitis. Using Bayesian reasoning, consider the history, physical, and CBC with diff (U/A and urine pregnancy test should both be unremarkable, although ureteral irritation sometimes occurs) to decide whether diagnosis needs to be made immediately, or have the patient return in 6–8 hours for a recheck. Abd CT for cases with high index of suspicion for appendicitis—not U/S!
   - Cysts >5 cm refer for gyn follow-up, for either aspiration (Br J Obstet Gynaecol 1989:1035), laparoscopy, or laparotomy

8.3 OVARIAN TORSION

Cause: Enlarged ovary (cyst) which twists on itself usually in a woman of childbearing age; perhaps tamoxifen as a risk (Gynecol Obstet Invest 1999:200); rarely due to leiomyomatosis peritonealis disseminata (Abdom Imaging 1998:640)

Epidem: Incidence ~7%; more common on the right side and in pregnancy (Int J Gynaecol Obstet 1989:21)

Pathophys: The enlarged ovary will asymmetrically grow in relation to its position in the meso-ovarium. This will allow it to twist on its axis, and this will threaten its blood supply, which may cause necrosis to the ovary

Sx: Pelvic pain, nausea, vomiting

Si: Pain upon palpation, palpable mass (80%)

Crs: Necrosis with nonviable ovary if not repositioned, with 50% gangrenous in OR

Cmplc: Loss of ovary

Lab: Check urine pregnancy test, and consider CBC with diff and U/A. X-ray: U/S with large and eccentric ovary, perhaps with Doppler to determine viability (Ultrasound Obstet Gynecol 1995:129); may also be seen with CT (J Reprod Med 1998:827)

GYNECOLOGY

ED Rx:
- IV access for parenteral antiemetics and narcotics if necessary
- Gynecologic consult

8.4 PELVIC INFLAMMATORY DISEASE

MMWR Morb Mortal Wkly Rep 1998:1

Cause: Chlamydia causes over half of mild cases (Ann Intern Med 1981:685); *Neisseria* gonococcus in 13–20% of cases (Am J Obstet Gynecol 1980:909); anaerobes (Clin Infect Dis 1999:S29); cytomegalovirus?; mycoplasma. All via sexual intercourse, especially with multiple partners. IUD use previously thought to increase risk but this is equivocal—presenting with febrile PID is probably higher in those with IUDs (Jama 1976:1851)

Epidem: ~1 million cases/year in U.S.; associated in those with induced abortion and harboring chlamydial or bacterial vaginosis (Am J Obstet Gynecol 1980:868), specific prophylaxis is helpful (Am J Obstet Gynecol 1992:100; Infection 1994:242)

Pathophys: Lower genital tract infections ascend cervical canal usually just before or during menses, with infection spreading to tubes and ovaries

Sx: Pain in lower abdomen, nausea, vomiting, anorexia, dyspareunia, dysuria, tenesmus, dysmenorrhea

Si: Adnexal mass (20%) and tenderness; cervical motion tenderness—chandelier sign; fever; cervical discharge; mild cases have no specific clinical criteria to aid in diagnosis (Sex Transm Dis 1986:119)

Crs: Bilateral tubal ligation is not protective (Ann Emerg Med 1991:344), but perhaps milder course (Am J Emerg Med 1997:271). Pregnancy is not protective in adolescents (J Pediatr Adolesc Gynecol 1996:129)

Cmplc: Infertility—15+ % with each episode; ectopic pregnancy; pelvic abscess; septic thrombophlebitis; surgical excision of reproductive organs

Diff Dx: Ectopic pregnancy; appendicitis—presentation to the ED in the latter 2 weeks of the menstrual cycle (Am J Emerg Med 1993:569), within 2 days of symptom onset, and with both nausea and vomiting may favor appendicitis (Am J Surg 1985:90); septic abortion; endometriosis; adenomyosis

Lab: CBC with diff, U/A, urine pregnancy test, GC and chlamydia screens, test for syphilis (Jacep 1978:93), consider HIV testing; consider ESR or CRP to follow for resolution (Arch Gynecol Obstet 1987:177). X-ray: Pelvic ultrasound or CT scan for abscess if clinically suspected

ED Rx: Initiate treatment based on pain and tenderness

Outpatients
- First: cefoxitin 2 g IM + probenecid 1 gram po, or ceftriaxone 250 mg IM; then tetracycline 500 mg po qid, or doxycycline 100 mg po bid × 14 days
- Second: ofloxacin 400 mg po bid + clindamycin 450 mg po qid or metronidazole 500 mg po bid × 2 weeks

Inpatients
Hospitalize if:
- Dx is uncertain, gyn consult for laparoscopy (J Reprod Med 1993:53)
- Mass is present
- Unable to keep po meds down
- Peritoneal signs present
- Outpt treatment failure
- Compliance is poor
- First: doxycycline 100 mg IV + cefoxitin 2 g IV q 6 hours, or cefotetan 2 g IV q 12 hours, or metronidazole 1 g IV bid
- Second: gentamicin + clindamycin IV until better, then f/u with po clindamycin for 14 days

Note: Treat partners

8.5 SEXUAL ASSAULT

Rev Infect Dis 1990:S682; Ann Emerg Med 1995:728; Emerg Med Clin North Am 1999:685, vii

Best if entire exam is done with dedicated nurse or forensic examiner (Ann Emerg Med 2000:353) present at all times since chain of evidence will need to be preserved. Sexual assault kits are available to help preserve the chain of evidence and guide you through key exam points. Breakdown is ~96% female and 4% male

Work Up:
- Medical history
- Exact detail of events, including times, names, recollection of physical area, and whether drugs, weapons, or threats were used
- Specifically ask if assailant ejaculated on victim's body, throat, vagina, or rectum, and ask whether a condom was used
- Evaluate and treat physical injuries—coincident trauma is common (Ann Emerg Med 2000:358)

For exam, some specifics are as follows—place all collected items in separate envelopes:
- Use Wood's lamp to look for semen on body. Use sterile gauze moistened with saline to collect any samples
- All of victim's clothes should be collected and placed in separate paper bags and taped closed
- Take 12 hairs from head and genital area
- Scrape under fingernails into envelope, and then clip nails into each envelope
- GC culture of throat
- DNA swab of oral mucosa
- Have pt spit on gauze and place in its own envelope
- Only saline for speculum exam, and collect DNA swab from vagina and rectum separately, as indicated, as well as GC and chlamydia cultures
- Photos of any specific injuries

Lab:

MMWR Morb Mortal Wkly Rep 1998:1

Consider testing for syphilis, HIV, hepatitis B_sAg and hep B_sAb, pregnancy, blood type. High incidence of coincident drug use in cases (J Anal Toxicol 1999:141), ETOH as most prevalent but including cannabinoids, cocaine, amphetamines, and gamma hydroxybutyrate (GHB = liquid ecstacy). GHB along with ketamine and rohypnol have been implicated as "date rape" drugs. Consider testing for these substances

ED Rx:

MMWR Morb Mortal Wkly Rep 1998:1

As above, but also include the following:
- "Morning after pill"—use one of the following: 2 each of 50-µg estradiol BCPs, or 35-µg estradiol BCPs po q 12 h × 2; or levonorgestrel 0.75 mg (Plan B) po q 12 h × 2 (Lancet 1998:428); (Med Lett Drugs Ther 2000;42:10)

- Prophylactic antibiotics if indicated or requested (Obstet Gynecol Surv 2000:5)—ceftriaxone 125–250 mg IM or spectinomycin 2 g IM; plus doxycycline 100 mg po bid × 7 days; or azithromycin 1 g po once + metronidazole 2 g po once
- Immunize with hep B vaccine and HBIG unless contraindicated
- Antiemetic of choice for ensuing nausea from treatment
- HIV counseling re AZT use prophylactically; useful for high-risk cases (Cmaj 2000:641)
- Rape support counseling
- Police report
- F/U with primary physician in 2–4 weeks

8.6 SEXUALLY TRANSMITTED DISEASES

MMWR Morb Mortal Wkly Rep 1998:1
This section on sexually transmitted diseases is appropriate when addressing female patients. Males are covered elsewhere.

Cause:
- *Chlamydia trachomatis*
- *Neisseria gonorrhoeae*
- Human papillomavirus—HPV or venereal warts as common name
- Herpes simplex types I and II (Jama 2000:791)
- Chancroid (J Am Acad Dermatol 1986:939)—*Haemophilus ducreyi*
- *Treponema pallidum* (syphilis)—see 10.9
- Human immunodeficiency virus—see 10.2
- *Trichomonas*—see 8.7

Epidem:
- All may be spread even when no active lesions
- GC and chlamydia coincident 15% of the time; GC may be present in girls <12 years of age who are Tanner Stage I without history of abuse but have vaginal discharge (Pediatrics 1999:e72)
- Chancroid associated with syphilis in 15% of cases
- HSV types I and II may both be venerally spread; active lesions associated with increased HIV transmission (Arch Dermatol 1999:1393); epidemics of type I among wrestlers is termed herpes gladiatorum (Jama 1965:993)
- HPV with higher prevalence in HIV + women and cause of laryngeal papillomas from aspiration at delivery of infant

Pathophys:
- GC infects membranes of genitourinary tract, with possible septicemia and rash secondary to systemic spread, and arthralgias secondary to immune complex disease—negative taps
- Chlamydia and GC commonly asymptomatic and difficult to diagnose clinically (Acad Emerg Med 1997:962)
- HPV present in normal as well as wart skin, highly infective
- HSV type I tends to be orolabial with complications of encephalitis, whereas type II tends to be genital and neonatal with complications of meningitis, but clinically full overlap exists

Sx:
- GC or chlamydia may present with sore throat with fellatio, labial tenderness, vaginal discharge, dysuria, abnormal vaginal bleeding associated with endometritis, and/or pelvic pain, or chlamydia may cause no symptoms
- HPV with 1–6 month incubation with pain at site
- HSV with sicker primary course, with fever, sore throat, and/or genital lesions
- Chancroid with painful ulcer after 2–15 day incubation

Si:
- GC or chlamydia may disclose pharyngitis, abdominal pain, cervical motion tenderness—chandelier sign, or pus on cervix
- HPV with warts on genitalia which are seen better with acetic acid swabbing
- HSV with adenopathy, gingivostomatitis, pharyngitis, cervicitis, external genital lesions that are painful; recurrent type with classic genital sores
- Chancroid with tender adenopathy—bubos; also with tender, necrotic ulcers

Crs:
- GC with 2–7-day or more latent period
- HSV with primary infection lasting 10 days, recurs 1–2 times/year lasting 4 days
- Chancroid with self-limited course

Cmplc:
- GC and chlamydia may go on to PID, endometritis, or sterility—higher chance of sterility with chlamydia
- GC (Br Med J 1970:420) with bacteremia with purpuric or vesicular pustule on broad erythematous base or hemorrhagic bullae; those with endocarditis will have 80% chance of arthritis as

well; Glisson's capsule inflammation—Fitz-Hugh–Curtis syndrome; polyarthritis; tenosynovitis; and newborns may acquire vertical transmission conjunctivitis
- Chlamydia may have perihepatitis analogous to Fitz-Hugh–Curtis syndrome
- HPV associated with cervical intraepithelial neoplasia often within 2 years of contagion; also associated with vaginal, endometrial, vulvar, anal, laryngeal, and conjunctival cancers
- HSV ocular keratitis by self-inoculation; colitis; aseptic meningitis— or recurrently as Mollaret's meningitis; urinary hesitancy and sacral paresthesias; disseminated forms with encephalitis

Diff Dx: (other than GC, chlamydia, syphilis, HSV, HPV, or HIV)
- GC and chlamydia: *Trichomonas*, *Candida*, Reiter's syndrome, appendicitis
- HPV: molluscum contagiosum
- HSV: erythema multiforme, hand-foot-mouth disease (where the base is not erythematous); monkey herpes in monkey handlers

Lab: Screen for associated STDs if STD suspected (syphilis (Ann Emerg Med 1991:627)), but specific tests listed below. Some results may not be available at end of visit and mechanism should be in place to assure treatment for positive test results (Sex Transm Dis 1999:496)
- GC (Cutis 1981:249): Gram's stain of D/C of cervix to look for >3 polys/hpf with intracellular gram-neg diplococci has a 67% sensitivity, 98% specificity. Culture or antigen screen (Am J Clin Pathol 1985:613), or DNA probe (J Clin Microbiol 1989:632) if negative
- Chlamydia: single swab culture is 100% specific, 66% sensitive (Genitourin Med 1994:300). Gram's stain shows 10 + polys/hpf (at 1000×) with 17% false positive, 10% false negative (Am J Epidemiol 1988:298). Monoclonal antibody immunofluorescence is 93% sensitive and 96% specific (N Engl J Med 1984:1146). Pap smear detection is unreliable (Obstet Gynecol 1986:691). ELISA on secretions or urine is 80% sensitive and 98% specific (APMIS Suppl 1988:35). PCR is accurate, but availability may be an issue
- HSV (J Med Virol 1998:177): Culture is 77% sensitive in primary herpes. Skin biopsy shows inclusion and giant cells; scraped Tzanck prep of skin lesion is sensitive and specific. Rapid slide prep kits <1 hr results, but culture if negative. PCR most sensitive.

- Chancroid culture is difficult and best with specialized media and sampling with sterile plastic loop (J Med Microbiol 1998:1023). PCR the best (J Clin Microbiol 1995:787)

ED Rx:

Med Lett Drugs Ther 1999:41:85

All partners should be tested, barrier methods for birth control recommended, report to State Public Health office if appropriate, and the specific following treatments:

GC

- Ceftriaxone 125–250 mg IM × 1 (Sex Transm Dis 1986:199), covers syphilis, and both pharyngeal and resistant GC, or
- Cefixime 400 mg po × 1 (Antimicrob Agents Chemother 1990:355), or
- Cefpodoxime 200 mg po × 1 (Pathology 1995:64), or
- Ciprofloxacin 250–500 mg po × 1 (Sex Transm Dis 1994:345), although no good vs. syphilis and resistance appearing, or
- Ofloxacin 400 mg po × 1, norfloxacin 800 mg po × 1 (Scand J Infect Dis Suppl 1988:49), or
- Second-line Rx with spectinomycin 2 grams IM × 1 (N Engl J Med 1977:889)—good if PCN allergy, but no good vs. syphilis or vs. GC pharyngitis; resistance developing in Army where used as first-line drug in Korea
- If complications with septicemia or arthritis, hospitalize, and tap joint—irrigate joint if clinically worsens. Give 10 million U aqueous PCN IV over 24 hours or divided bolus q 4 hours until afebrile × 3 days, then 7 days of cefoxitin 1 g qid IV, or spectinomycin 2 g bid IM
- Ceftriaxone and spectinomycin OK in pregnancy (Obstet Gynecol 1993:33)

Chlamydia

- Tetracycline 250–500 mg po qid × 7 days, or doxycycline 100 mg po bid × 7 days (Acta Derm Venereol 1981:273); or azithromycin (Zithromax) 1 g po × 1 (Eur J Clin Microbiol Infect Dis 1992:693); or ofloxacin 300 mg po bid × 7 days (Chemotherapy 1990:70); or minocycline 100 mg po qd-bid × 7–10 days (Med J Aust 1989:483)
- If pregnant, erythromycin 500 mg po qid × 7 days or × 3 weeks after treatment failure, nonestolated types OK in pregnancy

HPV

Clin Infect Dis 1995:S91

No therapy is outstanding

- Podophyllin soln, leave on 8 hours first time, 24 hours subsequently; or podophyllotoxin 0.5% cream (Condylox) (Lancet 1989:831); avoid in pregnancy because of fetal damage and even death with only 1–2 cc; use cryotherapy instead
- Trichloroacetic acid topically (Genitourin Med 1987:390)
- 5-Fluorouracil, 1% gel intravaginally (Int J STD AIDS 2000:371) or topical 5% ointment (Br J Dermatol 1970:218)
- Liquid N_2, although repeated applications at one visit with local reaction (Br J Vener Dis 1977:49)
- Imiquimod (Aldara) 5% cream topically 3×/week overnight × 3–4 months (Arch Dermatol 1998:25)
- Topical leukocyte interferon-α (Dermatology 1995:129) better than podophyllotoxin cream
- Interferon injections tid × 3 weeks; qd × 1 month then tid × 6 months helps for respiratory papillomas (Am J Obstet Gynecol 1990:348); consider doing this if surgery required on papillomas q 3 months

HSV
- Acyclovir 400 mg po tid or 200 mg po 5×/day (Lancet 1982:571) × 7–10 days for primary; or × 5 days for recurrent episode, then 400 mg po bid prophylaxis reduces recurrences by >50% long term (Jama 1991:747). Topical treatment is useless
- Famciclovir 125–250 mg po tid × 5 or 250 mg po bid days at first symptom of recurrence decreases shedding and duration/severity of outbreak (Jama 1998:887); or 500 mg po tid × 7 days for primary or severe infection
- Penciclovir 1% cream 5×/day for 7 days speeds healing and end of shedding × 1 day (Int J STD AIDS 2000:568)
- Valacyclovir 1 g po tid × 7 days or bid × 5 days (Sex Transm Dis 1997:481); 500 mg po daily to suppress herpes gladiatorum (Clin J Sport Med 1999:86)

Chancroid
- First choice: erythromycin 500 mg po qid × 7 days, or ceftriaxone 250 mg IM × 1, or azithromycin 1 g po × 1 (Clin Infect Dis 1995:409)
- Second choice: ciprofloxacin 500 mg po bid × 3 days (Sex Transm Dis 1998:293)
- Consider needle aspiration vs. I + D of fluctuant bubos, I + D may be better (Sex Transm Dis 1995:217)

8.7 VAGINITIS

Clin Obstet Gynaecol 1981:241; 1988:473; Obstet Gynecol 1998:757
Cause: Infectious with *Gardenerella vaginalis* and other bacteria—aka
   nonspecific bacterial vaginosis; *Candida albicans*; *Torulopsis
   glabrata*; *Trichomonas vaginalis*; or foreign body, e.g., tampon.
   Noninfectious such as atrophic in postmenopausal women,
   chemical irritant or traumatic. Atopic etiology.
Epidem:
   Acta Obstet Gynecol Scand 1994:802
   • Most common are *Gardenerella* and other co-inhabitants such as
     ureaplasmas and other anaerobes. All are endogenous flora that are
     not necessarily from a venereal etiology since they cause vaginitis in
     15% of virginal women
   • Risk factors for candidiasis are frequent sexual intercourse, oral
     contraceptives, spermicide use, previous infection, and black or
     other race than white (Am J Public Health 1990:329; Epidemiology
     1996:182). It is associated with diabetes, antibiotic use, steroids,
     blood dyscrasias, TPN, various endocrine conditions—
     hypoparathyroidism, hypothyroidism, and hypoadrenalism
   • *T. glabrata* may commonly be found in asymptomatic vaginitis as
     well as symptomatic females in ~30%—may be coincident finding
     (Obstet Gynecol 1990:651)
   • Trichomoniasis is considered a venereal disease; 10–25 % of adult
     females carry this asymptomatically, and it is present in 30–40% of
     male partners of infected women
   • GC may be present in girls <12 years of age who are Tanner
     Stage I without history of abuse but have vaginal discharge
     (Pediatrics 1999:e72)
   • Co-infection with more than one pathogen is not uncommon
Pathophys: Nonspecific bacterial vaginosis due to diminished presence
   of lactobacilli, with corresponding increase in pH leading to
   overgrowth with *Gardenerella* and others. Local conditions in
   vagina are influenced by birth control pills and IUDs such that
   anaerobes may predominate—this is not seen with use of barrier
   methods and condoms (Am J Obstet Gynecol 1986:520).
   Candidiasis is an opportunistic invasion
Sx: Vaginal discharge, dyspareunia except in nonspecific bacterial
   vaginosis

Si: Look for foreign body, erythema, evidence of trauma, and the following:
- Candidiasis shows lesions with white centers, erythematous bases, and satellite lesions and a thick white/cheesy discharge
- Nonspecific bacterial vaginosis shows a watery discharge with a vinegar-like smell, stronger smell with increased pH
- Trichomoniasis shows a watery discharge and an erythematous cervix ("strawberry" cervix with erythema and punctate hemorrhages <2% of those infected)

Crs: Protracted course at times, and consider other etiologies such as *Saccharomyces cerevisiae* (a yeast) (Clin Infect Dis 1993:93), which may require a prolonged and different therapy

Cmplc: Nonspecific bacterial vaginosis with increased incidence of premature labor and low birth weight infant (J Clin Microbiol 1994:176)

Diff Dx: Consider above etiologies, consider other STDs if considering trichomoniasis

Lab:
Clin Lab Med 1989:525
- Swab should be from vaginal pool, not the vaginal wall or cervix (J Adolesc Health 1994:245)
- Nonspecific bacterial vaginosis: vaginal smear shows >15–20% clue cells, which is considered 100%; pH >4.5–5.0; positive amine ("whiff") test, i.e., D/C smells of ammonia (70–80%) (Br J Vener Dis 1983:302); few polys; culture positive in 40%
- Candidiasis shows pseudohyphae 20% of the time on 10% KOH exam of vaginal D/C (J Fam Pract 1984:549); culture more sensitive but would advocate treat and recheck before going to culture initially; vaginal pH 4–4.5
- Trichomoniasis shows a motile 20-µ flagellate with axostyle undulating membrane on wet prep 50–70% sensitivity (Ann Emerg Med 1989:564); present on Pap smear in 60–70%, but false positives too; culture possible, rapid DNA and monoclonal antibody test 90% sensitivity and 99.8% specificity; vaginal pH 5–6, with amine smell on "whiff" test (Br J Vener Dis 1983:302)

ED Rx:
Nonspecific Bacterial Vaginosis
- Metronidazole (Flagyl) 2 g po qd × 1 with 75% cure (Lancet 1983:1379), or 500 mg po bid × 7 days with 95% cure; 30% recur in 1 month, at least if partner not Rx'ed, although partner Rx not

clearly helpful; or try metronidazole vaginal gel 5 g bid × 5 days
(Obstet Gynecol 1993:963), probably OK in pregnancy but avoid in
first trimester, or

- Clindamycin 300 mg po bid × 7 days (Obstet Gynecol 1988:799),
  or as vaginal cream 5 g qd × 7 days (South Med J 1992:1077)—
  preferred in pregnancy
- Sulfa and ampicillin are ineffective
- In pregnancy, Rx at least women at high risk for preterm labor
  since Rx decreases incidence from 50% to 30%

Candidiasis

- Miconazole (Monistat) 2% cream bid vaginally (Chemotherapy
  1982:73), or
- Clotrimazole (Lotrimin) 100-mg vaginal tab qd × 7 days, 2 tabs qd
  × 3 days, or 500 mg × 1 (J Fam Pract 1990:148), or
- Terconazole (Terazol) 80-mg vaginal tab qd × 3 or 7 days
  (J Fla Med Assoc 1992:693), or
- Nystatin topically (50% effective for vaginal candidiasis) or 5
  million U po biweekly for chronic prevention, implicating problem
  of intestinal reservoir (Am J Obstet Gynecol 1986:651), or
- Fluconazole (Diflucan) 150 mg po × 1 (Am J Obstet Gynecol
  1995:1263), or
- Ketoconazole (Nizoral) 400 mg po bid × 5 days, or qd × 14 days,
  then 100 mg po qd as prophylaxis
- Butoconazole (Femstat) (Mycoses 1993:379) and itraconazole
  (Sporonox) may also be options
- Perhaps boric acid for recalcitrant cases
- *Solanum nigrescens*, an ethnobotanical approach, has efficacy
  (J Ethnopharmacol 1988:307)

Trichomoniasis

- Metronidazole 2 g po × 1 to pt and partner, 90% cure (J Adolesc
  Health Care 1981:41); or 500 mg po bid × 7 days, 85–90% cure;
  local Rx no good (Sex Transm Dis 1998:176), or
- Tinidazole 2 g po × 1 (S Afr Med J 1985:455)
- In pregnancy: can use metronidazole after the first trimester;
  clotrimazole 100 mg vaginally qd × 7 days, is 50% effective
  (Minerva Ginecol 1975:348); Betadine douche to control symptoms
  no longer used due to suppression of fetal thyroid

9 Hematology/Oncology

9.1 ACUTE LEUKEMIA

Cause: Lymphocytic and nonlymphocytic varieties; this section will focus on acute lymphocytic (blastic) leukemia, or ALL. Two types of ALL, child and adult. Adult type is probably genetic, HLA-linked, autosomal recessive

Epidem: Adult type represents 15% of adult leukemias. Incidence of childhood type is 32/million/year. No increased incidence near power lines. Possible hydrocarbon exposure in parents as risk (Cancer Epidemiol Biomarkers Prev 1999:783)

Pathophys: CNS involvement more common (40%) than in AML (7%)
- 78% are B cells; 17% are T-cell types; 5% have no markers using monoclonal antibodies; some also have myeloid antigens, which correlate with worse prognosis. Prognostic factors for children not the same for T-cell and B-cell ALL (Leukemia 1999:1696)
- Associated with chromosome 9 deletion that has interferon α and interferon β genes
- Also associated with translocation of chromosome 11 in adults (Blood 1999:2072)

Sx: Malaise, fever

Si: Pallor, white plaque on lateral tongue (oral hairy leukoplakia (Oral Dis 1999:76)), hepatosplenomegaly, ecchymoses, petechiae; rarely leukemia cutis, which resembles a viral exanthem type eruption (J Dermatol 1999:216)

Crs: In children, now much higher cure rates, 70% 5-year survivals. In adults, prognosis is much worse than in children; T-cell types have worst prognosis, rest susceptible to Rx; 20–30% cure currently.

Cmplc: Varicella zoster disease with 7% mortality; 6% recurrence in testes, prevent with irradiation, which decreases testosterone later; *Pneumocystis carinii*; CMV; progressive multifocal

leukoencephalopathy; AML after chemotherapy in 4%; second
primaries in 0.5% of children; sterility; opportunistic infection

Lab: CBC with diff; metabolic profile including renal function, liver
function, Ca, Mg, Phos; U/A and urine culture, CXR, and consider
LP if looking for secondary infectious focus—consider PCR for
specific infections (Pediatr Infect Dis J 1999:395)

ED Rx:
- Treat secondary infections
- Order/transfuse appropriate blood products as necessary
- Consult patient's primary physician or hematologist/oncologist
(Med Pediatr Oncol 1999:1; J Clin Oncol 2000:547)

9.2 PRIMARY CNS AND SPINAL CORD NEOPLASMS

Am J Med 1978:4

Cause: Meningioma, lymphoma (Leuk Lymphoma 1995:223),
medulloblastoma, gliomas, ependymoma, craniopharyngioma

Epidem: Recent trends stable except for those >85 years of age
(J Natl Cancer Inst 1999:1382). Environmental risk factors
not well-proven (Cancer Epidemiol Biomarkers Prev 1994:197).
An increase in CNS lymphoma in those with AIDS has occurred
(J Natl Cancer Inst 1996:675)
- Adults: 50% gliomas, 25% meningiomas
- Peds: 50% gliomas, 25% medulloblastomas, 10% ependymomas,
5% craniopharyngiomas

Pathophys: Gliomas incorporate 4 subtypes— grade 1 is the
astrocytoma, grade 2 is the glioma, grade 3 is the astroblastoma,
aka anaplastic astrocytoma, and grade 4 is the glioblastoma.
Glioma class of tumors most commonly in cerebellum and pons
in peds, and spinal cord, cerebrum, and cerebellum in adults

Sx: Medulloblastoma may present with cerebellar signs such as ataxia;
all may present with seizures; less likely headache but possible
including other signs of increased intracranial pressure. *Spinal cord*
symptoms may be confined to one nerve root, or include "saddle"
anesthesia and/or incontinence of bladder or bowel

Si: Depends on location; craniopharyngiomas may present with
bitemporal hemianopsia, obesity, diabetes insipidus, growth

failure in children. Spinal cord findings may include anesthesia, pain, and loss of patella or Achilles reflexes; consider cauda equina syndrome if anesthetic in distribution of where one would sit in a saddle, overflow incontinence, lack of rectal tone, severe pain and loss of Achilles and patellar reflexes—usually gradual in onset and may have asymmetric findings

Crs:
- Meningiomas are benign yet can be recurrent
- Medulloblastomas are highly malignant with 30–70% 5-year remission, 92% 5-year survival, and perhaps 50% cure
- Glioma class tumors depend on grade; the higher the grade, the worse the prognosis
- Craniopharyngiomas are slow growing and at least 15-year survival with Rx

Cmplc: Panhypopituitarism with postop patients with craniopharyngiomas. Spinal cord tumors may present with isolated nerve root findings, but also as cauda equina (L1–S5) or conus medullaris (S2–5) problems

Lab: Neuroimaging with CT usually followed by MRI; check electrolytes, cortisol level, and TSH in those with pituitary locations

Note: MRI is procedure of choice if considering cauda equina or conus medullaris process, and should be done emergently. Also procedure of choice for diffuse brainstem glioma diagnosis (Neurosurgery 1993:1026, discussion, 1029)

ED Rx:
- Treat secondary symptoms of nausea and pain
- Consider glucocorticoids, such as dexamethasone (Decadron) 4 mg tid for mass effects
- Consider prophylactic antiepileptic such as phenytoin (Dilantin) if brain neoplasm, with or without seizures
- Neurosurgical consult, with arrangements for radiation Rx if cauda equina or conus medullaris problem

9.3 DIC MANAGEMENT

Emerg Med Clin North Am 1993:465; Bmj 1996:683

Cause: Two requirements: (1) reticuloendothelial system blockade by pregnancy, endotoxin, radiation, steroids, or colloid, and (2) clotting system activated by:
- Thromboplastin releaser, e.g., frozen tissue (hypothermia), placenta, tumors, trypsin, snake venom, open brain trauma, or renal transplant rejection, or
- Defibrination agent, e.g., amniotic fluid, or
- Platelet factor 3 (phospholipid) release, e.g., platelet clot, hemolysis, fat embolism, or immune reaction, or
- Activation of factor XII, e.g., by endotoxin

Epidem: More common than TTP. Increased incidence in ob pts esp. with septic abd, abruptio, eclampsia, hydatidiform mole, amniotic fluid embolus, missed ab, retained dead fetus, fatty liver of pregnancy; leukemia, cancer, and all cases of severe tissue damage; freshwater drownings; gram-negative sepsis (Jpn J Surg 1977:82)

Pathophys: Fibrinogen is low due to consumption and rapid lysis; tissue damage esp. in CNS, lung, and kidneys from thrombotic ischemia

Sx: Bleeding, coma; fever only if a secondary cause, unlike TTP

Si: Palpable purpuric rash; hypotension; oozing/bleeding at all sites; shock

Crs: Worse prognosis with extent of PT, PTT, platelet count, and/or thrombin time abnormalities (Thromb Haemost 1978:122); usually an acute and fulminant course, rarely chronic

Cmplc: Renal cortical necrosis, ATN, Sheehan's syndrome, acute cor pulmonale, adrenal insufficiency

Diff Dx: Vasculitis; implicated infections include "benign" viruses such as varicella (Infection 1998:306)

Lab: CBC with diff (microangiopathic anemia with helmet cells and other fragments); metabolic profile incl. liver and renal markers; ESR = 0 secondary to afibrinogenemia; PT/PTT (PT very sensitive); d-dimer and FDP markedly elevated; fibrinogen <40 mg% (Am J Hematol 1998:65); elevated AT III; U/A. Low levels of factors II, VIII, and V (<50% is diagnostic). Soluble fibrin as a pre-DIC marker (Acta Anaesthesiol Scand 1993:125)?

ED Rx:
- Treat underlying cause
- Replace factors—consider FFP and platelets
- Perhaps heparinize to break consumptive cycle, LMWH has proponents vs. unfractionated heparin (Thromb Res 1993:475; 1990:37); never do so in the face of liver disease, and only as a last resort if chronic cause and uncontrollable bleeding. Not advocated as a preventative therapy (J Emerg Med 1988:277)
- Use of dermatan sulfate (Thromb Res 1994:65)?

9.4 FEBRILE NEUTROPENIC PATIENT

Cancer Control 1996:366

Cause: Agranulocytosis (absolute neutrophil count <500/mm^3) due to:
- Allergic directly as with chloramphenicol or via lupus, e.g., from procainamide
- Autoimmune antibodies and occasionally, perhaps, killer T cells; idiopathic usually; ibuprofen-induced is reversible
- Direct drug toxic effect from chemotherapy, chloramphenicol

Epidem: Type of opportunistic pathogen changing from gram-negative to gram-positive organism (Clin Infect Dis 1999:495); autoimmune type associated with rheumatoid Felty's syndrome

Pathophys:
- Allergic type: delayed hypersensitivity T cells kill in marrow; drugs can act as hapten to induce
- Autoimmune type: antibodies esp. to HLA surface antigens

Sx: Malaise, fever, sore throat, cough

Si: Fever, pharyngitis, rash, pulmonary findings, recurrent infections in general

Crs: Idiopathic autoimmune type very benign—rarely progresses to sepsis

Cmplc: Sepsis

Diff Dx: Drug fever, pulmonary embolus, genetic cyclic neutropenia

Lab: CBC with diff; metabolic profile including liver markers; blood cultures × 2 with one from central line if present; U/A and urine culture; CXR—those with lower respiratory tract infection fare worse (Infection 1998:349); PT/PTT if sepsis suspected; consider LP; cultures of any wounds

ED Rx:
- Isolation
- IV access
- Treat fever, caution with acetaminophen or NSAIDs if liver dysfunction
- ABX: ceftazidime or imipenem alone, or with aminoglycoside (peds (Pediatr Hematol Oncol 2000:93)), e.g., amikacin; combination therapy of once daily ceftriaxone 80 mg/kg to 4 g max. and gentamicin 7 mg/kg (Arch Dis Child 1999:125); or aztreonam + vancomycin; low-risk patients may have oral ciprofloxacin and amoxicillin-clavulanate (N Engl J Med 1999:305)
- Low-risk children may have home therapy with oral ciprofloxacin (20 mg/kg daily divided bid) (Cancer 2000:1710)
- Perhaps GM-CSF for persistent or fungal etiologies in medium- to high-risk patients (Eur J Cancer 1999:S4)
- Consult medicine, hematologist/oncologist, or ID service

9.5 HEMOPHILIA AND REPLACEMENT FACTOR GUIDELINES

Emerg Med Clin North Am 1993:337

Cause: Hemophilia A is factor VIII deficiency and is genetic, sex-linked recessive. Hemophilia B is factor IX deficiency and may be genetic, sex-linked genetic, or acquired in nephrotics or those with amyloid. Not covered here are pseudo-hemophilia (von Willebrand's factor deficiency) and other more rare factor deficiencies such as factors I, II, V, VII, X, XI, and XIII

Epidem: Hemophilia A patients are 80% of all patients with lifelong bleeding diathesis; 1/7000–10,000 male births, only 1/3 have complete VIII deficiency. Hemophilia B has a prevalence of 1/10,000, and represents 16% of those with lifelong bleeding diathesis. Factor XI deficiency is common in Ashkenazi Jews, with 1/190 people in Israel affected—<1/million all others

Pathophys: Both with defective intrinsic system, hemophilia A secondary to defective factor VIII protein—thus present in plasma immunologically

Sx: Possibly chronic bruising, hematuria, no significant bleeding after minor cuts

Si: Bleeding after trauma, and hemarthroses possible

Crs: Lifelong, survival nearly comparable to normal population if don't get HIV, hep B, or hep C

Cmplc: Hemophilia A with flexion contractures of joints and intracranial bleeding cause of death in 25%

Diff Dx: Von Willebrand's disease or other factor deficiencies; acquired hemophilia (Haematologica 1994:550)—circulating antibody inhibitors due to SLE or multiple myeloma

Lab: CBC with diff, PT/PTT. Consider fibrinogen, fibrin split products, bleeding time, clotting time, tourniquet test—BP cuff at 100 mm Hg × 5 min; normal is no petechiae—this tests vessels and platelets. Factor levels and specific antibodies as dictated by screening workup. Factor VIII levels: none detectable = severe disease; 1–4% = moderate disease; 5–25% = mild disease

ED Rx:

If new and symptomatic diagnosis, consult hematology. Avoidance of ASA and NSAIDs. If known hemophiliac, determine desired factor level:

- For bleed of head, throat, neck, eye, abdomen (GI), lower back, groin, or hip—desired factor level for those with factor VIII deficiency is 80–100%, and those with factor IX deficiency is 60–80%
- For bleed of joints or muscles in arms and legs—desired factor VIII and factor IX levels are both 40%
- Bleeds of minor abrasions, bruises, minor lacerations, minor epistaxis, and minor mouth or gum bleeding may not require any factor replacement
- If in doubt, consider infusion and consult hematology
- Perhaps use of activated recombinant factor VII (Haemostasis 1998:93) in those with hemophilia A or B that have inhibitors in the perioperative period

If known diagnosis of factor VIII deficiency:

- Consider desmopressin (DDAVP) (Med Lett Drugs Ther 1984:82) 0.3 µg/kg over 30 minutes IV or nasal spray (Thromb Res 1979:775; J Pediatr 1983:228). This increases factor VIII transiently for uses such as post-traumatic or perioperative—probably induces release of factors from endothelium. Adequate alone in 80%
- Determine desired factor from above, and calculate factor VIII units (*The Hemophilia Handbook*, 1992:59): weight (lbs) ÷ 4.4 × desired factor level = number of units of factor VIII needed. Use all factor

from opened vials; it is better to infuse too much rather than too little

- Outpatient treatment may consist of recombinant DNA VIII; goal is to keep level >15%
- Follow-up in 24–36 hours if symptoms still persistent

If known diagnosis of factor IX deficiency:

- Determine desired factor from above, and calculate factor IX units needed (*The Hemophilia Handbook*, 1992:61): weight (lbs) ÷ 2.2 × desired factor level = number of units of factor IX needed. With factor IX, do not give more than the maximum dosage calculated
- Outpatient treatment may consist of alphanine or danazol 600 mg qd, which increases endogenous production; goal to keep levels 5–15% at all times, and >40% for surgery
- Follow-up in 24–36 hours if still symptomatic

9.6 SICKLE CELL CRISIS

Emerg Med Clin North Am 1993:365; Bmj 1997:656

Cause: Sickle cell anemia is genetic, autosomal

Epidem: In U.S. blacks, 7% are trait, 0.5% homozygous. Genetic distribution in world correlates with history, geography, and malaria

Pathophys:

Am J Epidemiol 2000:839

Valine substituted for glutamic acid in β chain leading to Hgb S, which is unstable at low O_2, leading to precipitation and sickling red cells. Sickled cells stick to vessel walls causing clots and infarctions. Splenic infarcts produce diminished antibody formation, which leads to increased infections. Hgb F ($\alpha_2\gamma_2$) may persist as survival mechanism into adult life. Heterozygous cells sickle only in severe hypoxia or if Hgb C or D present. Renal damage to medulla causes decreased concentration ability, K^+ loss, papillary necrosis, and ongoing renal disease. α-Thalassemia trait protects and vice versa

Sx: Painful crises arise in 60%; frequency correlates with worse prognosis

Si: Retarded growth and sexual maturation; frontal bossing; skin ulcers, especially lower legs; angioid streaking of fundi indicates neovascularization; pain may occur anywhere

Crs: 50% live to age 45 years, longer if fetal Hgb >8.6%; more severe disease in those with dactylitis, leukocytosis, and anemia <7 g/dL (N Engl J Med 2000:83)

Cmplc:
- Aplastic crises with severe pain most commonly secondary to infection with human parvovirus B19
- Pneumococcal and *Salmonella* infections, especially osteomyelitis, which can be difficult to differentiate from bony infarcts/necrosis (J Pediatr Orthop 1996:540)
- CVAs (Ann Intern Med 1972:643), which may be predictable by intracranial Doppler studies
- 25% have proteinuria that may progress to renal failure
- Gout
- Gallstones
- Sudden death rate with heavy exertion increased to 32/10,000 in heterozygotes in contrast to 1/100,000 in whites
- Myonecrosis and myofibrosis
- Priapism; impotence

Lab: CBC with diff, ESR low, sickled cells in peripheral smear; Hgb electrophoresis shows Hgb S + increased Hgb F. X-ray: Long bone infarcts/necrosis; "hair on end" skull; step fractures of vertebrae; acute chest syndrome (new pulmonary infiltrate) cannot be predicted on physical exam and CXR for all with sickle cell crisis who are febrile (Ann Emerg Med 1999:64). Perhaps U/S to help differentiate osteomyelitis from bony infarcts (J Pediatr Orthop 1998:552)

ED Rx:
- IV access; rehydration
- O_2 (N Engl J Med 1984:291)
- Parenteral narcotics and/or benzodiazepines; avoid using nitric oxide (potential neuropathy perhaps secondary to B_{12} deficiency (J Intern Med 1995:551)) (Clin Lab Haematol 1999:409)
- Possibly steroids (N Engl J Med 1994:733)
- Consider antibiotics; ceftriaxone OK in low-risk children (N Engl J Med 1993:472) and adults
- Transfusions, but Rx limited by sensitization, less with black blood donors

- Prevention with vitamin E 450 IU qd potentially helpful (Am J Hematol 1992:227); hydroxyurea 10–25 mg/kg/day gradually increased to just start suppressing polys—stimulates Hgb F production, but if used with erythropoietin, no benefit (N Engl J Med 1990:366); erythropoietin (Blood 1993:9; N Engl J Med 1993:73)

9.7 TRANSFUSION GUIDELINES

Transfus Med 1994:63; 1997:153

Cause: Whole blood, red cells, platelets, fresh frozen plasma (FFP), or cryoprecipitate needed for replacement due to consumption or external loss. Component therapy (the preceding list less whole blood) is preferred to maximize resources

Epidem: Use of these practices is common

Pathophys: Lack of or abnormal hematologic components may necessitate emergent replacement—the etiologies may be myriad. None of these products can be made completely pure, and platelets especially may be prone to bacterial contamination because they are stored at room temperature

Sx: Bleeding, shock

Si: Obvious bleeding source; shock; except for trauma, therapy guided by laboratory testing

Crs: Use of component therapy listed here usually necessitates admission

Cmplc: Febrile and allergic reactions may occur with use of these agents, as well as CMV and other viral transmissions

Lab: CBC with diff; metabolic profile; PT/PTT; blood bank tubes for appropriate agent replacement

ED Rx with Component Therapy:
Fresh Frozen Plasma
J Emerg Med 1998:239

1 mL of FFP contains one unit of coagulation factor activity. Use FFP for those who need replacement of multiple factor deficiencies—as seen in DIC, liver failure, massive blood or volume replacement, either due to symptomatic bleeding or those about to undergo an invasive procedure. Using an INR of 1.6 or higher may help guide the decision on those who may need FFP. The usual dose is 10–20 cc/kg which is ~4 units in an adult (220 cc/unit). A lesser dose

may be used—2 units—if supplementing the replacement of a vitamin K deficiency

Platelets

Transfus Med 1992:311

Composed of $>5.5 \times 10^{10}$/unit with some red cells and white cells and plasma unless leukocyte reduced where the final WBC is $<5 \times 10^6$ for final dose—less febrile reactions and CMV transmission with leukocyte reduced. May have HLA matched, which is a pheresis pack. One unit raises platelet count ~5000/µL in a 70-kg person; usual order is for a six-pack. Transfuse for bleeding due to thrombocytopenia or abnormal platelets, or consider empirically for platelet count <10,000/µL

Packed Red Blood Cells

J Emerg Med 1998:129

Composed of red cells at a hematocrit of ~75%, some plasma, WBCs, and platelets. May come prepared in different fashions to reduce allergic reactions, febrile reactions, and CMV transmission (Transfus Med 1998:59). Use in normovolemic patients with chronic anemia who may require increased oxygen-carrying capacity, such as those with symptomatic ischemia to any organ. In trauma, if patient not responding to a fluid bolus of 20 cc/kg of crystalloid, then should move to blood products if suspect hemorrhagic cause. Whole blood may be used, but the hypervolemia caused by rapid infusion and other fluid infusion has made packed RBCs the preferred replacement agent. Infusion of one unit of packed RBCs in an adult will increase hematocrit by ~3%

Cryoprecipitate

Ann Intern Med 1983:484

It contains factor VIII, fibrinogen, von Willebrand's factor, and factor XIII. When hemophilia A and von Willebrand's disease concentrates are not available, cryoprecipitate may be used. Fibrinogen will increase ~5 mg/dL for each unit, and an adult needs a level of >100 mg/dL to be hemostatic. For factor VIII replacement, the total number of bags required is the number of factor VIII units needed divided by 80—at least 80 IUs are in each bag. See 9.5 to calculate number of factor VIII units needed.

9.8 VENOUS THROMBOSIS

Arch Intern Med 1998:2315

Cause: Venous stasis as seen in long plane or car rides, or immobilization post fracture; intimal injury; coagulation abnormalities, for example as seen in some cancers; IVs are an occasional cause—2/3 due to particulates in IV, 1/3 chemical and/or needle irritation, <1% bacterial; and trauma pts have a 69% incidence, 18% is proximal DVT. Usually lower extremity although upper extremity DVT becoming more common and with similar causes (Surgery 1988:561). Inherited protein deficiencies: one of these four deficiencies is present in 31% of outpatients with lower and 9% with upper extremity DVT; a h/o DVT in the family or at a young age does not increase the likelihood

- Protein C deficiency or resistance; autosomal dominant, vitamin K dependent. Factor V (Leiden) mutation in 25–40% of pts with DVT; a heterozygous point mutation causing resistance to protein C is a separate inherited condition—possibly conferring higher risk of CVA. Screening asymptomatic population not cost effective since annual incidence of DVT is <1%
- Protein S deficiency is autosomal dominant, vitamin K dependent. Protein S is a protein C cofactor, and is associated with nephrotic syndrome. Can also occur as acquired autoimmune deficiency
- Antithrombin II deficiency; autosomal dominant
- Antiphospholipid antibodies—anticardiolipin, lupus anticoagulant. Seen in SLE, ITP, or primary antiphospholipid syndrome. Look for elevated PTT, manifest by arterial thrombi or DVT of any organ system (Ann Emerg Med 1992:207); get INR >3 on warfarin.

Epidem: Associated with major surgery, especially hip (AJR Am J Roentgenol 1996:659) or abdominal surgery (Br J Surg 1977:709) and previous thromboembolism (Arch Intern Med 2000:769). Association is high in hospitalized ICU patients (33%) who may be asymptomatic and despite >60% of patients receiving prophylactic treatment (Jama 1995:335). Association with occult cancer after one episode is equivocal (Arch Intern Med 1987:1907). Children (J Vasc Surg 1996:46, discussion, 50) and Asian/Pacific islander ethnic groups (Ann Intern Med 1998:737; Am J Cardiol 2000:1334) appear to have protective traits to avoid DVT.

Pathophys: As above

Sx: Calf pain; unilateral edema

Si: None; or Homan's sign, increased calf circumference, or warmth, which are all equivocal findings (Arch Surg 1976:34)

Crs: 75% 5-year survival; 25% recurrence over 5 years

Cmplc:

- Pulmonary embolus (14%), but incidence is decreased to <0.4% with Rx
- Chronic postphlebitic syndrome (edema, pain, stasis dermatitis, and ulcers) (Int J Dermatol 1987:14) in 30% after 5 years, incidence can be decreased by half with use of compression stockings × 2–3 weeks; Rx symptoms with herbal venastat 1 po bid, avoid in pregnancy. Thrombotic skin necrosis, especially of penis with protein C deficiency and warfarin Rx; Rx with vitamin K, avoid by using heparin Rx

Diff Dx:

Superficial phlebitis: Rx with local heat, ASA, NSAIDs (perhaps the same for upper extremity DVT, although some advocate same treatment as with DVT of lower extremity (J Vasc Surg 1997:853))

Lab: CBC with diff; PT/PTT; d-dimer (ELISA); fibrin split products— 5 minutes bedside d-dimer is 90–93% sensitive and 80–90% specific for proximal DVT compared to ELISA (Thromb Res 1997:93), may be helpful if negative in excluding people of DVT who have low risk—pro (Thromb Haemost 2000:191) and con (Ann Emerg Med 2000: 121)

Noninvasive Testing

- U/S: simple compressibility or duplex: noncompressibility with probe 91% sensitivity and 99% specificity or better (J Clin Ultrasound 1999:415); 6–10% of positives will be missed with single test, worse if pt is asymptomatic—repeat in 3–7 days if still suspicious (Circulation 1989:810). ED physicians may be able to do this if so trained with one study showing good concordance with noninvasive laboratory evaluation (Acad Emerg Med 2000:120)
- Impedance plethysmography (IPG) is not as good or as frequently used as U/S; valid in pregnancy if done in the decubitus position

Invasive

Venography, but 2% of the time it causes DVT—can trust a negative exam as true (Circulation 1981:622). Fibrinogen scans may diagnose the rare miss on venography (Jama 1977:2195)

ED Rx:
- Low molecular weight heparin (LMWH) protocol (Ann Intern Med 1998:299) as effective as IV unfractionated heparin (Haemostasis 1996:189). Enoxaparin (Lovenox) 1 mg/kg sc q 12 hours; all LMWHs are not the same! Begin warfarin on day 1. Oral heparins are on the horizon (Circulation 2000:2658)
- Heparin IV × 5 days + warfarin started on day 1
- Overlap heparin and warfarin with therapeutic INR (>2) at least for 2 days to avoid theoretical warfarin induced hypercoagulable state
- Continue warfarin for 6 months if no specific cause, for 1–2 months if specific transient cause, lifelong if recurrent idiopathic type or if due to hypercoagulable state
- Not thrombolysis, risk of systemic thrombolysis or procedural complications if catheter directed has not been shown to outweigh conservative treatment with anticoagulants, despite some literature (Can J Surg 1993:359)
- IVC filter to reduce pulmonary embolus rate from 4% to 1.5% but subsequent recurrent DVT is 20+% vs. 11%, and short- and long-term mortality is the same

10 Infectious Disease

Choice of antibacterial drugs, Med Lett Drugs Ther 1999;41:95; Drugs
for non-HIV viral infections, Med Lett Drugs Ther 1999;41:113

10.1 FOURNIER GANGRENE

Cause: Polymicrobial infection of scrotum from skin, urethral, or
perianal nidus

Epidem: Uncommon; mortality rate from 20–42% in adults; increased
risk in older age and those with chronic alcoholism (Eur Urol
1998:411)

Pathophys: Most commonly seen in those with diabetes mellitus or
other immunocompromised states; the scrotal area is at risk for
secondary or rapidly progressing infections

Sx: Scrotal pain, rectal pain, dysuria

Si: Hard and erythematous scrotum, diffuse tenderness, fever

Crs: May be protracted and lead to death; less ominous course in
children (Urology 1990:439)

Cmplc: May progress to abscess formation or necrotizing fasciitis;
acute renal failure; adult respiratory distress syndrome
(Br J Urol 1989:310)

Diff Dx: May arise from intra-abdominal processes (Urology 1994:779)

Lab: Glucoscan with serum glucose if elevated, HgbA1C if undiagnosed
diabetic, U/A, metabolic profile—metabolic abnormalities
correspond with severity of disease (J Urol 1995:89). X-ray:
consider scrotal U/S to R/O abscess or delineate extent of disease
(Radiology 1988:387)

ED Rx:
- IVF and parenteral antiemetics and/or pain meds if needed
- IV ampicillin/sulbactam, second-generation cephalosporin, or antibiotic combination to give coverage for gram-pos, gram-neg, and anaerobes
- Treat underlying metabolic disorders, such as hyperglycemia
- Topical unprocessed honey (Surgery 1993:200)
- Hyperbaric oxygen is controversial (J Urol 1984:918)
- Urologic referral if infected urine or abscess
- Next day F/U if no abscess, patient is not toxic, and patient is reliable

10.2 HIV

Adv Intern Med 2000:1; AIDS Read 2000:133 and the entire issue of *The AIDS Reader*; peds—Pediatr Clin North Am 2000:155

Note: This is a dynamic field; identify local experts and resources

Cause: Human immunodeficiency virus (HIV) type 1; rarely in U.S. but commonly in Africa is HIV-2; a retrovirus

Epidem: Spread via sexual intercourse; dirty/shared needles; blood products, e.g., screened blood transfusion 1996 risk = 1/500,000, factor VIII concentrates, and probably breast milk; rarely by casual or nonsexual familial contact, and percutaneous inoculation in health care workers—0.3% incidence, which increases with volume and HIV titer transmission enhanced by the presence of chancroid or other gential ulcers

Prevalence increased in gay males, drug users, hemophiliacs, female partners of infected males

90% of persons transfused with HIV-positive blood convert to positive themselves; 30% of babies from HIV-positive mothers who are untreated are positive at 6 months of age

Incidence decreasing in 1990s in U.S. as are AIDS-related deaths probably secondary to public health measures, drug treatment of HIV infection, and prophylaxis/treatment of opportunistic infections

Pathophys: AIDS defined by HIV infection and T4 count <200 (Semin Thorac Cardiovasc Surg 2000:130)

Increased suppressor T8 and decreased helper T4 cells (CD4); deficient production of interferon γ. Conversion rate of HIV positive to AIDS is approx. 2%/year in hemophiliacs, but is age-dependent so that 7% of HIV-positive young hemophiliacs have AIDS after 8 years, but 50% of those who are age 35–70 years will have AIDS after 8 years, and this is a similar pattern in homosexuals.

Billions of virons produced daily from infection with high viral RNA mutation rate that allows rapid selection of resistant organism in the face of treatment. Also sequestration of virus in lymphoid tissue (J Infect Dis 2000:354). Oxidative stress of illness appears to be reversed with effective therapy (J Acquir Immune Defic Syndr 2000:321)

Sx:

Primary HIV Infection

Mono-like syndrome 5–30 days after exposure lasting approx. 2 weeks; fever (95%), sore throat (70%), weight loss (70%), myalgias (60%), headache (60%), cervical adenopathy (50%)

AIDS

Diarrhea (60%), malaise, weight loss, fever adenopathy, dyspnea

Si:

Early

Lymphadenopathy; oral monilia/thrush (exudative, chelosis, or erythematous diffuse rash types) precedes overt disease often; dermatoses including warts and shingles; chronic fatigue syndrome

Later

Wasting syndromes; chronic diarrhea, Kaposi's sarcoma, hairy leukoplakia corrugations on sides of tongue due to reactivation of EBV

Crs: Variable RNA viral loads in first 4 months but worse course predicted by levels at 5–12 months from infection and by severity of primary infection symptoms

HIV Infection

Evolution to AIDS 10 years post-seroconversion varies from 0–72% inversely with RNA copies (viral load) at 12–18 months after seroconversion

AIDS

1997 mortality figures markedly improving with aggressive multidrug treatment based on viral loads, e.g., from 29 to 9/100 person years in patients with CD4 counts <100; older data were 50% 1-year survival, 15% 5-year survival, 5% 10+-year survival because of some viral attenuated pathogenicity; in pts with AIDS on AZT, 50% 1-year survival after CD4 count <50/mm^3; increased time to clinical AIDS and opportunistic infections (AIDS 2000:561). Prognosis (survival) worse with increasing age, but not associated with gender, IV drug use, race, or socioeconomic status

Cmplc:

- *Infections* with common bacterial pathogens as well as opportunistic organisms, esp when CD4 count <50, include the following (less since highly active antiretroviral therapy (J Acquir Immune Defic Syndr 2000:145)):
  - Pneumocystis or other pneumonias (J Infect Dis 2000:158)
  - Tuberculosis, and as a marker for HIV risk based on CD4 and CD8 ratio (AIDS Patient Care STDS 2000:79)
  - Atypical mycobacterium, especially *M. avium-intracellulare*, rarely *M. haemophilum* or *M. fortuitum* (Am J Med Sci 1998:50)
  - Herpes infections including tongue fissures: CMV, candida, aspergillosis, *Strongyloides*
  - Hepatitis B and C (Sex Transm Dis 1993:220)
  - *Nocardia*
  - *Mucor*
  - *Cryptococcus*, esp. meningitis
  - *Toxoplasma*
  - *Legionella*
  - *Chlamydia*; gonorrhea perhaps as marker for HIV risk (Aids 2000:189), and other STDs (Sex Transm Dis 2000:259)
  - *Monilia* and *Torulopsis*
  - Cryptosporidiosis
  - *Isospora belli*
  - *Listeria*
  - Cat scratch *Bartonella* (*Rochalimaea*) *henselae* or *quintana* causing bacillary angiomatosis and peliosis hepatitis
  - Syphilis with rapid (<4 years) appearance of neurosyphilis manifest by strokes, meningitis, and cranial nerve palsies and which is only transiently suppressed by penicillin regimens
- *Tumors* including the following:
  - Kaposi's sarcoma—HHV-8 coinfection, venerally spread among gay males. Sx/Si: Violaceous skin eruptions, ulcers on legs. Crs: 80% mortality. Diff Dx: bacillary angiomatosis. ED Rx: ID or

HIV specialist referral, to consider intralesional hCG, interferon, vinblastine
- Non-Hodgkins lymphoma, in 15% after 3 years of AZT treatment
- Burkitt's, EB virus-associated, in adults
- Leiomyosarcomas, EB virus-associated, in children
- Cervical cancer due to higher prevalence of HPV infection—pap q 6 months
- *Gastrointestinal*: upper GI hemorrhage; protease inhibitors helpful (Am J Gastroenterol 1999:358)
- *Hematologic*: ITP and aplastic anemia—both of these from parvovirus infection and diminished half-life and megakaryocyte infection
- *Metabolic*: insulin resistance with protease inhibitor therapy (J Biol Chem 2000:20251) and elevated lipid levels (*AIDS Read*; 2000:162, discussion, 171)
- *Myocardiopathy*
- *Neurologic* includes the following:
  - CNS degeneration leading to dementia
  - Progressive multifocal leukoencephalopathy (J Neurol 2000:134) associated with papovavirus, seen in transplant pts as well
  - Cord lesions
  - Meningitis (Arch Intern Med 1995:2231), lower risk with fluconazole use
  - Peripheral neuropathy
  - Cerebral toxoplasmosis
  - Cerebral lymphomas
- *Nephropathy*
- *Rhematologic* including Reiter's without conjunctivitis, and psoriasis with arthritis
- *Psychiatric* includes depression and suicide

Diff Dx:
- HTLV I infection—associated with paraparesis
- HTLV II infection—no disease association
- CD4 cell lymphopenia syndrome—rare and idiopathic disease

Lab:

Immunology
- Viral load, most important test; RNA by PCR, peripheral mononuclear cell viral m-RNA levels predict prognosis and treatment success; indicates rapidity of disease progression;

<10,000/cc good, 10,000–100,000/cc moderately OK, >100,000/cc bad

- T4 (CD4) <200/cc defines AIDS now and predicts opportunistic pneumonias, 200–500 = intermediate risk; a form of mile marker in disease progression
- ELISA with Western blot test, only 1.5% false positive in low-risk military population; if indeterminant, repeat in 1 month and should become positive if really HIV; if persistently equivocal, get PCR and viral culture. Tests negative for 4+ month incubation period. Peds with more variables (Pediatr Clin North Am 2000:39), peds referral
- Ora-Sure HIV-1 test from 2-minute swab between cheek and gum as specific as serum by ELISA/Western blot
- p24 nuclear antigen detection either of free antigen or dissociated form IgG antibody-antigen complexes; positive usually in early disease or in primary infection when ELISA still negative in 50%

Routine

If newly diagnosed, CBC with diff, metabolic profile, hep B status, syphilis serology, baseline Toxo and CMV titers, PPD plus controls, U/A warranted in that 10% have nephrotic syndrome. If known to be HIV positive, check other tests as warranted if evaluating secondary complaints. CXR if hypoxic or TB contacts (J Epidemiol Community Health 2000:64)

ED Rx:

Immediate

Public health, social service (Am J Public Health 2000:699), and medical AIDS specialist referral if AIDS defining diagnosis is present. If new diagnosis, consider the following:

- Prevention: condom use, AZT if pregnant—pre- and postpartum use decreases infant HIV positivity by 1/3. Protease inhibitors may predispose to low birth weight infants (Infect Dis Obstet Gynecol 2000:94)
- *Haemophilus influenzae* vaccine, Pneumovax, flu shot
- VZIG if exposed to chickenpox
- Fluconazole 200 mg po q week if local mucosal or systemic candidal infections

Treatment of Disease

A dynamic field and saves lives (Lancet 2000:1131), and common approach is the following: dual therapy is nucleotide reverse transcriptase inhibitor (NRTI) + protease inhibitor (PI); triple therapy is two NRTIs + PI for all pts with HIV viral load RNA levels >5,000–10,000/cc no matter what the CD4 count with doses increased to get RNA load levels <500/cc; and dual protease inhibitor therapy is as the name sounds (Annu Rev Pharmacol Toxicol 2000:649). Listing of available medications in *The Medical Letter: Drugs for HIV Infection* (Med Lett Drugs Ther 2000;42:1). *Note*: Avoid combinations of d4t + AZT; or ddC with ddI, d4t, or 3TC. Failure of treatment usually due to compliance and therapy potency (Jama 2000:205)

Specific Preventions

• Pneumocystis prophylaxis with CD4 counts 100–200 all 3 equally good so q 1 month pentamidine best since least toxic, but with CD4 counts <100, Tm/S better than dapsone which is better than pentamidine

• Tuberculosis prevention for those tuberculin positive with either 1 year of isoniazid or 2 months of rifampin/pyrazinamide (Jama 2000:1445)

• *M. avium* (MAI) prophylaxis if CD4 counts <100 with clarithromycin, azithromycin, or rifabutin

• Toxoplasmosis after encephalitis with sulfadiazine + pyrimethamine folate po qd or 3×/week (Eur J Clin Microbiol Infect Dis 2000:89); or if positive titer and CD4 <100 with Tm/S DS qd

• CMV infections with ganciclovir 1 g po tid if CD4 <50–100 decreases rate by 1/2?

• Cryptococcal with fluconazole, but no prolongation of survival

• Aphthous stomatitis with equal parts elixir of Mylanta: Benadryl: tetracycline: nystatin with 1 tsp qid swish and spit. Persistent cases—thalidomide 50–200 mg po qd × 2–4 weeks (Clin Infect Dis 1995:250); or topical granulocyte-macrophage colony-stimulating factor (Br J Dermatol 2000:171)

• Wasting syndromes may be treated with megestrol (Megace) 40 mg po qid, or marijuana, androgens, growth hormones, or thalidomide

• Diarrhea should be treated by finding the primary cause with consideration of the following: octreotide 50 mg sc q 8 hours, opiates, loperamide (Imodium), or diphenoxylate-atropine (Lomotil). Endoscopy for refractory cases with negative stool studies (Gastrointest Endosc 2000:427)

• Those responding to highly active antiretroviral therapies may be considered for discontinuation of secondary prophylaxis for opportunistic infections (AIDS 2000:383)

10.3 LYME DISEASE

Ann Emerg Med 1999:680

Cause: *Borrelia burgdorferi* spread by *Ixodes dammini* tick bite—same tick also spreads babesiosis.

Epidem: Deer tick also infests white-footed deer mice. Northeastern and northwestern U.S. HLA DR4 and DRw2 B-cell allotypes associated with increased CNS, cardiac, and arthritic involvement. Most common tickborne spirochetal disease in U.S.; attack rates up to 66% of people living in a highly endemic area over 7 years; annual incidence = 20–100+/100,000/year, depending on geographic locale (Jama 1997:112); also common in Northern Europe

Pathophys: Sometimes an immune complex disease, but organisms now identified in joints most of the time. Clinical syndromes very much like primary, secondary, and tertiary syphilis; but much overlap between stage 1 and 2 symptom complexes

Sx: Tick bite history in 80%; disease rare if tick on <24 hours, usually takes 72 hours and most ticks associated with disease have stayed on a week
- *Stage 1*: arthralgias (98%), malaise (80%), headache (64%), fever (60%), stiff neck, rash (77%)
- *Stage 2*: neurologic and cardiac
- *Stage 3*: arthritis; chronic neurologic changes

Si:
- *Stage 1*: fever, lymphadenopathy, erythema migrans—a warm "ringworm" around bite with median diameter 15 cm present in 60–80%
- *Stage 2*: neurologic: lymphocytic meningitis (15%) and meningoencephalitis, peripheral motor or sensory neuropathies, facial nerve palsies including Bell's palsy. And/or cardiac: myocarditis (8%), like rheumatic fever with heart block but valve disease rare or never; sometimes heart block is only symptom, no fever or even malaise; usually transient, ~6 weeks after primary infection
- *Stage 3*: recurrent polyarthritis at first, then 1–2 large joints; onset up to 4–6 months after skin rash with decreasing recurrences over years. Late keratitis

- *Peds*: presentation is variable, and usually diagnosis made with later stage findings (Pediatr Emerg Care 1998:356)

Crs: Stage 1 lasts 3–4 weeks. Symptoms and signs of stages 2 & 3 may be chronic and recurrent over months to years. Even after treatment, especially if given >3 months after symptoms, residual arthralgias, fatigue, memory problems may persist. Benign course in children

Cmplc: Chronic myocardiopathy. Neurologic: chronic encephalopathy in 90% of those who have stage 2 neurologic symptoms; cerebral vasculitis (Ann Emerg Med 1990:572); also chronic polyneuropathy and leukoencephalitis. Treatment and testing of those not meeting clinical criteria (Jama 1993:979; 1998:206)

Diff Dx: Ehrlichiosis, babesiosis as separate or concomitant infection(s)

Lab: CBC with diff and ESR with WBC <10,000 (92%), hematocrit >37% (88%), and ESR >20 mm/hr (53%) in those with disease. Serum IgG and IgM ELISA titer increased and positive Western blot; rare false positive with most occurring in low-prevalence populations, in syphilis, and SBE; ≤5% false negative especially in late stage, seen if early po antibiotic treatment or early in course, or with some labs that run 10–50% false negative and up to 25% false positive. Synovial fluid organisms positive by PCR. Path: positive silver stain or culture of rash edge for organism in 86%

ED Rx:

Med Lett Drugs Ther 2000;42:37

Prevention of tick bite with permethrin (Nix) treatment of clothing and DEET at 75+% concentration (Am J Hosp Pharm 1992:1164), and:

- Do tick checks and removal every 24 hours
- Prophylaxis after tick bite doubtful, perhaps 2 weeks of doxycycline in high-prevalence areas (N Engl J Med 1992:534)
- Consider vaccination with LYMErix (Med Lett Drugs Ther 1999;41:29) in highly endemic areas, a series of three shots at 0, 1, and 12 months—long-term safety and effectiveness is unknown (N Engl J Med 1998:209) (Med Lett Drugs Ther 3/26/99)

Stage 1: Decreases postrash arthritis and illness

- Tetracycline 250 mg po qid or doxycycline 100 mg po bid for 21 days; or amoxicillin 250–500 mg po tid for 21 days; or
- Second line with erythromycin 250 mg po qid for 10 days; or penicillin 20 million U qd IV for 10 days; or cefuroxime 500 mg po bid for 21 days

Stages 2 & 3:
- Doxycycline 200 mg po bid or amoxicillin as above but for 4–6 weeks or ceftriaxone 2 g IV/IM for 14–21 days, especially if bad arthritis or cardiac/neurologic findings, only 1/13 failures; or penicillin G 20 million U qd IV for 10–21 days for cardiac or neurologic abnormalities—incl. meningitis, cures 55% of arthritis. *Note*: Avoid intra-articular steroids

For *acute nonmeningitis disseminated disease*:
- Doxycycline 100 mg po bid for 21 days, equally effective as ceftriaxone 2 g IM qd for 14 days

For *heart block*: antibiotics and temporary pacer

For *chronic encephalopathy*: 60–85% improve with ceftriaxone treatment given even after several years

Note: If positive titers and chronic fatigue/fasciitis syndrome, no treatment

10.4 MENINGITIS

Cause: Different infectious causes in neonates, children, young adults, and the elderly:
- Neonates: first—group B streptococcus, second—*Listeria*, third—pneumococcus, fourth—*Escherichia coli*, vaginal flora, and *Staphylococcus epidermidis*
- Children 2–24 months of age (if vaccinated against *H. influenzae*): first—pneumococcus, second—*Neisseria meningitidis* (serotype Y > C > B > A), third—group B streptococcus, fourth—*H. influenzae*
- Children 2–18 years of age (if vaccinated): first—*meningococcus*, second—pneumococcus, third—*H. influenzae*
- Adults aged 20–60 years: first—pneumococcus, second—meningococcus, third—*H. influenzae*, fourth—*Listeria*
- Age 60 years +: first—pneumococcus, second—*Listeria*, third—all others

Epidem: Increased prevalence of meningococcal meningitis after influenza infection

Pathophys: Primary infection from bacteremia leading to a change/problem with blood-brain barrier. May also occur from direct extension or mastoiditis or otitis media, for example, or as a secondary site from a distant focal infection, such as pyelonephritis

Additionally, host factors of immune function may play a role, which is why the very young and very old have a different set of pathogens. Immunodeficiency associated with complement problems, or generalized decreased immune function from chronic disease or splenic problems, may also predispose to meningitis. Pathogens in these cases may be opportunistic (Lancet 2000:1426)

HIB (*H. influenzae* type B) vaccine has changed the major pathogens in pediatric meningitis (Lancet 1992:592)

Sx: Fever, change in mental status, stiff neck

Si: Fever, stiff neck, focal neurologic deficits, seizures, Brudzinski's sign—hip flexion elicited by active neck flexion, Kernig's sign—neck pain resulting from knee extension; petechial rash in *H. influenzae* and meningococcus; joint pain and erythema seen in meningococcal disease as well. Physical exam not helpful for peds <1 year of age (Ann Emerg Med 1992:910)

Crs: Death if bacterial meningitis not treated, high chance of mortality with treatment in both pneumococcal and meningococcal disease. Worse prognosis with change in mental status, hypotension, or seizure (Ann Intern Med 1998:862). Children with partially treated (previous antibiotics) meningitis may have no fever, no mental status change, and more URI signs and symptoms (Ann Emerg Med 1992:146)

Cmplc: CNS thrombophlebitis with focal seizures and deficits, cranial nerve neuropathies, communicating hydrocephalus, developmental problems

Diff Dx: Aseptic meningitis (predominant lymphocytes in CSF; if polys in first LP, re-do in 6–12 hours to look for change to lymphs (N Engl J Med 1973:571)):

- *Treatable*: tuberculosis, SBE, fungal (cryptococcosis), tumor, *Listeria*, herpes simplex, NSAIDs (Ann Pharmacother 1992:813), syphilis, subdural or epidural abscess, cysticercosis (*Taenia solium*), leptospirosis, partially treated bacterial, rheumatoid arthritis, rickettsia, Lyme disease, HIV, cat scratch fever, *Borrelia* (relapsing fever), high-dose immunoglobulin treatment
- *Untreatable*: sarcoid, viral including enteroviruses (polio, coxsackie, echo), mumps, mono, rabies, arbovirus, rarely benign recurrent aseptic meningitis (Mollaret's meningitis) (Arch Neurol 1979:657), rarely CMV (infants). Rarely anaerobic meningitis (in infancy),

from source such as pilonidal cyst abscess (Clin Neurol Neurosurg 1985:131)

Lab: CBC with diff although usually of little help (J Emerg Med 1988:33), CRP >1 in children (Ann Emerg Med 1991:36), serum procalcitonin level >0.2 ng/mL in adults with bacterial meningitis (Clin Infect Dis 1999:1313), metabolic profile, blood cultures, U/A and urine culture, CXR if suspected pulmonary component

- LP: CSF has >10 white cells/mm^3, usually (87%) >200, mostly polys; glucose <40 mg% (50%); protein >45 mg% (96%), usually >100 mg%; *H. influenzae* may have a paucity of abnormalities (Pediatr Emerg Care 1990:191); Gram's stain of CSF may show pathogen—gram-positive cocci in pairs in pneumococcus, intracellular gram-negative diplococci in meningococcus, coccobacillus in *H. influenzae*. Do fluid culture, consider bacterial antigen screen, if bloody tap, do cell counts on tubes 1 & 3 and look for xanthochromia. Perhaps PCR for enteroviral meningitis (J Pediatr 1997:393). Perhaps peds 1–3 years of age may be screened by those with <6 WBCs/mm^3 only requiring bacterial culture (98% sensitive, 75% specific (J Pediatr 1991:363)). CSF lactate level not much help (J Infect 1983:231)
- X-ray: head CT first before LP if focal signs including seizure, but do not delay antibiotic treatment

ED Rx:
- Give first dose of IV antibiotics in ED (Ann Emerg Med 1986:544; 1989:856)
- *Neonates*: ceftriaxone 100 mg/kg and ampicillin, consider gentamicin or cefotaxime
- *Age 6 months to 6 years*: ceftriaxone and ampicillin
- *Older children and adults*: ceftriaxone 2 g IV q 12 hours, add ampicillin if considering *H. influenzae* or *Listeria*. Cefotaxime, cefoperazone (Antimicrob Agents Chemother 1982:262), or rarely chloramphenicol may be used—if suspect resistance, better to use vancomycin
- If considering *Pseudomonas*, add ceftazidime and/or gentamicin
- Therapy may be altered depending on culture results
- Dexamethasone is controversial (J Emerg Med 1996:165), some studies have shown children have better hearing outcomes—pro (using CSF level of TNF-α >1000 pg/mL as level for initiation of dexamethasone (J Infect 1999:55)) and con (Eur J Pediatr 1999:230; J Antimicrob Chemother 2000:315), dose is 0.15 mg/kg

IV 20 minutes before antibiotic, then q 6 hours × 4. No benefit in adults (Intensive Care Med 1999:475)

- Ketorolac also controversial as used to prevent hearing loss (J Infect Dis 1999:264)

Prevention: Treat household and day care contacts of those with meningococcus or *H. influenzae*, use either rifampin or ciprofloxacin

- For meningococcus, rifampin 600 mg po qid for 2 days or ciprofloxacin 500 mg bid for 2 days if an adult. For children, rifampin 10 mg/kg bid for 2 days
- For *H. influenzae*, rifampin 600 mg po qd for 4 days or ciprofloxacin 500 mg po bid for 4 days if an adult. For children, rifampin 20 mg/kg qd for 4 days

10.5 PERIORBITAL CELLULITIS

Head Neck Surg 1987:227

Cause: *S. aureus*, pneumococcus, and *H. influenzae*—*H. influenzae* now rarer with vaccine (Ann Emerg Med 1996:617). Rarely mucormycosis (Clin Exp Neurol 1994:68)

Epidem: Young children have higher risk of periorbital disease, or those who are not immunocompetent (J Rheumatol 1988:840)

Pathophys: Extension to periorbital area from underlying sinusitis, from hematogenous spread or from external trauma such as eyebrow plucking (Am J Ophthalmol 1986:534)

Sx: Facial pain, fever

Si: Periorbital tenderness, erythema, sinus tenderness

Cmplc: Abscess formation or meningitis

Diff Dx: Allergic reaction, trauma, orbital cellulitis, conjunctivitis, insect bite

Lab: CBC with diff, blood culture, ESR if diagnosis somewhat equivocal. TSH if bilateral proptosis in someone adolescent age or greater. LP should be considered in those <6 months of age, or in anyone with symptoms of meningeal disease, but not necessary as part of routine evaluation (J Pediatr 1993:355). X-ray: CT of orbit and sinuses if unilateral proptosis, cranial nerve or visual field/acuity deficit—to R/O abscess or tumor

ED Rx:
- IV access if systemically ill, and consider ampicillin/sulbactam or ceftriaxone
- Outpatient treatment of dicloxacillin or cephalexin, with next day follow-up

10.6 PERITONITIS (BACTERIAL)

Cause: Inflammation of peritoneal cavity; the most common bacteria in these settings are bowel flora and *Streptococcus* sp., but many other pathogens have been found as well

Epidem: Unknown, no identifiers for localized versus "frank" peritonitis, and definition of localized with negative cultures (if done) is not well characterized

Pathophys: Inflammation of peritoneal surfaces, specifically the parietal peritoneum from either blood, infectious causes, gastric acid, digestive enzymes, or release of pancreatic enzymes. Free blood in the peritoneal cavity should be suspected if peritoneal signs in a traumatic or suspected aneurysmal condition. Infectious causes may be spontaneous as seen with spontaneous bacterial peritonitis (SBP) in those with end-stage liver disease, or as a secondary complication of peritoneal dialysis, intraperitoneal chemotherapy (Am J Med 1985:49), hollow viscus perforation such as appendiceal rupture (Pediatrics 1979:36), or previously unrecognized intra-abdominal abscess. Rarely due to congenital abnormalities such as infected urachal cysts (Arch Surg 1984:1269)

Pancreatitis may cause release of enzymes into the peritoneum, with resultant tissue self-degradation

Peritonitis in those with chronic ambulatory peritoneal dialysis is not uncommonly due to a process other than the dialysis intervention (Ann R Coll Surg Engl 1998:36)

Sx: Abdominal pain, fevers, chills, spasm of abdominal muscles causing inability to straighten up

Si: Pain with palpation; cough tenderness (pain with coughing) (Bmj 1994:1336); peritoneal signs such as rebound, percussion, or heel strike tenderness, as well as involuntary guarding or rigidity of the abdomen

Crs: Spontaneous bacterial peritonitis and peritonitis from pancreatitis have a high morbidity and mortality. Hemorrhagic causes are variable depending on the degree of hemorrhage and a patient's individual physiologic response

Cmplc: Sepsis or septic shock. Those with peritoneal dialysis may need to have site changed or go onto hemodialysis

Diff Dx: Sclerosing peritonitis in those with CAPD (Am J Kidney Dis 1994:819); colitis such as from *Clostridium difficile* (Arch Surg 1985:1321); ruptured AAA; hemoperitoneum from any cause, such as ruptured ectopic pregnancy or hemorrhagic ovarian cyst

Lab: CBC with diff; amylase; lipase; blood cultures × 2; peritoneal fluid for cell count, Gram's stain, culture, protein, glucose, and LDH, although turbidity most consistent finding if secondary to chronic ambulatory peritoneal dialysis (Perit Dial Int 1989:179). Finding of *Candida* on ascitic smear in a patient without chronic ambulatory peritoneal dialysis, recent abdominal surgery, or suggestive disseminated candidiasis by medical history is associated with bowel perforation (Am J Gastroenterol 1980:305). Consider glucoscan for DKA or EKG for MI evaluation. X-ray: Consider CXR for lower lobe pneumonia; plain films rarely show free air with SBP (Jama 1983:921), but may show with bowel perforation from any cause; abd CT may help delineate anatomy for abscess, or perhaps carcinomatosis vs. infectious etiology (AJR Am J Roentgenol 1996:743)

ED Rx:
- IV access
- Parenteral narcotics and/or antiemetics as needed
- *If infectious* etiology, consider paracentesis. IV antibiotics, consider third-generation cephalosporin
- *If hemorrhagic* cause, surgical consult and abd CT if pt stable—resuscitate pt if not stable, and consider bedside ultrasound
- *If from pancreatitis*, consider gallbladder ultrasound, and obtain GI consult
- *If unknown* cause and pt is stable, consider abd CT to elucidate cause

10.7 RABIES

Ann Emerg Med 1983:217; Am J Emerg Med 1993:279

Cause: Rabies virus, a rhabdovirus

Epidem: From saliva of infected animal, inhaling infected guano in bat caves, or corneal transplant. Bats may be reservoir since not killed by it, whereas uncommon in mice and squirrels as carriers since they probably die quickly. Cats are most commonly affected domestic animal. Most common wild animals affected are foxes, skunks, raccoons, and prey species like rabbits and woodchucks; possible in domestic animals such as goats, horses, and cows

Pathophys: Spread along nerves to CNS

Sx: History of animal bite except in bat rabies where often no bite or contact history. Pain/paresthesias at site; difficulty swallowing; fever; priapism; nausea; vomiting

Si: Guillain-Barré–like syndrome; tonic contractions, especially on throat with minimal stimulation—thus the presumed hydrophobia

Crs: 15–60-day incubation period, rarely up to 6 years later—depends on nerve length from CNS. Fatal unless treated before symptoms, usually, although some severe cases now recovering with intensive supportive care

Complc: Actual disease complications more common in third world countries; in the U.S., we seem to vacillate between under- and overtreating postexposure scenarios (J Emerg Med 1996:287; Public Health Rep 1998:247)

Diff Dx: Guillain-Barré

Lab: CSF shows elevated protein after 1 week—cells are a mix of lymphs and polys, 6–300/mm^3. Serology shows half positive after 1 week of symptoms, 2/3 after 1 1/2 weeks, all positive by 2 weeks of symptoms. Brain pathology shows Negri bodies

ED Rx:

For prevention (Ann Emerg Med 1999:590), vaccinate with human diploid cell vaccine—HDCV (Imovax)—OK in children with HIV disease (Clin Infect Dis 2000:218):

- Primary series postexposure: HDCV on days 1,3,7,14,28
- Pre-exposure: days 1,7,28
- Booster q 2 years to veterinarians and other high-risk people; chloroquine malaria prophylaxis may prevent adequate immunization

For acute single exposure: HDCV as above + HRIG (immune
globulin) 20 IU/kg, 1/2 in wound and 1/2 IM deltoid—not gluteal!
Perhaps purified chick embryo cell vaccine (Bull World Health
Organ 2000:693) in the future
Note: Use liberally in bat exposures even with no bite

10.8 SEPSIS

Ann Emerg Med 1993:1871; Emerg Med Clin North Am 1996:185

Cause: Most commonly gram-negative shock, but many occur
secondary to any infectious etiology. Postsplenectomy at risk
for encapsulated organisms (e.g., pneumococcus) (Br J Surg
1989:1074). Intravenous drug users may have soft-tissue nidus in
descending order of frequency—wrist/forearm, antecubital fossa,
fingers/hand, and thigh/groin (Br J Addict 1990:1495)

Epidem: Septic shock in 25% of those who present with sepsis;
septic shock mortality 34% at 28 days and 45% at 5 months
(Jama 1997:234)

Pathophys: Important to differentiate the different levels of infection
and their responses (Chest 1992:1644). Bacteremia may lead to
systemic inflammatory response (SRS) which is defined by the
following: P >90, RR >20, T >36–38.0°C (96–99°F), PCO_2 <32,
WBC >12,000 or <4000. SRS that is due to infection is the sepsis
syndrome. This may progress to severe sepsis, which is laboratory
evidence of end-organ dysfunction. When hypotension ensues with
inadequate end-organ perfusion, this is septic shock. Cytokine and
nitric oxide production may be mechanisms that can be treated
with inhibitors—exact role in sepsis is controversial (Ann Emerg
Med 2000:26)

Sx: Fever, localized discomfort, dyspnea, mental status changes

Si: Fever, possible rash or other localized findings

Crs: Severe sepsis identified in ED is difficult to prognosticate, and
does not mimic the mortality seen for inpatients with severe
sepsis (Acad Emerg Med 1998:1169); not influenced by antiseptic
central lines—not preventive for line sepsis (Arch Surg 1996:986);
preoperative antibiotics and antiseptic prep do prevent wound
sepsis in abdominal surgery that carries high risk of peritonitis
(Arch Surg 1984:909)

INFECTIOUS DISEASE

Cmplc: Encephalopathy correlates with severity of sepsis and Glasgow coma scale score

Lab: ABG; CBC with diff; metabolic profile; ESR if suspect bony origin; blood cultures; U/A and urine culture; consider DIC profile if evidence of end-organ damage; tumor necrosis factor α (TNF-α) (Crit Care Med 1999:1303) and procalcitonin levels (Crit Care Med 2000:950) with persistent elevation may identify those who will do worse; consider LP for CSF evaluation; perhaps tympanocentesis by ENT for infants with sepsis and unknown organism (Laryngoscope 1989:1048); consider EKG if hypotensive or if cardiac history or if age >60 years. X-ray: CXR; specific bone X-ray if considering osteomyelitis; spinal MRI if suspect disciitis; abd CT if suspect intra-abdominal process

ED Rx:
- IV access with fluid bolus
- IV antibiotics to cover *Staphylococcus* and *Pseudomonas* like third-generation cephalosporin + aminoglycoside
- Foley catheter and consider endotracheal intubation
- Consider pressors and ionotropes if needed, see 2.10
- NSAIDs help fever but no survival advantage
- Unless adrenal suppression, steroids of no help and may worsen situation
- Experimental monoclonal anti-endotoxins of no help
- Tumor necrosis factor receptor treatment is of no help

10.9 SYPHILIS (LUES)

Clin Microbiol Rev 1999:187

Cause: *Treponema pallidum*

Epidem: Incidence = 20+/100,000 in U.S., increasing since 1985; spread via direct contact (venereal) with primary (1°) or secondary (2°) lesion; screening all young adults presenting to EDs for any reason during epidemics will diagnose ~4% more cases (Ann Emerg Med 1993:1286). Strongly associated with HIV positivity (Sex Transm Dis 1990:190)

Pathophys: In 2°, marked bacteremia is present. Tertiary (3°) (Acta Derm Venereol 1969:336) probably represents a hypersensitivity reaction since few organisms are present. Gummas from

endarteritis obliterans which cause necrosis, e.g., in aortic media.
Three types of neurosyphilis:

- Tabes dorsalis
- Meningovascular
- General paresis of the insane, primary parenchymal involvement

All 3° complications are increased in AIDS (Genitourin Med 1996:176)

Sx:

- *1°*: painless chancre
- *2°*: rash, round with pigmented center; fever; headache, alopecia, eye pain from iritis

Si:

- *1°*: chancre with edema (looks like a squamous cell CA), and nonsuppurative lymphadenitis
- *2°*: macular/papular/pustular rash with pustules, annular-appearing as it ages, on palms and soles and split papules at mouth corners and other moist body areas (condyloma latum) (Br J Dermatol 1975:53); diffuse lymphadenopathy; meningitis
- *3°*:
  - Neurosyphilis: Argyle-Robertson pupils (small, unequal, reactive to accommodation not light); general paresis dementia; meningovascular, strokes, meningitis, and cranial nerve palsies most commonly seen within 3–4 years of primary infection especially in AIDS pts, tabes dorsalis with motor long tract and sensory losses in lower extremities
  - Vascular including aortitis with AI and aneurysms in 10%
  - Gummas in 15%; 75% are cutaneous
- *Congenital*: onset at age 14+ weeks even if seronegative at birth. Look for rash, fever, hepatosplenomegaly, rhinitis, lymphadenopathy, elevated LFTs, CSF cells, and protein; notched permanent (Hutchinson's) teeth in 25%; interstitial keratitis in 50%; saddle nose

Crs:

- *1°*: 9–90 days, 20–30% develop secondary syphilis
- *2°*: months if no Rx

Cmplc:

- *2°*: obstructive pattern hepatitis; nephrosis from immune complex disease
- *3°*: cirrhosis

Diff Dx: Herpes and chancroid—both with painful ulcers. The rash may resemble an allergic reaction, pityriasis rosea, guttate psoriasis, or numular eczema. The meningitis and encephalitis may resemble those reviewed in 10.4 and 13.5

- Bejel (Br J Vener Dis 1984:293) and pinta (J Am Acad Dermatol 1993:519, quiz, 536) from *Treponema carateum*, spread by skin-to-skin contact with lesions, as well as by flies in pinta. Bejel in Arabia, pinta in Central and South America. Primary disease consists of a nonulcerating papule; secondary, of pigmented skin lesions later becoming depigmented and hyperkeratotic; tertiary, of cardiovascular and nervous system involvement. Rx with PCN
- Yaws (J Am Acad Dermatol 1993:519, quiz, 536) from *T. pertenue*, spread skin to skin in many tropical areas, especially affecting children. Ulcerating papules with "strawberry" scar formation. Rx with PCN

Lab:

J Emerg Med 2000:361

- VDRL or RPR is positive in 76% of 1° cases (if negative, dark field still positive), 100% of 2° cases, and 75% of 3° cases; false positive (>1/16) in mononucleosis, malaria, collagen vascular diseases, sarcoid, leprosy, yaws, pinta. TPI is positive in 50% of 1°, 98% of 2°, and 90% of 3° cases. FTA is positive in 90% of 1°, 98% of 2°, and 98% of 3°; false positives in only 30% of VDRL false positive patients, some with yaws, pinta, or in 10% of those with lupus but is atypical; remains positive for life
- Bacteriology may show a dark field exam with bacteria with 8–14 spirals, ~7 μm long: false positives in mouth from normal treponema flora
- CSF: do LP 1 year post Rx of 1° and 2° types if VDRL or FTA still positive; in meningovascular syphilis elevated protein and cells are present; VDRL positive in 50% but can be negative even if bacteremia present, thus FTA better (J Neurol Sci 1988:229). Probably best just to Rx for 3–4 weeks without LP if asymptomatic, except for those with AIDS (do LP) (Genitourin Med 1996:176)
- X-ray: congenital type has lytic areas (bites) in long bones, subperiosteal (J Bone Joint Surg [Br] 1989:752)

ED Rx:

MMWR Morb Mortal Wkly Rep 1998:1

- Partner and public health notification

- Early disease (1°, 2°, or latent <1 year): first, benzathine PCN (Bicillin) 2.4 million units IM × 1; or second, doxycycline 100 mg po bid × 14 days; or third, erythromycin 500 mg po qid × 14 days
- Late, short of neurosyphilis: first, benzathine PCN 2.4 million units IM weekly × 3; or second, doxycycline 100 mg po bid × 4 weeks
- Neurosyphilis: PCN G 2–4 million U IV q 4 hours × 10–14 days, or procaine PCN 2.4 million U IM + probenecid (Benemid) 500 mg po qid × 10–14 days
- Congenital: PCN G 50,000 U/kg IM/IV q 8–12 hours × 10–14 days, or procaine PCN 50,000 U/kg IM qd × 10–14 days
- If PCN allergy: ceftriaxone IM qd × 10 days, or tetracycline 2 g qd or doxycycline 100 mg po bid × 15 days or erythromycin 2 g qd × 10 days (30 days for 3°)—12% failure rate for both erythromycin and doxycycline. Rx for 28 days if late latent disease
- Less than 1% relapse; follow VDRL, goes negative in 3–6 months; with CNS lues, follow CSF results; Jarisch-Herxheimer reaction (endotoxin symptoms with fever) within hours after PCN. Longer Rx in AIDS where early neurosyphilis develops and PCN Rx only transiently effective since long-term cure normally depends on immunity

10.10 TETANUS

Ann Emerg Med 1986:1111; 1987:1181; Am J Surg 1974:616; Bull Am Coll Surg 1992:22

Cause: *Clostridium tetani*, via wound contamination with dirt

Epidem: Present in most soils; <120 cases/year in U.S. (Morb Mortal Wkly Rep CDC Surveill Summ 1992:1); mainly in southern states with Texas having 56%; highest incidence in those inadequately immunized, such as born outside of U.S., older age (Ann Emerg Med 1990:1377), fewer years of formal education, and female gender—history is not reliable (Am J Emerg Med 1989:563); increased incidence in "skin popping" drug addicts

Pathophys: Exotoxin production and transport both via circulation to CNS (probably most significant in humans), and along motor nerves to CNS (but cannot correlate wound distance from CNS with morbidity and mortality in humans). Meticulous wound care helps prevent exotoxin production

Sx: Puncture wound or lacerations, or postpartum, postsurgery, or skin ulcers

Si: Spastic paralysis; tonic convulsive contractions precipitated by intrinsic or extrinsic muscle movement—lockjaw; facial muscles pulled tightly into smile—risus sardonicus; rarely any fever

Crs: 1–54 day incubation period, median of 8 days with 88% within 14 days; short incubation period in patients under age 50 is poor prognostic sign. 60% mortality

Complc: EDs tend to overimmunize which can lead to toxoid reactions (Ann Emerg Med 1985:573)

Diff Dx: (1) Neuroleptic malignant syndrome; (2) "stiff man syndrome"—autoimmune antibodies against GABA neurons inducing muscle spasms over years, seen with hypopituitarism, IDDM, Graves' and other endocrinopathies; occasionally is an autoimmune paraneoplastic syndrome in breast cancer

Lab: A clinical diagnosis with laboratory studies usually unhelpful (J Emerg Med 1998:705). Bacteriology studies show smears with gram-positive bacilli; culture shows fastidious anaerobe, positive in 32% of proven cases. Protective serum level of antibody is 0.01 IU/mL

ED Rx:

- *Prevent* with toxoid vaccine primary series, after 4 or more injections the protection is for at least 12 years after last injection and too many injections may cause toxoid reaction (N Engl J Med 1969:575); some argue that routine Td booster is unnecessary in adults; booster of Td is enough >5 years since last injection for dirty wound (perhaps still to frequent (Arch Emerg Med 1988:4)) and >10 years for clean wound
- For *dirty wounds with no primary series completion*, tetanus human immune globulin 250 U IM (J Hyg (Lond) 1978:267) with coincident vaccine administration in different area
- For *clean wounds with no primary series completion*, DPT or DT in those <7 years of age and Td in all others
- If *active tetanus*
  - Metronidazole 500 mg IV q 6 hours (J Appl Bacteriol 1968:443; Br Med J (Clin Res Ed) 1985:648)
  - Tetanus human immune globulin
  - Intubate and place on ventilator if inadequate ventilation/respiration

11 Metabolic

11.1 ACIDOSIS

Am J Med Sci 1999:38; Postgrad Med 2000:249, 253, 257, passim

Cause: Ketosis from DKA; isopropyl alcohol poisoning; lactic acidosis (Am J Med 1994:47)—ETOH (Hum Exp Toxicol 1996:482), septic shock, metformin treatment, hypotension, respiratory failure, liver failure, or short bowel *Lactobacillus* overgrowth; salicylate; acetaminophen (Ann Emerg Med 1999:452); ethylene glycol, methanol, isopropyl alcohol, paraldehyde, or toluene poisoning; severe diarrhea, D-lactate produced by gut flora, pancreatic fistulas; uremia, RTA; ileal conduit? Non-anion gap in those with asthma secondary to prolonged hypocapnia, not lactic acidosis (Crit Care Med 1987:1098)

Crs: In trauma, severity of metabolic acidosis correlates with development of acute lung injury (Crit Care Med 2000:125)

Lab: Metabolic profile, ABG (venous pH OK if low suspicion, do ABG if pH < 7.3), salicylates, acetaminophen, ketones, ETOH, measured vs. calculated osmoles, lactate level; Wood's lamp evaluation of urine to assess for ethylene glycol

ED Rx:
- Address the primary disease
- Treatment with any alkali, even sodium bicarb may paradoxically worsen the physiology (Metabolism 1966:1011) even if pH < 7.2 although helpful in "low" (normal) anion gap acidoses, especially if not associated with tissue hypoxia (Br J Anaesth 1991:165)
- Dichloroacetate no help in lactic acidosis (Am J Med 1994:47)
- TRIS buffer (Resuscitation 1998:161) no help in acidosis, even during CPR

11.2 CALCIUM DISORDERS

Emerg Med Clin North Am 1989:795

Cause:

- *Hypocalcemia* (J Clin Endocrinol Metab 1995:1473) seen in hypoparathyroidism post-thyroidectomy (Arch Surg 2000:142) seen in first 48 hours; spontaneous/sporadic (Am J Med Sci 1989:247); acquired through renal failure; pancreatitis; hypomagnesemia—seen post-thyroidectomy (World J Surg 2000:722); alcoholism—by hypomagnesemia or direct suppression of PTH; major/minor abdominal surgery (J Clin Endocrinol Metab 1999:2654); sepsis (Crit Care Med 2000:93); and consuming soft drinks with phosphoric acid, F > M (J Clin Epidemiol 1999:1007)

- *Hypercalcemia* (J Clin Endocrinol Metab 1993:1445) seen in hyperparathyroidism via renal calcitriol production; cancers (Int J Oncol 2000:197)—especially lung, breast, hepatoma; granulomatous diseases—sarcoid, talc granulomas (Chest 2000:1195), chronic TB, coccidioidomycosis; Hodgkin's lymphoma; non-Hodgkin's lymphoma; cat scratch disease; vit D intoxication—including the milk-alkali syndrome (Yale J Biol Med 1996:517); immobilization (Clin Orthop 1976:124); thyrotoxicosis; thiazides—rarely; vit A intoxication; benign familial hypocalciuric hypercalcemia—autosomal dominant; and adrenal insufficiency

Epidem: Hypoparathyroidism associated with Addison's disease, pernicious anemia, Hashimoto's thyroiditis, DiGeorge syndrome (third and fourth pharyngeal pouches)

Pathophys: For parathyroid physiology, PTH is necessary for an osteoclastic response to low calcium, renal tubular calcium resorption, renal tubular phosphate excretion, and vit D activation. Lack of parathyroid glands or PTH results in hypocalcemia and hyperphosphatemia. An ensuing alkalosis is due to blocked PTH stimulation of organic acid production in bones in hypoparathyroidism. Hypercalcemia may be due to excess PTH or PTH-like proteins—as seen in some T-cell leukemias/lymphomas, secretion of other bone-resorbing substances, tumor conversion of 25-OH vit D to 1,25-OH vit D (calcitriol), local osteolytic metastases, or other causes as seen on the list above

Sx:

- *Hypocalcemia*: circumoral paresthesias, carpopedal spasms, stridor, seizures—brief and mild, bronchospasm, GI cramps, anxiety, cataracts
- *Hypercalcemia*: fatigue, weakness, sleepiness, nausea/anorexia, constipation, polyuria/polydipsia, and volume depletion

Si:

- *Hypocalcemia*: tetany (carpopedal spasm, Chvostek's and Trousseau's signs), hyperreflexia, cataracts, ophthalmoplegia (Am J Emerg Med 1999:105), vascular corneal opacities, psychiatric changes, dystonias, and dyskinesias
- *Hypercalcemia*: confusion, delirium, drowsiness, and coma

Cmplc: Patients with hypoparathyroidism may have pustular psoriasis and dermatitis herpetiformis. Patients with hypercalcemia are at increased risk for pancreatitis and digoxin toxicity.

Lab: Metabolic profile to include calcium, albumin, magnesium and phosphate, TSH, amylase, lipase; consider ABG; EKG—special attention to QT interval (J Pediatr 2000:404; J Clin Psychopharmacol 2000:260); urine for calcium in hypocalcemia

ED Rx:

Hypocalcemia

- First: vit D_3 50,000–100,000+ U qd; or 1,25-$(OH)_2$ vit D (Rocaltrol), expensive; narrow margins of safety for hypercalcemia
- Second: Calcium po or IV; Calcium gluconate 10% 10 cc IV or calcium chloride 10% 5 cc IV—repeat PRN q 5 minutes
- Third: Chlorthalidone 50 mg po qd or other thiazide, with low-salt diet, voids renal stones of vit D treatment

Experimental use of synthetic PTH

Hypercalcemia

Acute Rx for Ca >13 mg%:

- Normal saline 2.5–4 L/24 hours IV to assure intravascular volume adequately replaced (CVP or Swann-Ganz monitoring); avoid furosemide initially, but often needed after volume replaced to prevent volume overload and accelerate renal clearance
- Pamidronate (Aredia) 60–90 mg IV over 24 hours, or 4–8 mg/hr

Chronic Rx:

- Biphosphonates, e.g., pamidronate (Aredia) 60–90 mg IV infusion over 8–24 hours or 1200 mg po qd × 5 days
- Steroids primarily for sarcoid patients, e.g., prednisone 20 mg po tid or IV 3–4 days

- Calcitonin 4 U/kg q 6 hours sc or IM, relatively weak agent alone
- Indomethacin (rarely helpful if due to cancer)
- Gallium nitrate IV infusion, experimental 200 mg/M^2 in 1-L continuous infusion qd × 5 days

11.3 MAGNESIUM DISORDERS

Emerg Med Clin North Am 1989:795; Can Med Assoc J 1985:360

Cause:
- Hypomagnesemia seen with GI fluid and electrolyte loss treated with Mg-free fluids; malnutrition; diabetes mellitus (Arch Intern Med 1996:1143); fistulae; burns; diuretics; cisplatinum-induced renal disease; cyclosporine use in transplant recipients (J Am Coll Cardiol 1992:806), and commonly associated with hypokalemia (Clin Chem 1983:178), hypophosphatemia, hyponatremia, and hypocalcemia (Arch Intern Med 1984:1794)
- Hypermagnesemia seen in renal failure often parallels potassium; chronic Mg-containing antacid and laxative use (Ann Emerg Med 1996:552). Enemas, especially in megacolon, with Mg-containing soaps

Epidem:
- Hypomagnesemia associated with large GI fluid losses and malnutrition, e.g., with ulcerative colitis, regional enteritis, chronic alcoholics, toxemia of pregnancy, primary hypo/hyperparathyroidism, primary hyperaldosteronism, thyrotoxicosis, RTA, diuretic phase of ATN
- Hypermagnesemia is much less common

Pathophys: Average daily intake of Mg is 20–40 mEq. Total body stores are 2000 mEq, half in bones, half intracellular. Low Mg inhibits PTH secretion, which in turn causes hypocalcemic signs and symptoms. ETOH also inhibits PTH secretion

Sx:
- Hypomagnesemia causes cramps
- Hypermagnesemia causes difficulty with defecation and urination; nausea; drowsiness at pharmacologic doses only

Si:
- Hypomagnesemia causes carpopedal spasm, Chvostek's sign, Trousseau's sign, delirium, muscle tremor, bizarre movements, convulsions, hypotension
- Hypermagnesemia causes depressed DTRs and hypotension

Crs: Ventricular arrhythmias can be abolished with magnesium supplementation in those with hypomagnesemia (J Intern Med 2000:78). Ataxias in hypomagnesemia take months to clear. No correlation of hypomagnesemia with degree of cardiac distress in those with chest pain (Arch Intern Med 1991:2185)

Cmplc:
- Hypomagnesemia pt may have hypocalcemia and/or hypokalemia in cisplatin type
- Hypermagnesemia may go on to heart block and respiratory paralysis, and hypocalcemia as well (N Engl J Med 1984:1221)

Lab: Metabolic profile to include magnesium, calcium, albumin, and phosphate; EKG

ED Rx:
- Hypomagnesemia requires 40–80 mEq of $MgSO_4$ (10 cc of a 50% hydrated soln, 1 g = 8 mEq) IV in 1 L D_5NS or D_5W over 3 hours
- Hypermagnesemia requires calcium gluconate 5–10 mEq (10–20 cc of 10% soln IV) (N Engl J Med 1984:1221)

11.4 PHOSPHOROUS DISORDERS

Crit Care Clin 1991:201; Endocrinol Metab Clin North Am 1993:397

Cause: Hypophosphatemia seen in sepsis (Am J Med 1998:40); malnutrition (J Pediatr 1998:789) or drugs such as aluminum-binding antacids, IV glucose, catecholamines, β-agonists, $NaHCO_3$, or acetazolamide (Ann Pharmacother 1994:626)—think COPD (Chest 1994:1392); renal tubular damage from hypokalemia; osmotic diuresis; or rarely Fanconi's anemia or hyperphosphaturia from vitamin D intoxication (Ann Intern Med 1966:1066). In types without cell injury like acute DKA, hyperalimentation, or acute respiratory alkalosis, no bad consequences occur because total body PO_4 depletion has not occurred

Hyperphosphatemia may be seen in renal failure (Clin Nephrol 1977:138), hypoparathyroidism, exogenous phosphate loading via po or enema, ketoacidosis, rhabdomyolysis, and rarer causes such as tumor lysis syndrome

Epidem: Hyperphosphatemia much more uncommon than hypophosphatemia

Pathophys: Hypophosphatemia can be classified as follows: mild is 2.3–3 mg/dL, moderate is 1.6–2.2 mg/dL, and severe is <1.5 mg/dL (Crit Care Med 1995:1504)

Sx: Hypo—confusion, weakness

Si: Both—nothing specific

Cmplc: Hypo—bleeding (impaired platelet function) and infections (impaired granulocyte function) (J Lab Clin Med 1974:643); rhabdomyolysis (Am J Med 1992:458). Hyper—complications secondary to induction of hypocalcemia (see 11.2)

Lab: Metabolic profile with phosphorous, calcium, and magnesium

ED Rx:
Hypophosphatemia: 2.5 mg elemental phosphorous/kg in NS over 12 hours via IV or po with Neutra-Phos. *Hyperphosphatemia*: Oral phosphate binders to decrease phosphate absorption in the GI tract

11.5 POTASSIUM DISORDERS

HYPOKALEMIA

J Am Soc Nephrol 1997:1179

Cause: Loop diuretics—most common; GI losses with persistent vomiting, diarrhea, or other drainage; β-agonist medications (Pediatr Emerg Care 1998:145; Pediatr Pulmonol 1999:27)— such as nebulized meds; renal tubular acidosis—Type I; hyperaldosteronism; ion shifting with $NaHCO_3$ or insulin and glucose administration IV; malnutrition; hypercalcemia; and hypomagnesemia. Rarely thyrotoxic periodic paralysis (Am J Emerg Med 1989:584), theophylline overdose (since this overdose is now more uncommon) (Am J Emerg Med 1988:214), or acute leukemia; in children IVF resuscitation (Pediatr Emerg Care 1990:13) or head trauma (J Pediatr Surg 1997:88)

Epidem: Common in those using loop diuretics

Pathophys: K^+ levels <2.5 mEq/L considered severe; <2.0 mEq/L may induce respiratory paralysis
- Paradoxical aciduria
- Nephrogenic DI with severe dehydration
- Glycosuria
- Increased ammonia production

Sx: Fatigue; nonspecific

Si: Fatigue; nonspecific

Crs: Worse with accompanying ventricular ectopy

Cmplc: Coincident digitalis (Digoxin) use necessitates higher threshold for normal, with K^+ preferably >4.0 mEq/L

Diff Dx: Bartter's syndrome; Liddle syndrome (pseudohyperaldosteronism)

Lab: Metabolic profile with Ca, Mg; EKG—low voltage, flat T-waves, widening QRS, prominent U waves. Urine K^+ levels <20 mEq/L suggest chronic etiology

ED Rx:
- Continuous monitoring
- IV KCl with no more than 40mEq/ hour, put in 250-cc IV bag
- KCl 20 mEq po if possible
- Consider coincident Mg correction with 2 g IV, especially if arrhythmias present
- Consult for admission if necessitating ongoing IV replacement, serum level severe/critical or symptomatic

HYPERKALEMIA

Semin Nephrol 1998:46

Cause: Renal failure, hemolysis, rhabdomyolysis, freshwater drownings, Addison's disease, ACE inhibitor use, NSAID use (Am J Kidney Dis 1994:578), Tm/S use especially in AIDS patients

Epidem: Unsure

Pathophys: Worsening or inability of kidneys to excrete K^+, versus overwhelming cell lysis as seen in hemolysis or freshwater drowning

Sx: Palpitations or nonspecific constitutional complaints

Si: Nonspecific

Crs: Variable

Cmplc: Lethal arrhythmias may manifest

Diff Dx: "Pseudo"-hyperkalemia due to thrombocythemia, increased white cells, fist-clenching (causing hemolysis) with blood draw, or delay in processing blood specimen

Lab: Metabolic profile; EKG shows tall peaked T waves, which may evolve to wide QRS, then evolve to sine wave as K^+ increases—do not base diagnosis on EKG findings (PPV 65% and NPV 69%) (Ann Emerg Med 1991:1229)

ED Rx:
Conn Med 1999:131
- IV access
- Calcium gluconate 10% 10 cc IV or calcium chloride 10% 5 cc IV—repeat prn q 5 minutes for cardioprotective effects
- $NaHCO_3$ 1–2 amps IV, lowering plasma H^+ will force H^+ out of cells with trade-off of K^+ going into cells
- Regular insulin 10–30 units IV, give along with amp (50 cc) of D50 if sugar is normal, low, or unknown—this will drive K^+ into cells
- Albuterol nebulizer 10–20 mg over 30 minutes
- In children, may consider Salbutamol 5 µg/kg IV D_5W over 15 minutes (Clin Nephrol 1996:67), may give nebulized if IV access a problem
- K^+-resin binder po such as Kayexalate, may give along with sorbitol
- Consider dialysis or hemofiltration (Child Nephrol Urol 1988:236)

11.6 SODIUM DISORDERS

Emerg Med Clin North Am 1989:749; Clin Lab Med 1993:135; Pediatr Ann 1995:23

HYPONATREMIA

Am J Emerg Med 2000:264

Cause:
- Elevated antidiuretic hormone (ADH) from (1) SIADH or tumor; (2) drugs such as vincristine, Cytoxan, clofibrate, narcotics, nicotine, isoproterenol, or tricyclic antidepressants; or (3) hypovolemia

- Increased renal ADH sensitivity due to (1) first- but not second-generation hypoglycemics; (2) NSAIDs; (3) thiazides; or (4) carbamazepine
- Lab error (pseudohyponatremia) due to elevated triglycerides, proteins, glucose, mannitol, or post-TURP glycine
- Free water replacement of isotonic emesis, diarrhea, blood, serum; or seen as idiopathic cause postoperatively
- Dehydration in extreme athletes (Clin J Sport Med 2000:52) or prolonged heat exposure with exertion (Am J Emerg Med 1999:532)
- Hypothyroidism, Addison's disease
- Psychiatric patients with polydipsia, SIADH, and decreased renal free water excretion
- Alcoholics, especially if only nutrition is ETOH (Ann Emerg Med 1986:745)
- Postop for 1–3 days, equal sex ratio, 1% incidence; caused by high ADH levels and hypotonic or sometimes even isotonic IV fluids, but respiratory arrest and mortality much higher in menstruating women

Epidem: Females > males

Pathophys: Free water replacement/conservation without regard for sodium

Sx: Confusion

Si: Altered mental status; seizures (especially infants <6 months of age (Ann Emerg Med 1995:42))

Crs: Variable based on cause—morbidity/mortality usually based on underlying cause, with hyponatremia usually a poor prognostic sign

Cmplc: Mortality increased 60 × in hospitalized patients when Na <130

Lab: CBC with diff; metabolic profile with Na < 125; uric acid <5 mg% with ADH-producing tumor or SIADH: if fever, pursue ID eval with blood cultures, urine culture, and consider LP and CXR

ED Rx:

Acutely

- Stop drugs
- IV NS and furosemide—if developed slowly, correct at <2.5 mEq/hr, not >10 mEq/day vs. not >20 mEq/day with iso- or perhaps hypertonic saline (3% NaCl), and possibly IV furosemide, then go slowly to avoid pontine demyelination; or go slowly over days, no

benefit from rushing or using twice normal saline even when Na$^+$ <110 unless symptomatic or very acute (Am J Med 1985:897)
- Consider dialysis with hypertonic solution and intraperitoneal site as first choice

For Chronic Cases
- Restrict water and give liberal salt diet or tablets
- Consider salt tablets plus loop diuretic
- Consider demeclocycline (Declomycin, a tetracycline) 0.6–1.2 g/day
- Consider lithium 300 mg po tid or qid
- Possible future use of vasopressin antagonist

HYPERNATREMIA

Endocrinol Metab Clin North Am 1993:411
Cause:
- Central and nephrogenic diabetes insipidus (DI)—see 4.3
- Dehydration from inability to drink, Betadine Rx of burns, or diminished urine concentration and diminished thirst in elderly esp. in the setting of adult onset diabetes mellitus—this may lead to a nonketotic hyperosmolar state

Epidem: Pregnancy may unmask DI
Pathophys: See 4.3 for DI; dehydration as per etiology
Sx: Excessive thirst and urination; confusion
Si: Altered mental status; hypotension; dehydration
Crs: Infantile dehydration may lead to mental retardation
Cmplc: Mortality >40% in elderly; infantile
Diff Dx: Psychogenic water drinker who can partially concentrate urine with fluid restriction
Lab: CBC with diff; metabolic profile; serum osmoles; U/A; urine osmoles—look for Na >150
ED Rx:
- Acutely replace water but not >12 mEq/24 h secondary to cerebral edema
- Calculate water deficit and treatment for DI (see 4.3)

12 Nephrology

12.1 ACUTE RENAL FAILURE

Am Fam Physician 2000:2077

Cause:

- *Prerenal*: hypovolemia, anemia
- *Renal*: drug toxicity (e.g., NSAIDs (Am J Epidemiol 2000:488)—even topical (Bmj 2000:93)); acute tubular necrosis (ATN)—as seen in shock, crush injuries, hypothermia, heavy metal toxicity, snake venom toxicity, organic solvent toxicity, intravascular hemolysis; rhabdomyolysis from drug abuse, such as ETOH, IV heroin, and more recently IV temazepam (Qjm 2000:29); IV dye reaction in those with underlying renal insufficiency; multiple myeloma (Nephron 2000:96); HIV with many etiologies such as interstitial nephritis (Am J Kidney Dis 2000:557)
- *Postrenal*: obstruction

Epidem: Community-acquired is much more common (3×) in the black population compared to whites (Arch Intern Med 2000:1309), with possibly higher mortality rates

Pathophys: Many physiologic effects from cellular death and ATP depletion, many competing theories of most significant mechanism (Semin Nephrol 2000:4). Ensuing acidosis, Ca/P imbalances, hyperkalemia, anemia, hypertension, peripheral and autonomic neuropathy from PTH, delayed hypersensitivity immune suppression, pruritus probably from histamine

- Uremia may lead to sallow skin, pericardial effusion

Sx: Lassitude, pruritus, nausea/vomiting, anorexia, muscle cramps, sleep disturbance

Si: Uremic breath, increased pigmentation, postural hypotension or hypotension, absent tendon reflexes and other peripheral neuropathies—reversible

Crs: Variable, even straightforward causes (e.g., hypovolemia) may progress to a chronic process; poorer prognosis with increased age, recent MI, CHF, requiring respiratory support, or liver dysfunction (Clin Nephrol 2000:10)

Cmplc: Chronic renal failure; secondary infection (Nephrol Dial Transplant 2000:212)

Lab: CBC with diff; metabolic profile including Ca, Mg, Phos; U/A; urine culture; venous pH/ABG; type and screen; EKG. X-ray: renal U/S

ED Rx:
- Hold all potentially offending drugs
- Consider IV fluid bolus for hypovolemia (Drugs 2000:79), correction of anemia
- Place indwelling catheter
- Treat underlying arrhythmias/hyperkalemia as warranted
- Thyroxine of no help in euthyroid patients (Kidney Int 2000:293)
- Dialysis to prevent complications and death (Kidney Int 1972:190)

12.2 DIALYSIS PATIENT ISSUES

J Emerg Med 1992:317

Cause: Patients receiving either peritoneal dialysis or hemodialysis have a time-intensive commitment, but those with hemodialysis have less flexibility and more side effects

Pathophys: Continuous ambulatory peritoneal dialysis (CAPD) with similar biochemical results as hemodialysis (HD) (Arch Intern Med 1986:1138)

Adverse effects: Similar in the two types of dialysis patients
- Folate deficiency (Br Med J 1969:18)
- EKG artifacts from fistula/cannula arm
- Pericarditis (Am J Med 1977:874)
- Pneumonia, atelectasis, and pleural effusion from CAPD (Lancet 1966:75)
- Mortality = 10–20%/year, 5% per year from peritonitis in those with CAPD (Perit Dial Int 1997:S15)
- Zn deficiency (Am J Clin Pathol 1971:17) causes primary gonadal impairment, reversible with 2.5 mg po qd
- Amyloidosis (Kidney Int Suppl 1993:S78)

- Rare antacid Mg intoxication
- Rare Cu intoxication from tubing (N Engl J Med 1967:1209)
- Fe deficiency
- Increased ASHD (Lancet 1980:276)
- Gynecomastia (Plast Reconstr Surg 1982:41)
- Hepatitis C (Nephron 1993:40)
- $CaPO_4$ deposits in joints (Contrib Nephrol 1984:58)
- Catheter displacement in those with CAPD (Clin Nephrol 1999:124)
- CVA (Stroke 1974:725)
- Secondary hyperparathyroidism with change in bony structure (Kidney Int Suppl 1993:S116)
- Bleeding complications, secondary to platelet dysfunction and perhaps exacerbated by heparin use in those with hemodialysis (J Am Soc Nephrol 1991:961)
- Infection at central catheter or shunt site in hemodialysis; tunnel infection and peritonitis in peritoneal dialysis (Arch Surg 1984:1325)
- Scrotal swelling if patent processus vaginalis in those receiving peritoneal dialysis (Br J Surg 1984:477)

12.3 RENAL CALCULI

Emerg Med Clin North Am 1988:617

Cause: Calcium oxalate (75%), from hyperparathyroidism (~10%) but probably most idiopathic hypercalciuria—rarely sarcoid—which is genetic in most cases with autosomal dominant inheritance; struvite (10–15%), from UTIs with urease-producing organisms; urate (5%); hydroxyapatite or brushite (5%); cystine (1%). Protease inhibitor (indinavir) stones possible (Urology 1997:508), these are radiolucent

Epidem: Incidence = 100/100,000 men, 36/100,000 women; 3–5% of U.S. population will get sometime in life; incidence higher in Southeast U.S. Increased risk with vasectomy (Am J Kidney Dis 1997:207) and associated with medullary sponge kidney (Clin Radiol 1982:435)

Pathophys: 80% of stones are calcium type, associated with a red blood cell and probable renal tubular oxalate excretion defect or a deficit of the Ca/Mg pump; another 10% are associated with hyperparathyroidism

- Increased calcium absorption may also play a role, either primary or by bringing out deficits like those above, e.g., in sarcoid. Uric acid stones may also precipitate calcium on themselves
- Calcium oxalate stones are increased in colectomy, blind loop syndrome, and intestinal bypass patients due to bacterial breakdown of bile salts leading to absorption of glycolytic acid
- Struvite stones are caused by ammonia from urea-splitting *Proteus* in patients with chronic UTIs due to indwelling Foley and/or quadriplegia

Sx: Pain radiating into groin; urine may appear normal, tea-colored, or bloody

Si: CVA tenderness; usually nontender abdomen despite severe pain

Crs: Recurrence after first stone is 15% at 1 year, 35% at 5 years, 50% at 10 years

Cmplc: Secondary infection; renal failure

Diff Dx: AAA in elderly patient, which may also have laboratory evidence of microscopic hematuria secondary to dissection into renal arteries; renal artery embolism pain; rarely primary hyperoxaluria with oxalosis as renal failure develops

Lab: Hematuria; BUN/Cr; consider CBC with diff and urine culture if febrile or other concerns for complicated UTI; stone analysis. IVP if young patient and diagnosis not certain, and in elderly—renal U/S if renal failure concerns; CT without contrast better than IVP in some centers (Urol Radiol 1992:139; Radiology 1998:308)

ED Rx:

- Pain control, usually requires IV access with narcotic/antiemetic
- Consider IV NSAID, such as ketorolac (Toradol) 30 mg; IV or IM administration with possible benefit for acute pain relief (Br J Urol 1990:602; Am J Emerg Med 1999:6)
- Consult for admission if secondary infection or pain control issues

Outpatient Regimen

- Pain control with po NSAID (all equivalent) and po narcotic; consider po or pr antiemetic for pain control synergism with narcotic and to better tolerate narcotic
- Primary care follow-up, urology if high-grade obstruction
- Strain all urine
- Increase po fluid intake—caffeine and ETOH do help; reduce salt and protein intake; avoid phosphoric acid–containing soft drinks

- Avoid calcium supplements but further restriction not helpful because calcium decreases oxalate and urate absorption
- Drug regimens: depending on 24-hour urine, metabolic evaluation, or stone type in peds (Pediatr Nephrol 1992:54) and adults (J Urol 1989:760); thiazide diuretics, allopurinol, Polycitra K, sodium cellulose phosphate, acetohydroxamic acid, pyridoxine, or cholestyramine may be prescribed
- Potential benefit of modest ETOH (beer) intake, low-fat diet, or weight reduction to reduce risk of nephrolithiasis (Am J Kidney Dis 1996:195)
- Cystoscopic stone retrieval, lithotripsy, or surgical removal may be required for stones causing persistent problems

12.4 URINARY RETENTION

Emerg Med Clin North Am 1988:419; Pediatr Emerg Care 1993:205

Cause: Medications (sympathomimetic agonist); voiding avoidance such as a long car trip in someone with borderline obstruction; mechanical obstruction due to mass or stricture such as seen in prostatic hypertrophy, bladder carcinoma, or urolithiasis; blocked indwelling catheter; postoperative due to catecholamine release or perhaps due to spinal/epidural anesthesia; infection; systemic disease such as hypothyroidism; or neurologic etiologies such as trauma, spina bifida, or multiple sclerosis

Epidem: ~5% in postop surgical patients, >50% in those with genitourinary surgery; suggested that males have a higher incidence coincident with the lunar cycle (on the new moon) (Bmj 1989:1560)

Pathophys: As above, either inability to pass urine around a fixed lesion, or due to inability to control bladder neck muscles

Sx: Lower abdominal pain

Si: Palpable bladder; assess for obvious mechanical problem such as stenotic urethral opening or imperforate hymen (J Accid Emerg Med 1999:232); overflow incontinence

Crs: Drainage is therapeutic and diagnostic

Cmplc: Postobstructive diuresis; secondary infection (if frank pus, pyocystis)

Diff Dx: Rarely due to acute abdominal processes such as ectopic pregnancy (Am J Emerg Med 1999:44) or appendiceal abscess (Ann Emerg Med 1993:857), pathophysiology uncertain

Lab: Urine for culture if infection suspected

ED Rx:

- Access with 16F Foley; coudé catheter if necessary. Diagnosis made with residual >500 cc
- If cannot access, filiforms and followers or urologic consult
- If postoperative or secondary to chronic process requiring intermittent catheterization, OK to remove catheter after drainage if urine clears with irrigation
- IV access with narcotic analgesic if pain uncontrollable and cannot quickly access bladder
- If new acute problem, chronic disease with new manifestation, or urine not clearing with irrigation, leave catheter in place and leg bag for home. Urology follow-up in 2–3 days if not sooner
- Consider antibiotics if secondary infection suspected
- Urologic consult for admission if continuous irrigation necessary secondary to pyocystis or recurrent catheter obstruction secondary to blood clots
- Also consider admission if symptomatic postobstructive diuresis (Br J Urol 1989:559)—profuse passage of urine, hypotension, dizziness, or tachycardia

12.5 URINARY TRACT INFECTION

Emerg Med Clin North Am 1988:403; Infect Dis Clin North Am 1997:551; Pediatr Clin North Am 1999:1111, vi

Cause: Infectious cystitis/urethritis in females due to coliforms 70% of the time, with other pathogens such as *Staphylococcus saprophyticus*, *Proteus*, or STDs such as *Chlamydia trachomatis*, gonorrhea, or herpes simplex

Epidem: Incidence ~20% of all women each year, increased with catheters, sexual activity (Epidemiology 1995:162), cervical cap or diaphragm use, and previous UTI (Am J Epidemiol 1986:977; N Engl J Med 1996:468). Not prevented by various hygiene habits except voiding after sex. Unknown rate in children <2 years of age but suspect it is common among females, especially in those with

fever without origin, and URI and OM do not exclude this
diagnosis (Pediatrics 1998:e16)

Nosocomial risks include catheter, diabetes mellitus, coincident
infection, not free draining catheter, and renal insufficiency
(Am J Epidemiol 1986:977)

Recurrence within 6 months associated with initial *Escherichia coli*
infection (Am J Epidemiol 2000:1194)

Pathophys: Most likely ascending disease; thus women are more prone
secondary to short urethra. Recurrent disease, due to a possible
inherent defect in epithelial cell membrane leading to easier
adherence by bacteria

Sx: Dysuria, urgency, frequency; stuttering onset over many days
with *Chlamydia*; cystitis with internal pain (Arch Intern Med
1978:1069) or pain at end of urination

Si: Pain superior to symphysis pubis with cystitis

Crs: Many resolve without Rx; catheter-induced UTIs have 2–4 times
the mortality of non-catheter-induced UTIs and only 1/3 resolve
after removal without Rx, and 90% will resolve with single dose
or 10-day Rx

Cmplc:

• Pyelonephritis: possibly secondary to ascending infection, may also
be due to hematogenous seeding. Increased incidence in neonates,
infants up to 18 months, females of childbearing age, and those s/p
GU instrumentation. Increased cases in papillary necrosis as seen in
sickle cell disease and diabetes. Look for fever, flank pain, and CVA
tenderness

• Evaluate for reflux in children with first case with renal U/S and
VCUG—outpt w/u (AJR Am J Roentgenol 1994:1393)

• Emphysematous cystitis, seen usually in those with diabetes mellitus

Diff Dx: Urolithiasis; vaginitis (Pediatrics 1982:299), herpes, and
chronic interstitial (idiopathic) cystitis (Curr Opin Obstet Gynecol
1990:605)

Lab:

• U/A—dipstick nitrite with high false positive; although nitrite
and leukocyte esterase are sensitive if we think the patient has the
disease and they are positive, otherwise less reliable (Ann Intern
Med 1992:135); rapid urine catalase test (Uriscreen) with 100%
sensitivity and thus, high negative predictive value and could be
used to predict those who do not have UTI (Pediatrics 1999:e41);
number of WBCs/hpf only useful depending on pretest probability

—symptomatic and >5–6 WBCs/hpf as threshold with10% false
negative and 50% false positive; urine Gram's stain of unspun urine
highly predictive of UTI (Ann Emerg Med 1995:31; J Clin
Microbiol 1982:468); hematuria may be present

- Urine culture if neonate, infant (Pediatrics 1998:E1), child, or those
with potentially complicated UTI (this includes pregnancy)—10^5
organisms only in 50% of infected women, 10^2 better criterion
when symptomatic. Consider CBC with diff and blood cultures
if considering pyelonephritis. Need catheter urine in children
<2 years of age, and first drops of specimen should be discarded
(Pediatr Emerg Care 2000:88)
- IVP and cystoscopy of no value to work-up of recurrent UTIs in
adult women

ED Rx:

Uncomplicated UTI

- Sulfisoxazole 500 mg po qid, Tm/S single or double strength bid,
ciprofloxacin 100 mg po bid, ofloxacin 200 mg po bid (Am J Med
1999:292), or amoxicillin 250–500 mg po tid for 3–5 days; but
consider 5–7 day Rx with nitrofurantoin (Macrobid) 1 pill bid
(J Antimicrob Chemother 1999:67)
- Single-dose regimens (Ann Emerg Med 1984:432): Tm/S DS 1–2
pills (Rev Infect Dis 1982:444), amoxicillin 2–3 g po, sulfisoxazole
1–2 g po, or ciprofloxacin 500 mg po—more frequent recurrence
- Phenazopyridine (Pyridium) 200 mg po tid × 2 days prn for
pain, turns urine dark orange and prolonged use may lead to
methemoglobinemia (Acta Urol Belg 1967:465)
- Encourage fluids, specifically cranberry juice (Epidemiology
1995:162)—complexes with *E. coli* so that bacteria do not "stick"
to bladder epithelium
- Asymptomatic bacteriuria is not an indication for treatment (J Am
Geriatr Soc 1996:293), and is generally not improved with Rx
- Infants should be treated if any suspicion, and have treatment and
follow-up based on urine culture

Catheter-Related

- Remove catheter if possible, Rx if symptomatic—will not clear UTI
with persistent indwelling catheterization

Prophylaxis

- Postmenopausal women may benefit from estriol 0.5 mg cream
(Ovestin) qd × 2 weeks then biweekly if no contraindications

- Tm/S 1/2 single-strength pill qd hs or postcoital is cost effective if ≥3 UTIs/year

Complicated UTI (Includes UTI in Pregnancy)
- Consider first dose of antibiotics IV/IM, such as ceftriaxone 1–2 g IV; oral ciprofloxacin 500 mg po as expedient as IV medication, and effective (Cmaj 1994:669). Cefazolin 1–2 g IV and ampicillin 1 g IV safe in pregnancy
- Control pain, vomiting, and dehydration issues
- If outpt, 2-week course of treatment with Bactrim DS bid or ciprofloxacin 250–500 mg po bid; if allergic to the former, use amoxicillin 500 mg po tid or cephalexin (Keflex) 500 mg tid for 10–14 days
- Pregnancy (Ann Pharmacother 1994:248): simple bacteriuria with single dose amoxicillin or cephalexin; symptomatic UTI with 3 days of amoxicillin or cephalexin at above doses; upper tract infection with 10–14 days of amoxicillin or cephalexin. All with repeat culture 1 week after finishing therapy
- If septic or cannot control secondary symptoms (such as vomiting), consult for admission

NEPHROLOGY

13 Neurology/ Neurosurgery

13.1 ACUTE SEROTONIN SYNDROME

J Psychopharmacol 1999:100

Cause: MAO inhibitors (*Hypericum perforatum*, aka St. John's wort, is a weak MAO inhibitor), SSRIs (selective serotonin reuptake inhibitors), and nonselective 5-HT receptor agonist/antagonist, specifically *meta*-chlorophenylpiperazine (*m*-CPP) (Psychiatry Res 1998:207), as leading causes, with increased likelihood when combined with meperidine (Acad Emerg Med 1999:156), dextromethorphan, venlafaxine (Neurology 1998:274), bromocriptine, levodopa, buspirone, lithium, cocaine, amphetamines, ecstacy (Ann Emerg Med 1998:377), tramadol (J R Soc Med 1999:474), or other serotonergic drugs (Med J Aust 1998:523). Equivocal data for combination with sumatriptan (Ann Pharmacother 1998:33)

Epidem: Not uncommon, with symptoms occurring within hours or days when increasing the dose of or adding a serotonergic drug

Pathophys: Increased activity at the postsynaptic serotonin receptors in the brain (Pediatr Emerg Care 1999:440)

Sx: Agitation, anxiety, shakiness, nausea

Si: Mental status changes; tremors; seizures; autonomic instability with tachycardia or dysrhythmias, hyperthermia, hypertension, diarrhea, salivation, rigidity, dysarthria, ataxia, myoclonus, or localized neuro signs or deficits

Crs: Most recover within 24 hours; this may be a difficult diagnosis when confounded with drugs of abuse—have a high index of suspicion

Cmplc: Rhabdomyolysis with subsequent myoglobinuria; fatalities rare but possible

Diff Dx: NMS, drug abuse or withdrawal, malignant hyperthermia, meningitis, encephalitis, heat stroke, MAO inhibitor interactions, acute lethal catatonia, central anticholinergic crisis that responds to IV physostigmine, thyroid storm

Lab: Clinical diagnosis when other etiologies excluded—CBC with diff; metabolic profile with Ca and Mg; U/A with myoglobin; CPK; aldolase; panculture if suspect infectious etiology; TSH if suspect endocrine source; consider LP. X-ray: head CT or MRI if suspect bleed, focal deficit, or other CNS concerns

ED Rx:
- Hold all meds, especially serotonergic agonists—listed above, also avoid codeine
- Supportive care, and IV fluids, mannitol, IV NaHCO$_3$ if rhabdomyolysis
- Consider serotonin antagonists such as cyproheptadine 0.5 mg/kg/day divided into q 4–6-hour dosing at a maximum dose of 32 mg/day—usually 4–8 mg po q dose (Pediatr Emerg Care 1999:325; J Emerg Med 1998:615); methysergide; and propranolol
- Benzodiazepines may be used to lessen discomfort—nonselective serotonin antagonists

13.2 ACUTE STROKE SYNDROME

Am J Epidemiol 1999:1266; Stroke 1996:1711; Ann Emerg Med 1999:244

Cause: Cerebrovascular accident (CVA) classified according to 3 groups, and all types associated with hypertension and smoking (Jama 1999:1112):
- Thrombotic CVA due to atherosclerosis (Cerebrovasc Dis 2000:102); hypotension—this may be transient and physiologic as seen in sleep; homocystinuria; crack cocaine abuse; migraine; high-dose estrogen birth control pills; arteritis caused by radiation, collagen vascular diseases (Lupus 1997:420; Arthritis Rheum 1998:1497), drug use, including ETOH in males (Alcohol 1999:119); infection leading to venous thrombosis or carotid occlusion; trauma to carotid or head that may cause

spasm—associated with history of migraines; hematologic causes such as polycythemia, sickle cell disease (Blood 1998:288), TTP, DIC, or dysproteinemias. Associated with anabolic steroids (Neurology 1994:2405) and immediate postpartum period

- Embolic CVA due to proximal arterial atherosclerotic plaque; left-sided cardiac lesion as seen in SBE, left atrial myxoma, or clot (mitral stenosis or mitral valve billowing, prosthetic valve, sustained or intermittent atrial fibrillation (J Am Coll Cardiol 2000:183), post-MI mural thrombus); paradoxical embolus from right heart, fat emboli, or venous system if patent intracardiac (foramen ovale—40% of pts <55 years of age with CVA have this open) right-to-left shunt. Associated with homocystinuria

- Hemorrhagic CVA is further subdivided into intraparenchymal vs. subarachnoid. *Subarachnoid* CVAs due to aneurysm or AV malformation; associated with ETOH use in females (Alcohol 1999:119). *Intraparenchymal* CVAs are 50% due to HTN, 17% from amyloid angiopathy, 10% from anticoagulation Rx, 5–10% from brain tumors, 5% from smoking, 5% from crack cocaine use

Epidem:

- Thrombotic CVAs comprise 34% of all CVAs in large vessel type, and 19% of all CVAs in lacunar CVAs; 3% are patients <40 years of age

- Embolic CVAs comprise 31% of all CVAs, with 5× increased incidence in atherosclerotic Afib, and 17× increase in rheumatic Afib. 35% lifetime increased incidence in Afib, 3/4 are embolic

- Subarachnoid hemorrhages comprise 7% of all CVAs and 1% of all adults have aneurysm. 2% of all with subarachnoid bleed and aneurysm have polycystic kidneys; associated with IV cocaine use; sometimes familial; sometimes with Ehlers-Danlos syndrome, Marfan syndrome, and Type I neurofibromatosis

- Intraparenchymal bleeds comprise 9% of all CVAs

- Black Americans with 2× risk for intracerebral hemorrhage compared to whites (Neurology 1999:1617)

- Possible Southeastern U.S. stroke belt (Am J Med Sci 1999:160)

- Increased risk with either surgery or radiotherapy of pituitary adenoma (Int J Radiat Oncol Biol Phys 1999:693)

- Livedo reticularis may be noted on physical exam in those with CVA who have antiphospholipid syndrome (Sneddon's syndrome) (J Eur Acad Dermatol Venereol 1999:157)

Pathophys: Thrombotic CVAs usually affect a watershed area in anterior circulation or vertebral basilar syndrome. Hypertension is a marker for stroke risk, but CVAs in these patients is a multifactorial issue, genetically determined (Cardiologia 1999:433). Hyperglycemia linked to delay in calcium recovery in ischemic stroke (J Cereb Blood Flow Metab 1992:469), and degree of hyperglycemia linked to size of infarct (Schweiz Arch Neurol Psychiatr 1993:233) and worse outcome (Stroke 1993:1129). Increase in superoxide dismutase (Life Sci 1994:711) in ischemic stroke, perhaps secondary to oxygen radicals causing problems

Sx:
- *Thrombotic*: TIA history in 80%; nocturnal onset in 60%
- *Embolic*: very abrupt onset; seizures occasionally
- *Subarachnoid bleed*: severe headache of sudden onset which is frequently preceded by milder sentinel headache, nausea, vomiting, possible loss of consciousness, possible neck and back pain
- *Intraparenchymal bleed*: cerebellar with ataxia, headache, vomiting, nausea; cerebral with decreased level of consciousness, sudden onset, headache, nausea, vomiting

Si: Lateralized neurologic findings
- *Carotid occlusion* or significant stenosis may be elucidated with flow reversal through the supraorbital artery which one feels, and then occludes the facial artery as it wraps anterior to the inferior border of the mandible just anterior to the angle of the jaw—if lose pulse, then flow is reversed
- *Thrombotic and embolic* with specific occlusion patterns:
  1) Middle cerebral: face and arm motor; expressive aphasia (Broca's)
  2) Carotid watershed: parietal aphasias, weakness arm > face > leg
  3) Posterior cerebral: homonymous hemianopsia, hemisensory loss, memory loss
  4) Lateral medullary plate syndrome—posterior inferior cerebellar artery: ipsilateral pain and temperature loss on face, contralateral for rest of body, hoarseness, swallowing dysfunction, Horner's, singultus (hiccups/hiccoughs), ipsilateral cerebellar signs
- *Subarachnoid bleed*: hypertension, stiff neck, Parinaud's sign— upward gaze paralysis; subhyaloid retinal hemorrhage
- *Intraparenchymal bleed*
  1) Cerebellar: awake, alert even with ophthalmoplegias; acute hypotonia; conjugate gaze paresis, skew deviation

NEUROLOGY/NEUROSURGERY

2) Cerebral: motor and always sensory deficits; 13% have seizure within 48 hours

3) Brain stem: early loss of consciousness; brain stem signs including involvement of cranial nerves V, VII, VIII, IX, X, XI, XII; quadriplegia

Crs: Nonhemorrhagic CVAs with 15% 30-day mortality; hemorrhagic CVAs with worse prognosis if large bleed in putamen or thalamus with hypertension, whereas subcortical, cerebellar, and pontine bleeds without correlation to blood pressure (Stroke 1997:1185)

Cmplc: Pulmonary emboli, aspiration pneumonia, UTIs, poststroke depression, possible conversion of nonhemorrhagic CVA to hemorrhagic CVA

Diff Dx:
- Transient ischemic attack (TIA)—CVA symptoms that last less than 24 hours, with anterior circulation symptoms including amaurosis fugax; and posterior circulation symptoms including bilateral blindness, diplopia, and quadriplegia. Carotid bruit correlates poorly with symptomatic disease. Risk of subsequent CVA is 8% in first month, 5% per year for 3 years, 3% per year thereafter; 41% will die of MI
- Reversible ischemic neurologic deficit (RIND)—lasts longer than 24 hours but less than 72 hours
- Migraine headache
- Benign vertigo
- Tumor
- Carotid artery dissection
- Vertebral artery dissection
- Segmental mediolytic arteriopathy in young patients with CVA (Cardiovasc Surg 1994:350)

Lab:
- CBC with diff; PT/PTT; metabolic profile including immediate glucoscan; EKG—cardiac markers if abnormal
- X-ray: Consider CXR; head CT without contrast—contrast given if lesion noted except bleed because may elect to do angiography if bleed noted. CT ability and readings moving towards delineating area and size of ischemia to correlate thrombotic vs. embolic—still being developed (Stroke 1992:1748). MRI will determine ischemic CVAs within hours whereas CT will show in days. MRI or MRA for AVM evaluation

- U/S: consider emergent carotid studies or echocardiogram if embolic source entertained. Leg studies if paradoxical embolus suspected
- LP: do LP if high suspicion for subarachnoid bleed, CT will miss up to 3–10% of these (Acad Emerg Med 1996:16; Ann Emerg Med 1998:297)

ED Rx:

- Stabilize airway
- Control/resuscitate blood pressure (Stroke 1998:1504); this is controversial and a "double-edged sword"—if hypertensive, get systolic BP around 180 mm Hg since the hypertensive response is to maintain flow to the brain, which may be experiencing local edema, but even relative hypotension may decrease cerebral perfusion; if hypotensive, get systolic BP >110 mm Hg to maintain flow to brain
- IV meds for pain/nausea/vomiting

Nonhemorrhagic CVAs

Drugs Aging 1999:11

Consider ASA, heparin, and thrombolytics

- 4 baby ASA chew and swallow (Stroke 2000:1240)
- Unfractionated heparin IV with weight-based protocol or low molecular weight heparin (LMWH) sc, no help for CVA in progress but perhaps help in 6-month survival—*when* to anticoagulate is the difficult decision—pro (Cochrane Database Syst Rev 2000) and con (Cochrane Database Syst Rev 2000). With Afib, controversy of ASA vs. LMWH (Lancet 2000:1205)
- Limit blood draws/procedures if possible if considering thrombolytics (N Engl J Med 1995:1581). Complete HIHSS stroke scale (Stroke 1999:2347) (See Table 13.1)
- The decision to perform thrombolysis should be made within 3 hours of symptom onset, BP <185/110 with minimal pharmacologic help, no mild or dense deficits, and moderate deficits should not be improving. Should have no recent major surgery or dental work within 2 weeks, no recent trauma, no GI bleed, and no history of cancer. Relative contraindications are those associated with embolic phenomenon such as Afib, carotid stenosis, prosthetic valve, DVT with suspected patent foramen ovale, etc. Use TPA, not other agents—TPA 0.9 mg/kg given as a 10% bolus, and 90% over next 60 minutes, ~6% chance of bleed into CVA (Stroke 1997:2109)
- Equivocal data of glucose-insulin-potassium (GIK) for those with mild to moderate hyperglycemia (Stroke 1999:793)

Table 13.1. Current Form of the NIHSS (Stroke 1993;30:2349)

Item	Name	Response
1a	Level of consciousness	0 = Alert 1 = Not alert, arousable 2 = Not alert, obtunded 3 = Unresponsive
1b	Questions	0 = Answers both correctly 1 = Answers one correctly 2 = Answers neither correctly
1c	Commands	0 = Performs both tasks correctly 1 = Performs one task correctly 2 = Performs neither task
2	Gaze	0 = Normal 1 = Partial gaze palsy 2 = Total gaze palsy
3	Visual fields	0 = No visual loss 1 = Partial hemianopsia 2 = Complete hemianopsia 3 = Bilateral hemianopsia
4	Facial palsy	0 = Normal 1 = Minor paralysis 2 = Partial paralysis 3 = Complete paralysis
5a	Left motor arm	0 = No drift 1 = Drift before 10 seconds 2 = Falls before 10 seconds 3 = No effort against gravity 4 = No movement
5b	Right motor arm	0 = No drift 1 = Drift before 10 seconds 2 = Falls before 10 seconds 3 = No effort against gravity 4 = No movement
6a	Left motor leg	0 = No drift 1 = Drift before 5 seconds 2 = Falls before 5 seconds 3 = No effort against gravity 4 = No movement
6b	Right motor leg	0 = No drift 1 = Drift before 5 seconds 2 = Falls before 5 seconds 3 = No effort against gravity 4 = No movement

Table 13.1. (*cont'd*)

Item	Name	Response
7	Ataxia	0 = Absent 1 = One limb 2 = Two limbs
8	Sensory	0 = Normal 1 = Mild loss 2 = Severe loss
9	Language	0 = Normal 1 = Mild aphasia 2 = Severe aphasia 3 = Mute or global aphasia
10	Dysarthria	0 = Normal 1 = Mild 2 = Severe
11	Extinction/inattention	0 = Normal 1 = Mild 2 = Severe

- Permissive hypothermia is currently investigational (J Neurosurg 2000:91)
- Consult primary physician/neuro

Hemorrhagic CVAs

- Consult neurosurgery
- Control of systemic hypertension does not influence cerebral flow unless pt made hypotensive (Crit Care Med 1999:965), but better blood pressure control with better morbidity and mortality outcomes (Stroke 1995:21). Consider use of nitroprusside, clonidine, labetalol, or ACE inhibitors
- Consider nimodipine 60 mg po q 4 hours × 21 days—prevents arterial spasm
- Hypertonic saline as effective as mannitol, and neither influences cerebral blood flow (Neurosurgery 1999:1055, discussion, 1063)
- EACA (ε-aminocaproic acid) equivocal, but may reverse TPA
- Dexamethasone no help
- Hemodilution to hematocrit of 32% with colloid after phlebotomy helps limit damage in spasm?

13.3 BELL'S PALSY

Cause: Controversial and many proposed etiologies—idiopathic seventh cranial nerve palsy is prototypical Bell's palsy; diagnosis of exclusion after considering differential diagnosis

Epidem: Possibly increased in diabetics, or possibly due to diabetic nerve infarcts. Seen in all ages with congenital in children (J Otolaryngol 1997:80), sarcoid as most common cause of seventh cranial nerve palsy in young adults (Sarcoidosis Vasc Diffuse Lung Dis 1997:115), and a myriad of etiologies with increasing age

Pathophys: Peripheral cranial nerve VII dysfunction with drooling and inability to completely close eye as possible consequences

Sx: Facial weakness; pain; increased noise sensitivity from lack of stapedial muscle tone

Si: Cranial nerve VII weakness sparing the forehead since nerve fibers cross from the contralateral side; absence of taste on the anterior 2/3 of the tongue if lesion proximal to chorda tympani

Crs: 90% recover completely. If residual motion on affected side, patient always recovers

Cmplc: Corneal ulceration—Rx is to tape lid; errors in nerve regeneration—1) jaw wrinkling; 2) orbicularis oculi with ori, and vice versa; and 3) parasympathetic nerve problem with eye tearing when good food tasted, aka crocodile tears

Diff Dx:
Otolaryngol Clin North Am 1991:613
Herpes zoster (Ramsay-Hunt syndrome)—only 50% recover; EB virus; sarcoid; Lyme disease; tumor; basilar skull fracture; otitis media; birth; syphilis; HIV, but most likely multiple cranial nerve palsies

Lab: EMG at 2 weeks if still fibrillation; MRI in 6 weeks if not resolving

ED Rx:
- Protect eyes with Lacrilube gtts and taping—especially HS
- Consider prednisone 60 mg taper over 10 days, data equivocal (Pediatr Neurol 1999:814). Perhaps high-dose steroids in those with complete paralysis (J Accid Emerg Med 1999:445)
- Consider acyclovir, pro (Ann Otol Rhinol Laryngol 1996:371) and con (J Neurol Sci 1999:19)

- Surgery initially no help, consider surgery if EMG flat at 2 weeks, if persistently abnormal electroneurographic pattern (Otolaryngol Head Neck Surg 2000:290), or if MRI at 6 weeks with lesion—rare consequences. Pro (Am J Otol 2000:139) and con (Arch Otolaryngol Head Neck Surg 1998:824)

13.4 INCREASED INTRACEREBRAL PRESSURE

Cause: Tumor (see 9.2), infection (see 13.5), bleed (see 13.7), cerebral venous sinus thrombosis (Lancet 1996:1623), or idiopathic—pseudotumor cerebri (Am J Emerg Med 1999:517)

Epidem: Pseudotumor cerebri associated with anemia; vitamin deficiencies and intoxications—especially vitamin A; chronic hypoxia; postconcussive state; post–otitis media, hypoparathyroidism; start of thyroid replacement in myxedematous patients; steroid replacement and withdrawal (Addison's); lateral sinus thrombosis. Mostly in young, overweight women—BCPs?

Pathophys: Unknown

Sx: Headache; nausea; vomiting; visual field losses; no impairment of consciousness

Si: Enlarged blind spot; central vision losses; later, inferior quadrant defects/visual field constrictions. Papilledema without hemorrhages or exudates

Crs: Variable but concern for intracranial hypertension necessitates ICP monitoring (Surg Neurol 1978:371); worse prognosis with initial unconsciousness, subarachnoid bleed, shift of midline structures, elevated blood pressure, elevated serum glucose, and vomiting (Stroke 1997:1396)

Cmplc: Visual loss, monitor with quantitative visual perimetry

Lab: LP is diagnostic—high pressures of >20 cm, normal CSF otherwise—neuroimaging to R/O lesion, will see small or normal ventricles

ED Rx:

Pseudotumor Cerebri

- IV access for pain and nausea control if necessary
- Take off CSF to get pressure to 20 cm, may need to repeat in ~1 week

- Consider 2–6 weeks of steroids
- Consider diuretics; acetazolamide (Diamox) used to be favored, but loop diuretics such as furosemide OK
- Surgical shunt rarely needed

Increased Intracranial Pressure with Mass Effect (Abnormal Neuroimaging)

- Keep head of bed elevated
- Avoid IV fluid overload
- Intubation with hyperventilation
- Consider mannitol 1 gm/kg, although as effective as hypertonic saline with no change in cereberal blood flow in those with intracerebral hemorrhage (Neurosurgery 1999:1055, discussion, 1063)
- Consider dexamethasone 1 mg/kg or methylprednisolone 10 mg/kg; efficacy equivocal (Neurology 1972:56)
- May treat hypertension with labetalol 20 mg IV q 10–20 minutes, prn; or nitroprusside drip 5–20 μg/kg/min; avoid overtreatment since systemic hypertension is a response to maintain cerebral blood flow, and relative hypotension will adversely affect this (Neurol Res 1997:169)
- Neurosurgical consult for consideration of ICP monitor or shunting

13.5 ENCEPHALITIS

Adv Neurol 1978:197; Neuroimaging Clin N Am 2000:333

Cause: Arboviruses—1) St. Louis (Arch Neurol 2000:114), 2) eastern equine, 3) western equine, 4) La Crosse (Pediatr Infect Dis J 2000:77, 5) West Nile encephalitis (Emerg Infect Dis 2000:370); herpes viruses—1) HSV type 1, 2) HSV type 2, 3) varicella, 4) Epstein-Barr virus (mononucleosis), 5) cytomegalovirus (CMV); paramyxovirus—rubeola (measles) (AJNR Am J Neuroradiol 2000:455); rubella virus (German measles); *Mycoplasma pneumoniae* (Ann Emerg Med 1994:1375)

Epidem: Tick-borne encephalitis is usually a milder illness in children vs. adults (Infection 2000:74). Regional epidemics may be predicted by estimating snow melt water run-off since this has some relation to mosquito population (J Am Mosq Control Assoc 2000:22). Previous dengue virus infection conveys some protection against

St. Louis and West Nile encephalitis (Proc Soc Exp Biol Med 1970:573)

- *St. Louis*: urban *Culex* mosquito from birds (including birds that may be domestic (J Wildl Dis 2000:13)) and invertebrates. Incidence increased in adults >40 years of age, many cases unapparent
- *Eastern equine*: mosquitoes (incl. *Aedes albopictus* (Science 1992:526)) or ticks from wild birds, and snakes? In eastern U.S., incidence up after rainy winter; <100 cases in literature; kills horses by the thousands and children age <10 years
- *Western equine*: rural *Culex* mosquito, from birds and snake reservoirs. Incidence in infants and adults >50 years of age is 3000 cases in 1959; endemic in Columbia River basin; many cases unapparent
- *La Crosse*: spread by *Aedes triseriatus* mosquitos; usually causes mild disease in children, although severe illness has occurred
- *West Nile*: 1999 U.S. epidemic, exact transmission unsure although birds, mosquitoes, and ticks hypothesized (MMWR Morb Mortal Wkly Rep 1999:845) and originating in Israel (Science 1999:2333); 1996 epidemic in Europe (Lancet 1998:767)
- *Herpes simplex types 1 and 2*: occurs in babies under age 3 months born of mothers with active disease or to asymptomatic but viral shedding mothers; or those who are immunosuppressed or atopic—such as those with eczema
- *Varicella*: a complication of chicken pox or zoster. Chicken pox with 14-day incubation period; may return to school/day care when lesions are crusted. Zoster is more common in the elderly, or those with HIV or cancer but not a sign of occult malignancy
- *EB virus*: 18% of adults are asymptomatic; spread by intimate contact with carrier
- *CMV*: congenital via transplacental acquisition; newborn via vaginal infection at birth; blood products; organ transplantation; increased in homosexual males
- *Rubeola*: spread via direct contact with patient in day 2 or more of incubation period with 12–14 day incubation period; common worldwide, higher in vitamin A–deficient patients. Encephalitis in 0.1% with 65% of these having neurologic residue—subclinical in 15–20%
- *Rubella*: carrier is newborn infant

Pathophys:
- *Arboviruses*: humans and horses do not develop enough viremia to transmit these diseases
- *HSV types 1 and 2*: see 8.6
- *Varicella*: same organism first causes chickenpox, and then zoster
- *EBV*: lives only in B-lymphocytes and oral epithelial cells, only replicates in epithelial cells of mouth
- *CMV*: ubiquitous, may be congenital or acquired and found in all body fluids of carrier
- *Rubeola*: respiratory tract involved, viremia within 2 days of contact; Koplik's spots and skin lesions are areas of local intracellular viral replication. Encephalitis is a hypersensitivity reaction, not infectious
- *Rubella*: a mild virus, damages without killing the fetus

Sx: Fever, severe headache, nausea, vomiting; herpes viruses may also have herpetic rash, gingivostomatitis; rubeola, rubella, and West Nile with maculopapular rash

Si: Change in mental status, meningismus, adenopathy, frontal lobe release signs, cranial nerve palsies, seizures. May resemble anticholinergic crisis (J Toxicol Clin Toxicol 1997:627)
- *Varicella*: chicken pox with herpetic rash of various ages, zoster (shingles) with dermatomal eruption
- *EBV*: tonsillitis, posterior adenopathy
- *CMV*: mild hepatitis and splenomegaly
- *Rubeola*: Koplik's spots on buccal mucosa—white on red base opposite molars; palpebral conjunctivitis; vascular spiders on soft palate; the rash is "brown paint spilled over head and neck," starts around ears and can be on palms and soles when severe
- *Rubella*: conjunctivitis, splenomegaly, and sore gums; rash is on face first and spreads in 3 days

Crs:
- All arbovirus encephalitis patients with moderate to high neurologic morbidity risk and the following mortality risks—St. Louis with 16% mortality, 66% if seizure; eastern equine with 36% mortality; western equine with 10% mortality
- Herpes encephalitis with about 70% mortality
- Rubeola with a 2–10% mortality in developing countries
- Rubella with severe neurologic sequelae including mental retardation and deafness

Cmplc: A myriad of problems possible, including multiorgan secondary infections or some degree of failure

Diff Dx: Meningitis, human granulocytic ehrlichiosis (J Infect 2000:55), syphilis, anticholinergic crisis; other childhood exanthems—roseola, scarlet fever, erythema infectiosum (fifth disease)

Lab: CBC with diff; blood cultures; metabolic profile; U/A and urine culture; CSF with specific viral serologies and look for increased protein, white cells, and red cells, PCR may be helpful (J Neurol Sci 1993:213; J Clin Microbiol 2000:1527; J Clin Virol 2000:31) —if neuro deficit, do CT scan first to look for mass lesion or bleed. MRI may show more abnormalities consistent with encephalitis (J Neurol Sci 2000:3). EEG may be helpful in subacute encephalitis (Clin Electroencephalogr 1989:1)

ED Rx:

Give coincident meningitis treatment as diagnosis is developing, and specifically the following:

- Arbovirus infections require supportive care
- Herpes virus infections use acyclovir 5 mg/kg q 8 hours IV for 5–7 days (Brain Inj 1999:935), foscarnet, or vidarabine. Corticosteroids of equivocal efficacy, but at least not detrimental (J Neurovirol 2000:25)
- Rubella patients should have contacts immunized or titers tested if immunization status not up to date
- Rubeola with vitamin A 200,000 IU × 2 increases survival in developing countries

Prevention

- Cochrane Data Base of available vaccines (Cochrane Database Syst Rev 2000)

13.6 EPIDURAL ABSCESS

Neuroimaging Clin N Am 2000:333; Rev Infect Dis 1987:265

Cause: Infection of epidural space after surgery or invasive procedure such as epidural catheter for analgesic or other medicine infusion (J Neurol 1999:815), from remote or contiguous primary site with extension, or spontaneous. Skin pathogens such as *Staphylococcus* sp. or *Streptococcus* sp. most likely, but also possibly *Escherichia coli* or TB. Less likely intracranial

Epidem: Uncommon, ~0.2–1.2/10,000 admissions to tertiary care centers (N Engl J Med 1975:463)

Pathophys: Causes compression of cord with long tract signs below level of lesion

Sx: Fever, pain, paresthesias

Si: Hyperreflexia, bladder and rectal sphincter incontinence, paraplegia or quadriplegia, percussion tenderness

Crs: Usual presenting progression is spinal ache followed by neuropathic pain followed by neuro deficit

Cmplc: Paralysis

Diff Dx: Epidural hematoma, cauda equina syndrome, conus medullaris syndrome, possibly meningitis or vertebral osteomyelitis if no neurologic deficits

Lab: CBC with diff; ESR; blood cultures. X-ray: CT, MRI better (Scand J Infect Dis 1988:323; Arch Neurol 1992:743) of suspected level; if myelogram performed, do not violate infected area

ED Rx:
- Removal of catheter if necessary
- CSF sampling if possible, not through inflamed site
- IV antibiotics, consider third-generation cephalosporin with vancomycin
- Immediate neurosurgical consult (Neurosurgery 1990:185)
- Steroids equivocal

13.7 HEAD TRAUMA

Curr Opin Pediatr 1998:350; Emerg Med Clin North Am 1999:9, vii

Cause: Myriad of adult causes, consider shaken baby syndrome in infants

Epidem: Helmets prevent brain morbidity and overall mortality, and do not increase the risk of C-spine injury (Eur J Emerg Med 1998:207). Half the deaths due to trauma are from head trauma in those <44 years of age, where trauma is the leading cause of death, such as car accidents, assault, bicycle and motorcycle accidents. Height >3 feet is significant in those <2 years of age (Arch Pediatr Adolesc Med 1999:15). Falls in the elderly can cause significant damage even from a standing height, although more significant if falling down stairs (J Emerg Med 1998:709)

Pathophys: Our concern is skull fractures and intracranial injuries, although significant scalp lacerations and facial trauma can also be concerns. Primary brain injury is when we speak of neuronal and axonal injury at time of injury, and secondary brain injury is due to delayed physiologic changes that may be treatable—hypoxia, cerebral edema, intracranial hemorrhage, hypercarbia, etc.

- *Minor head traumas* may be classified as those with a normal neurologic exam, no evidence of CNS penetration on physical exam, and with no or fleeting loss of consciousness, and a normal head CT if one was performed

- A *concussion* is a closed head injury where loss of consciousness may have occurred, the neurologic exam is normal, a head CT does not show a subarachnoid or other bleed but a clinically insignificant subarachnoid bleed has probably occurred, especially in those who go on to a postconcussive syndrome in which the headaches can last for weeks to months. Different grading scales exist, but a useful one is by Cantu (Sports Med 1992:64) and outlines the following: mild (Grade 1)—no LOC, and amnesia less than 30 minutes; moderate (Grade 2)—<5 minutes LOC or amnesia >30 minutes; and severe (Grade 3)—>5 minutes LOC or amnesia >24 h

- *Severe head injuries* may be seen with skull fractures from blunt or penetrating trauma, cerebral contusions, subarachnoid bleeds, intraparenchymal bleeds, epidural hematomas (arterial bleed, usually middle meningeal artery), and subdural hematomas. Subdural hematomas can be acute or chronic, and are venous in nature due to tearing of bridging vessels between the subarachnoid space and dural sinuses. These are more common in the elderly, especially if they are on anticoagulants, and can result from even minor trauma

Sx: Change in mental status; nausea; vomiting; headache; neck pain

Si: Obvious skull trauma; periorbital ecchymosis (raccoon eyes); postauricular ecchymosis (Battle's sign); focal neurologic deficit; seizure; decreased mental status; Cushing's reflex—hypertension and bradycardia

Crs: Severe head trauma with only ~40% functional recovery. Those with minor head trauma, GCS of 15, and lack of headache, nausea, vomiting, and depressed skull fracture do not need head CT (J Emerg Med 1997:453). Loss of consciousness is an equivocal finding for predicting a positive head CT (Am Surg 1994:533, discussion, 535). Evaluating those who are intoxicated is difficult, and our clinical history, GCS, and neuro exam criteria will not predict those who have intracranial pathology who present with minor head trauma (Acad Emerg Med 1994:227)

Cmplc: Severe head trauma with 35% mortality. Long-term psychological disability in adults (Ann Emerg Med 1989:9). Children with minor head trauma rarely have long-term physical disability—parental reassurance is key (Pediatrics 1986:497). Children with severe head trauma present difficulties in evaluating the abdomen—CT OK and useful (J Pediatr Surg 1987:1117). Adults with severe head trauma can have abdominal CT or diagnostic peritoneal lavage (Lancet 1980:759) as options to evaluate for intra-abdominal injuries

Lab:

- CBC with diff; PT/PTT; metabolic profile—transient and mild hypokalemia in children (J Pediatr Surg 1997:88); ABG; ETOH; liver function tests; consider amylase; U/A; urine toxic screen; EKG
- X-ray: plain films of C-spine if severe head/neck injury, or if clinically suspect injury in the conscious and alert adult patient based on exam since in these circumstances it is rarely an occult injury (Am J Surg 1986:643); chest and pelvis X-rays in severe trauma; head CT without contrast for all but minor head trauma; consider CT of C-spine if unable to clear with plain films. Plain skull X-rays with no benefit, yet does not miss intracranial lesions in low-risk patients because they probably did not need imaging (N Engl J Med 1987:84). Facial fractures are not uncommon in even minor head trauma (Injury 1994:47)

ED Rx:

- *Minor head trauma* may go home after period of observation if appropriate, and with reliable observers. First-time concussions of Grades 1 or 2 may return to sports after 1 week of no symptoms; all others should follow up with their primary physicians in 1 week before returning to sports
- *Moderate head trauma* will deserve a prolonged interval of observation at the least, and should consider neurosurgical consult for observation/admission
- *Severe head trauma* deserves the following:
  1) Maintain airway, consider rapid sequence intubation—pretreat with either topical lidocaine to back of tongue or 1.5 mg/kg IV push to prevent acute increase in cerebral pressure. Hyperventilate

2) If other comorbid conditions, address those first—even prior to head CT. The comorbid conditions/injuries (usually intra-abdominal hemorrhage (J Trauma 1993:40, discussion, 44)) are usually more significant than the intracranial problems (J Trauma 1995:154; Surg Gynecol Obstet 1993:327)

3) Maintain IV fluids for shock but do not overload

4) Phenytoin (or fosphenytoin in phenytoin equivalents) 20 mg/kg IV bolus for seizures—fosphenytoin is loaded faster; attempt primary control with lorazepam 1–2 mg IV push

5) Permissive hypothermia to 32–33°C is experimental (J Neurotrauma 1995:923)

6) Meningitis can occur despite prophylactic antibiotics for basilar skull fracture (Am J Emerg Med 1983:295)

7) Neurosurgery consult for patients with fractures; mild head injuries but cannot be safely monitored at home; or those with moderate head trauma or worse

13.8 LOW BACK PAIN

Spine 1997:2128; Ann Emerg Med 1996:454; Emerg Med Clin North Am 1999:877, vi–vii; Curr Opin Rheumatol 1999:151

Cause: Ruptured herniated intervertebral disc; musculoligamentous strains/trauma; osteoarthritis of facet joints; perhaps leg length discrepancies; in elderly, vertebral compression fractures (Pain 1984:105) or multiple myeloma if no trauma

Epidem: 65% of the population have low back pain symptoms at some point in their lifetime

Pathophys: Myofascial, skeletal, disc, or ligamentous entrapment/compression of nerve conduction or vascular flow; this causes secondary edema, spasm and contracture, or hypersensitivity or paresthesias

Sx: Segmental pain with distal radiation of burning or shooting pain, or perhaps paresthesias; decreased range of motion due to pain or muscular restriction

Si: Abnormalities of the following give approximate level—patellar reflex is L4 root; Achilles reflex is S1 root; extensor hallucis longus and first web sensation are L5 root. Leg length discrepancy is

≥5 mm for significance in literature; most use 1 cm practically speaking

Crs: Over 90% improve with conservative therapy over several days to weeks and no workup is required unless motor loss is present and does not improve, or actually worsens. 2/3 have recurrence within 1 year, and pain lasts 2 months on average

Cmplc: Worker's compensation—those with this as part of the history have an extended course (Spine 1997:2016)

Diff Dx: AAA in elderly; spinal stenosis—pain, pseudoclaudication, numbness, worse with hips extended such as walking downhill, bilateral in 2/3; fibromyalgia; myofascial syndromes; anorectal abscess (Ann Emerg Med 1994:132); duodenal ulcer (Arch Phys Med Rehabil 1998:1137); retroperitoneal hemorrhage (Arch Phys Med Rehabil 1997:664)

Lab:

- CBC with diff looking for anemia and metabolic profile & U/A for renal insufficiency if considering multiple myeloma
- X-ray: Consider plain films empirically in those ≤18 years of age or ≥50 years of age if no history of minor trauma; most do not require X-ray evaluation (Ann Emerg Med 1986:245; Spine 1995:1839). CT/MRI is good if observed abnormality correlates with clinical exam, but 1/3 of CTs have abnormal finding, and in normal and asymptomatic people we find bulges (50%) and protrusions (25%) on MRI. *Scanograms* for leg length are only accurate measurement—rarely needed. Tape measuring is inaccurate

ED Rx:

- Appropriate level of pain management with acetaminophen, NSAIDs, and narcotics as scheduled (not prn) and time-limited (Drugs 1994:189; Spine 1996:2840, discussion, 2849); antiemetics as needed. Ibuprofen po as efficacious as ketorolac IM (Ann Pharmacother 1994:309; Acad Emerg Med 1998:118)
- Consider muscle relaxant if crampy or spasm component in history (Spine 1989:438); may not be appropriate if oversedation is an issue
- Resume normal daily activities with pain limited caution for lifting (N Engl J Med 1995:351)
- Consider manipulative therapy through osteopaths (N Engl J Med 1999:1426), physical therapy, or chiropractors—physical therapy (Phys Ther 1988:199) and chiropractic data shows higher pt satisfaction with no difference in clinical outcome

- Hard bed/mattress
- Prolonged bed rest unhelpful (N Engl J Med 1986:1064); steroids of no help
- Exercise not helpful for acute, but good for chronic back pain
- Consider MRI or primary care consult if persistence >2 weeks; neurosurgical consult if abnormal MRI or exam

13.9 MIGRAINE HEADACHE

Ann Emerg Med 1996:448

Cause: Possibly genetic

Epidem: In U.S. 17.6% of females and 5.7% of males with migraine headache each year, associated with lower-income household in females (Jama 1992:64). Possibly autosomal dominant with incomplete penetrance; 80% have positive family history. Higher incidence in obsessive/compulsives, patients with family history of epilepsy, after psychological trauma, and in patients who had motion sickness as children

- *Common and classic*: female/male ratio = 3–4:1; in women on oral contraceptives incidence increased × 9, 10% have each year, 15% lifetime risk
- *Cluster*: male/female ratio = 10:1

Pathophys: Angiographically documented cerebrovascular constriction, shunting; perhaps from 5-HT–induced vascular changes; perhaps sludging leads to brain ischemia, which causes vasodilatation and pain especially in external carotid distribution

Sx:

- *Common* (80%): slow onset over 4 hours, no scotomata or other aura; prodrome of yawning, euphoria, depression; usually bilateral; lasts 4–72 hours
- *Classic* (10%): precipitated by bright light, sound, or idiopathic; usually unilateral headache follows 20–30 minute scotomata, which spread then recede, or other sensory, speech, or motor aura. Headache lasts 4–72 hours; associated with nausea, vomiting, diarrhea, polyuria, and hemiplegias—hemiplegias all on opposite side of headache and scotomata. Consistently on one side 90% of the time

- *Cluster* (10%): "a migraine packed into 1 hour." Clusters of several/week for ~1 month; precipitated by vasodilators like alcohol, nitroglycerin during cluster period only; sweating, tearing, flush, salivation, rhinorrhea; nocturnal; severe episodes may precipitate suicide

Si: Ergotamine trials help most but not all
- *Common*: eye tearing, face and neck muscle stiffness
- *Classic*: on affected side, small pupil, external carotid pain; carotid sinus pressure temporarily relieves headache
- *Cluster*: Horner's syndrome

Crs: *Classic*: after attack, ~1 week immunity from recurrence

Cmplc: CVA

Diff Dx: Tension headache (may mimic common migraine signs); subarachnoid hemorrhage; meningitis/encephalitis; glaucoma—distinguished by cupped discs; epilepsy—scotomata last longer with migraine; trauma/tumor—in migraine no permanent scotomata except in very old, varies to opposite side 10% of the time, headache no worse with Valsalva; carotid artery (face pain) or vertebral artery (neck pain) dissection

Lab: Serum tests not necessary if considering headache of migraine or tension physiology; CT/MRI not necessary if classic symptoms, although CT abnormalities have been noted in previous case reports (Headache 1987:578); EEG shows spike patterns (Clin Electroencephalogr 2000:76)

ED Rx:
Common or Classic
- Rest in a quiet and dark room
- Prochlorperazine (Compazine) 5–10 mg IV, or droperidol 0.625 mg IV or 2.5 mg IM (Am J Emerg Med 1999:398), or chlorpromazine 25 mg IV (Ann Emerg Med 1989:360; 1990:1079); metoclopramide 10 mg IV is second-line therapy (Acad Emerg Med 1995:597; Ann Emerg Med 1995:541)
- ASA 900 mg + metoclopramide 10 mg po as effective as po sumatriptan
- Caffeine/ergotamine 1 mg po or 2 mg pr up to 6 mg/24 hours or 10 mg/week; overdose can cause vascular occlusion especially when on β-blockers or erythromycin
- Dihydroergotamine 0.5–1.0 mg IV/IM/sc (Ann Emerg Med 1998:129); nasal spray (Novartis) 1 inhalation each nostril and may repeat in 15 minutes

- Sumatriptan (Imitrex—5-HT analog) 6 mg sc × 1 helps 90% within 2 hours; or 100 mg po × 1 helps 50% within 2 hours; or as nasal spray 5–20 mg/dose helps within 15 minutes like sc (Cephalalgia 1998:532); may precipitate coronary artery disease. Similarly zolmitriptan (Zomig) 2.5 mg po, can repeat in 1 hour; rizatriptan (Maxalt); and naratriptan (Amerge) 1–2.5 mg, may repeat × 1 after hours and takes 4 hours to work. With all of these, beware drug interactions with MAO inhibitors, SSRIs, ergots, BCPs, and cimetidine
- Narcotics to "break the cycle," such as meperidine 1.5 mg/kg (Ann Emerg Med 1998:129)
- Butorphanol (Stadol) 1 nasal spray, may repeat × 1 in 4 hours (Am J Emerg Med 1997:57)
- Lidocaine 4% intranasally decreases headache by 50% in 50% of patients in 15 minutes (Jama 1996:319)
- All NSAIDs equal, no benefit of parenteral ketorolac (Ann Pharmacother 1994:309; Acad Emerg Med 1998:118)
- Nitrous oxide 50:50 over 20 minutes (Am J Emerg Med 1999:252)
- Dexamethasone 10 mg IV; data is anecdotal (Headache 1994:366)

Cluster

- Prednisone 40–60 mg po qd × 7 days; chlorpromazine 100–700 mg qd; indomethacin; sumatriptan as above

Prevention

- *Common and classic* patients should stop BCPs, and may have prophylaxis with 1 ASA daily, β-blockers, methysergide, calcium channel blockers, valproate, or riboflavin (Headache 2000:30)
- *Cluster* patients should avoid vasodilators and may be maintained on lithium

13.10 NEUROLEPTIC MALIGNANT SYNDROME (NMS)

J Clin Psychiatry 1980:79; 1987:328

Cause: Use of neuroleptic drugs (major tranquilizers) including phenothiazines, butyrophenones, thioxanthenes, loxapine, and rarely clozapine; or withdraw of dopamine agonist such as bromocriptine or levodopa

Epidem: ~0.5% of patients given these drugs will develop NMS, unrelated to dose; 96% of cases within one month of starting drug. Incidence increased with dehydration, exhaustion, and organic brain syndrome

Pathophys: Diminished CNS dopamine

Sx: 1–3 day onset, up to 5–10 days after drug has stopped, or 10–30 days after IM deposited doses. Agitation, confusion, disorganization, and catatonia as risk factors for developing NMS (Biol Psychiatry 1998:748)

Si: Fever in 87%; rigidity; hypertonia; mental status changes; autonomic instability such as pallor, diaphoresis, hypotension, hypertension, tachycardia, arrhythmia; akinesia; tremor; perhaps choreoathetoid-type movements

Crs: 10% mortality in 3–30 days

Cmplc: Respiratory failure, myoglobinuric renal failure, cardiovascular collapse, arrhythmias, pulmonary embolus

Diff Dx: Heat stroke, malignant hyperthermia, acute serotonin syndrome, antibiotic (aminoglycoside)-induced neuromuscular blockade—usually postoperative, idiopathic acute lethal catatonia (Am J Psychiatry 1989:324), drug interactions with MAO inhibitors, central anticholinergic crisis that responds to IV physostigmine, tetanus, tick paralysis, stiff man syndrome, myotonia, meningitis, encephalitis, thyroid storm

Lab:
- CBC with diff; metabolic profile including Ca, Mg, and phosphorous; CPK; aldolase; U/A with myoglobin—67% have myoglobinuria; consider panculture if infectious etiology; consider LP if considering meningitis or encephalitis
- X-ray: head CT or MRI if bleed suspected, focal deficit, or other CNS concerns

ED Rx:
Am J Emerg Med 1991:360
- Hold all neuroleptics
- Dantrolene (Dantrium) 1–2 mg/kg IV initial dose, then up to 10 mg/kg/day IV or po divided in q 6 hour doses—beware of concomitant Ca channel blocker use. Controversial (Br J Psychiatry 1991:709), as is bromocriptine
- Bromocriptine 2.5–10 mg po tid (J Clin Psychiatry 1987:69), or amantidine 100 mg po bid
- Consider L-dopa

- Nitroprusside IV (Ann Intern Med 1986:56) and minoxidil po are a case report success
- Rx myoglobinuria with IV fluids most important (Ren Fail 1997:283); $NaHCO_3$ IV may prevent damage by myoglobin (J Biol Chem 1998:31,731); mannitol of equivocal efficacy

13.11 GRAND MAL SEIZURE/STATUS EPILEPTICUS

Emerg Med Clin North Am 1994:1027; 1999:203, ix

Cause: 20% idiopathic; 80% due to organic disease; trauma (subdural, scar), infection, neoplasia, vascular (AV malformation, CVA), degenerative disease (MS, Alzheimer's), metabolic (intoxications including cocaine (Ann Emerg Med 1989:774), anoxia, hypoglycemia, fever, hyponatremia, alkalosis, hypomagnesemia, hypocalcemia). Neonates/infants include congenital malformations and drug withdrawal. Pregnancy includes eclampsia (Emerg Med Clin North Am 1994:1013). Failure to take antiepileptic medications

Epidem: Not a significant cause of car accidents, but clinically more serious if they occur as a result of a head injury (Ann Emerg Med 1983:543)

Pathophys: Crosses midline; functional brain transection at midbrain (decerebrate)

Sx: Auras, Jacksonian progression, and postictal Todd's paralysis all indicate focal onset/origin; precipitated by menses

Si: Tonic decerebrate posturing evolving to clonic phase after 1–2 minutes; postictal amnesia, confusion, often Todd's paralysis

Crs: No decrease in IQ due to seizures unless complicated by status epilepticus

Cmplc: Status epilepticus—seizures >10–20 minutes in duration or failure to awaken between tonic-clonic seizures causes brain damage after 1 hour even with normal vital signs; death hypothesized as due to cardiac arrhythmias as the terminal event (Epilepsia 1984:84)

Diff Dx: Cardiac etiology with syncope—arrhythmias including prolonged Q-T syndrome (Ann Emerg Med 1996:556)

Febrile seizures—ages 6 months to 6 years; recurrence risk factors include first seizure at young age, febrile seizure history in first-degree relative, low-grade fever in ED, and short time interval between onset of fever and seizure (Arch Pediatr Adolesc Med 1997:371); no increased risk for bacteremia or UTIs, and rare to have bacterial meningitis if not evident on initial laboratory tests (LP results) (Pediatr Emerg Care 1999:9)

Hysterical seizures—longer and less precise onset, more pelvic thrusting, side-to-side head movement, eyes tightly shut, and alternating movements of limbs; Lennox-Gastaut syndrome in children

Lab:

- Immediate glucoscan; CBC with diff; metabolic profile including Mg^{++} and Ca^{++}—rarely helpful in pediatric (Pediatr Emerg Care 1992:65; 1992:13) or adult (Ann Emerg Med 1985:416) patients unless clinically suspect metabolic abnormalities; PT/PTT if likely intracranial bleed; consider ETOH; urine toxic screen; EEG abnormal in 30–50% and increases to 60–90% with repeated studies

- X-ray: Head CT to check for bleed emergently, even consider in those with "other" cause for seizure such as alcohol intoxication/withdrawal (Epilepsia 1980:459) or cocaine use (Ann Emerg Med 1992:772) if patient not recovering from seizures or other evidence of abnormal neurologic exam; MRI to assess for organic cause

Children with simple febrile seizures or fever with new onset seizure that does not fit the definition of simple febrile seizure rarely have significant lesions on head CT if nonfocal seizure and nonfocal neuro exam after postictal state (J Pediatr 1998:664); children at higher risk for intracranial lesion if <6 months of age, seizure >15 minutes long, history of malignancy, neurocutaneous syndrome, recent closed head injury, recent shunt surgery or abnormal neuro exam postrecovery (Ann Emerg Med 1997:518)

Prehospital Rx:

- Protect patient from self-injury
- Airway, O_2, suction
- Administer benzodiazepine, such as buccal midazolam 10 mg or rectal diazepam 10 mg if IV access is not available (Lancet 1999:623)

ED Rx:

If Actively Seizing/Status Epilepticus

Epilepsia 1989:S33; J Child Neurol 1998:S23, discussion, S30

- Empiric thiamine 100 mg IV and glucose bolus if glucoscan not immediately available
- Maintain airway, intubate if necessary
- Lorazepam (Ativan) 0.05 mg/kg IV with usual adult dose 2–4 mg IV; or diazepam (Valium) 0.1 mg/kg IV, double this pr, usual adult dose 5–10 mg IV; or midazolam (Versed) 0.2 mg/kg IV
- Fosphenytoin 20 mg/kg of phenytoin equivalents IV over 10 minutes—may use phenytoin if 30-minute bolus OK; repeat 10-mg/kg bolus if still seizing. Perhaps not effective in ETOH-related seizures (Ann Emerg Med 1994:513)
- Phenobarbital (first line for children) 10 mg/kg at 100 mg/min with usual adult dose of 0.7–1.5 g IV—may give an additional 10 mg/kg if not successful—*be prepared to intubate secondary to respiratory depression*
- Consider barbiturate coma, such as pentobarbital 100 mg IV bolus prn; must be intubated for this

Patient with AIDS

- Neuroimaging and lumbar puncture in ED or as inpatient for new onset seizures (Acad Emerg Med 1998:905)

If Patient with Self-Limited/Easily Controlled Seizure

- Consider outpatient treatment with phenytoin (Dilantin)—300–400 mg po qd after loading dose; carbamazepine (Tegretol)—400–1200 mg po qd; or valproic acid—1–3 g po qd divided
- More likely to treat adults than children after first seizure; especially if child has simple febrile seizure or no cause found
- Phenytoin usually first line for adults; phenobarbital—0.6 mg/kg po qd first line for children

13.12 SPINAL CORD INJURY

Surg Neurol 1978:71; 1978:60; 1978:64; Bmj 1990:34; 1990:110;
J Neurotrauma 1992:S385

Cause: Usually traumatic, may be due to a transient shock to the cord,
prolonged ischemia, cord contusion, or direct trauma

Epidem: Most commonly a male in the third decade of life; usual
mechanism of MVA, falls, and firearms in descending order of
frequency

Pathophys: Transient and permanent cord lesions are possible, as well
as complete or partial cord syndromes (J Neurosurg 1991:15).
Cord injury may occur without obvious bony fracture in children
(SCIWORA—see 26.2) (J Trauma 1989:654) or others with
underlying laxity of the vertebral column (Spine 1990:466)

- *Spinal shock* is a lower motor neuron problem (areflexia) where a
flaccid quadriplegia may last hours to months. If this is transient,
usually turns into a spastic paralysis with return of reflexes in
~24 hours. Also manifests with autonomic instability (paralytic ileus
and urinary retention, e.g.) and hypotension with bradycardia in the
face of adequate urine output. Important to assess for significant
cardiac and hypovolemic event

- *Anterior spinal cord syndrome* is a problem with motor function
(paralysis) and sensory input of temperature and some degree
of pain loss distal to the lesion—temperature is lateral columns,
whereas pain is lateral columns and posterior columns. The
motor loss should show areflexia at the level of the lesion, and
hyperreflexia/spasticity (upper motor neuron lesion) distal to the
injury. Due to injury or occlusion of the anterior spinal artery, or
the cord itself

- *Central cord syndrome* is another partial cord syndrome where the
involved portion affects first the hands, then the upper extremity,
and then the legs—this is exactly the anatomic positioning from the
center of the cord outward. Usually a hyperextension injury with
possibly some degree of predisposition (congenital stenosis, e.g.);
ischemia to the cord center is implicated

- *Brown-Séquard's syndrome* is a cord hemisection with a motor
loss and the senses of vibratory, gross proprioception and some
pain loss on ipsilateral side at the level of the lesion, and sensory
loss of temperature and some pain loss two levels lower on the

contralateral side—the lateral columns carry fibers up two levels before they decussate to travel back to the brain, whereas the posterior columns and motor fibers decussate above the spinal cord

Sx: Back pain; localized weakness; obvious external trauma

Si: Spinal exam crepitus, ecchymosis, abnormal curvature; paralysis; sensory deficits; loss of sphincter tone; spasticity

Crs: Variable, "time will tell." Children usually fare well independent of coincident fracture or subluxation (J Neurosurg 1988:18)

Cmplc: Permanent dysfunction; syringomyelia

Diff Dx: Transverse myelitis

Lab: X-ray with plain films to find obvious fractures—do the whole spine; MRI if available; CT is an option but less definitive for cord injury. If in shock, do whole trauma evaluation before focusing on the spine—CBC with diff; PT/PTT; type and cross; metabolic profile; ETOH; liver function tests; U/A; urine toxic screen; EKG; plain films of chest and pelvis as well; consider head and abdominal CT

ED Rx:
- Treat shock—airway, IV resuscitation, control bleeding, keep warm
- Maintain spinal stability; best way to do this has not been elucidated. Whether holding in-line traction conveys any benefit over C-collar and sandbag head immobilization is not clear
- IV fluids at 20 cc/kg bolus × 2 if needed; consider cardiac evaluation
- Pressors (e.g., dopamine) if still in shock (see 2.10)
- Methylprednisolone 30 mg/kg IV bolus over 15 minutes followed by 5.4 mg/kg/hour drip if spinal cord injury—data is equivocal (Vet Surg 1995:128; J Trauma 1998:1088) and therapy may not be benign with increased infection and hospitalization (Ann Surg 1993:419, discussion, 425)
- Many experimental therapies such as U-50488H, an opioid kappa receptor agonist (Brain Res 1993:45)
- Neurosurgery consult

14 Obstetrics

14.1 ABDOMINAL TRAUMA/UTERINE RUPTURE

Clin Obstet Gynecol 1990:432; Obstet Gynecol Clin North Am 1999:419, vii

Cause: Multiple causes, but usually motor vehicle accidents; uterine rupture may be spontaneous in those with normal labor; as a result of previous uterine surgery such as myomectomy (Hum Reprod 1995:1475) or previous C-section (Am J Obstet Gynecol 1991:996)—high risk if previous classical C-section; from cocaine abuse (Am J Obstet Gynecol 1995:243); or in those with Asherman's syndrome (Obstet Gynecol 1986:864)

Epidem: Most maternal traumas are found to be minor, and fetal health is directly related to maternal well-being. Even those with minor maternal trauma, though, may have a problem with significant fetal injury or death. Three-point restraints—low-lying seatbelt with shoulder harness—convey the most protection to mother and fetus if they were to suffer a motor vehicle accident

Pathophys: Although uterine rupture can occur with abdominal trauma, it happens <1% of the time and it is more common to get retroperitoneal hemorrhage, splenic lacerations, liver lacerations, or kidney lacerations from abdominal trauma in the gravid patient. Placental abruption may also be a factor in ~4% of minor traumas and up to 50% of major traumas

Sx: Uterine rupture presents with a diffusely tender abdomen

Si: Shock, unable to determine uterine fundus or fetal lie

Crs: Timely diagnosis of a surgical abdomen is paramount

Cmplc: Maternal hemorrhage causing shock or fetal distress or death

Lab:
- CBC with diff; PT/PTT; medical blood type for consideration of RhoGAM; Kleihauer-Betke; consider type and cross; consider DIC profile if significant maternal/fetal transfusion suspected

- X-ray: U/S for uterine and fetal imaging (Am J Perinatol 1996:177), and evaluation of intra-abdominal free fluid, and imaging of kidneys, liver, spleen, and retroperitoneum if possible
- Fetal heart: 10 minutes with Doppler if <20 weeks' gestation, and 20 minutes of monitoring with contraction monitor if >20 weeks' gestation and patient is stable; longer periods of monitoring for more severely injured patients with 4 hours being the standard of care if patient is significantly injured

ED Rx:
- IV fluids and O_2
- Doppler to listen for fetal heart tones
- Patient on left side if fetal distress
- Do not limit maternal evaluation during trauma due to pregnancy status—standard of care is the same as for a nongravid patient
- Immediate OB consult; general surgical consult as deemed appropriate

14.2 ECTOPIC PREGNANCY

Acad Emerg Med 1995:1081; 1995:1090

Cause: Implantation of embryo other than in uterus

Epidem: ~2% of all pregnancies with increasing incidence; 95% are tubal, but also can be ovarian, cervical, intra-abdominal (0.5%). Post-tubal ligation rate is 1/1000 over 10 years; it is 30/1000 if electrocoagulation tubal performed. Increased in urban populations due to PID, previous pelvic surgery such as previous ectopic, IUD, and other reasons (Ann Emerg Med 1999:283); those in rural populations tend to have no risk factors (Fam Med 1996:111)

Pathophys: Scarred tubes have a slow transfer rate and the blastocyst implants wherever it is on day 6

Sx: Nearly all in first trimester; report of missed period, although withdrawal bleeding may mask this. Abdominal/pelvic discomfort similar to menstrual pains, referred pain to shoulder may be a sign of diaphragmatic irritation from intraperitoneal bleeding

Si: Nonspecific (Ann Emerg Med 1999:283), palpable pain or cervical motion tenderness may not be present; hypotension may be present

Crs: Without surgery, death in 2/1000 of the population

Cmplc: Shock, surgical sterility

Diff Dx: PID, spontaneous abortion (threatened), septic abortion, appendicitis, ruptured ovarian corpus luteum or follicle cyst, endometriosis cyst

Lab:

- CBC with diff; serum β-HCG, with level <1000 mIU/mL with 4-fold higher risk (Ann Emerg Med 1996:10); type and screen (consider type and cross if in shock); progesterone levels not wholly reliable but should be <20–25 ng/mL in ectopic (Am J Obstet Gynecol 1989:1425, discussion, 1428); subunit of β-HCG, the core fragment, may be predictive of ectopic if <100 μg/L in the urine—data dredging (J Clin Endocrinol Metab 1994:497). Urine pregnancy test positive when serum level >50 U, thus 90+% positive at first missed period. Serum CK not helpful (Br J Obstet Gynaecol 1995:233). Serum amylase is not helpful (Am J Emerg Med 1988:327)

- X-ray: U/S with transvaginal is the gold standard in radiology (Fertil Steril 1998:62) and combined with serum β-HCG shows a sensitivity of 100% and specificity of 99.9% for ectopic pregnancy diagnosis (Obstet Gynecol 1994:1010)—intrauterine pregnancy (IUP) with an ectopic twin is rare phenomenon. U/S by U/S-trained ED physicians with 90% sensitivity and 88% specificity for right diagnosis (Ann Emerg Med 1997:338), but the discriminatory zone was a serum β-HCG of 2000 mIU/mL, whereas other sonographers with discriminatory zone of 1000 mIU/mL or less (J Emerg Med 1998:699). Look for thin endometrial stripe (Fertil Steril 1996:474) and is best when serum β-HCG <1000 (Acad Emerg Med 1999:602); even indeterminate scans should be subclassified as low-, intermediate-, or high-risk (Acad Emerg Med 1998:313)

ED Rx:

- *If equivocal data*, repeat serum β-HCG in 48 hours—highest risk for ectopic is empty uterus and β-HCG rising <66%, followed by empty uterus and β-HCG decreasing less than 50%, followed by empty uterus and β-HCG rising more than 66%. If β-HCG decreased more than 50%, low risk for ectopic irrespective of U/S findings (Ann Emerg Med 1999:703). Discuss with obstetrician

- *If positive but stable*, OB consult. Consider methotrexate if fetal tissue <4 cm in diameter, no fetal heart beat (Fertil Steril 1989:435), and serum β-HCG <5000 mIU/mL (Am J Obstet Gynecol 1996:1840, discussion, 1846), or laparoscopic salpingostomy

- *If positive and unstable*, 2 large-bore IVs, type and cross performed, OB consult for laparotomy
- Culdocentesis not commonly performed, but will show nonclotting blood from hemoperitoneum along with positive serum β-HCG in 99.2% if ruptured ectopic (Obstet Gynecol 1985:519). Laparoscopy (diagnosis and therapy) has replaced paracentesis in these cases as well

14.3 PERIMORTEM DELIVERY

Cause: Trauma, chronic pulmonary or cardiac conditions, pulmonary embolus, substance abuse (e.g., toluene (Obstet Gynecol 1991:504)), or other etiologies that may cause maternal death

Epidem: Rare, but increases with increasing maternal age (Obstet Gynecol 1983:210) and previously higher frequency in adolescents (Clin Obstet Gynecol 1978:1191)

Pathophys: Fetus at risk with maternal resuscitation, emergent stratification as follows:
- Gestational age
- Length and quality of resuscitation
- Underlying maternal health
- Prenatal problems, such as oligohydramnios, abnormal triple markers or level II U/S, etc.

Sx: Shock

Si: Shock

Crs: More than 20 minutes of resuscitation unlikely to have good outcome, with each 5-minute increment from 0 to 20 ranging from good to poor prognosis

Cmplc: Fetal demise

Lab: None specific since this is a clinical decision—usual trauma labs on mother, remember CBC with diff and glucose on child

Rx:
- Resuscitate mother
- Immediate C-section
- Obstetrics and neonatology consults immediately

14.4 PLACENTAL ABRUPTION

J Perinatol 1988:174

Cause: Previous history, hypertension, spontaneous, trauma, and drug use (cigarettes (Am J Epidemiol 1996:881), ETOH, cocaine, amphetamine) are the major causes

Epidem: ~1% of pregnancies; recurrence rate of ~10%; associated with increasing maternal age

Pathophys: Separation of placenta prior to delivery of fetus, with <100 cc of blood loss and no other problems as mild, 100–500 cc of blood loss with fetal distress and uterine contractions as moderate, and hemorrhagic shock with imminent fetal demise as severe

Sx: Painful peripartum third-trimester bleeding

Si: Tender and large uterus; uterine contractions; signs of shock; fetal distress

Crs: Varies

Cmplc: Maternal hemorrhage, shock, fetal distress

Diff Dx: Cervical bleeding, marginal sinus bleeding, uterine rupture, vaginal trauma, bloody show, hematuria

Lab: CBC with diff; type and cross; PT/PTT

ED Rx:
- IV fluids, O_2, patient on left side if fetal distress
- Blood products as appropriate if demonstrated coagulopathy (see 9.7)
- Delivery, OB consult emergently for anything more than minor bleeding

14.5 PLACENTA PREVIA

J Perinatol 1988:174

Cause: Low-lying placenta about the cervical os

Epidem: 1/150–200 deliveries; increases with maternal age, history of previous previa, and with previous uterine scar

Pathophys: Vessels of placenta will be exposed and prone to bleeding if trying to implant in the cervical region

Sx: Painless peripartum third-trimester bleeding

Si: U/S before digital exam—manipulating cervical os region may cause hemorrhage; signs of shock; careful speculum exam with clear speculum (watching as advancing the speculum) is probably OK as long as you remove it once you confirm bleeding from cervical os

Crs: Most low-lying placentas found on U/S during pregnancy migrate from the cervical os by the third trimester

Cmplc: Maternal hemorrhage

Diff Dx: As for placental abruption (see 14.4)

Lab:
- CBC with diff; consider type and cross
- X-ray: U/S, and transvaginal is OK

ED Rx:
- IV fluids, O_2, patient on left side if fetal distress
- OB consult for C-section delivery

14.6 PRECIPITOUS DELIVERY

Cause: ?

Epidem: ?

Pathophys: Delivery occurs within 3 hours from the onset of true labor

Sx: Contractions every 2–3 minutes, urge to defecate, spontaneous rupture of membranes

Si: Uterine contractions, cervix widely dilated with complete effacement, crowning

Crs: Fast and imminent delivery

Cmplc: Uterine atony with postpartum hemorrhage

Lab: Fetal heart monitoring will usually show deep variable decelerations—increased vagal tone from head compression—look/listen for fetal heart rate accelerations that are appropriately tachycardic (150–160 bpm) as soon as the contraction eases

ED Rx:
- IV access
- OB consult
- Deliver the neonate (skills to be developed with 1:1 mentoring), but remember to put hands on either side of neonate's head with thumbs towards the nose, bulb suction mouth and then nares, deliver the anterior shoulder with gentle downward pressure followed by upward pressure delivering the posterior shoulder,

slide hand along back and gently grasp the thigh so that the baby does not slip
- Hand baby off for warming, drying, and stimulation
- Anticipate *postpartum hemorrhage* (Int J Gynaecol Obstet 1998:79)—

1) Uterine massage or breast feeding if uterine atony; 2) assess for retained products of conception, and remove if necessary; 3) examination of cervix, vagina, and perineum for repairs; 4) oxytocin 20–30 U in 1 L of IVF and run at 100 cc/hr; 5) Methergine 0.2 mg IM; 6) prostaglandin 15-methyl (PGF_{2a}) 0.25 mg IM or intrauterine injection (Obstet Gynecol 1980:665); 7) misoprostol 1000 µg pr (Obstet Gynecol 1998:212); 8) gemeprost (PGE_1 analogue) pessary 1 mg intrauterine (Br J Obstet Gynaecol 1993:691), intravaginal, or per rectum (J Perinat Med 1999:231)

14.7 ABNORMAL PRESENTATIONS

J Perinatol 1991:297

Cause: Occiput anterior is the preferred position for presenting fetal portion at perineum. Occiput posterior, transverse, brow presentations, face presentations, and asynclitism (parietal bone presenting) are probably variations that occur as the fetus proceeds through the birth canal. Breech and transverse lie presentations are more common in those with preterm labor and uterine anomalies (e.g., fibroids) (Obstet Gynecol 1976:427)

ED Rx:
- All deliveries should be performed in a hospital birthing center. Those with known or suspected problems should be encouraged to be checked as soon as labor onset is questioned
- If the appropriate delivery staff is not available, it may be necessary to perform a delivery in the setting of precipitous delivery or perimortem delivery. This book is not a substitute for appropriate mentoring and training, but a refresher guide. For breech and limb presentation and prolapsed cord, please read on.

BREECH PRESENTATION

Curr Opin Obstet Gynecol 1992:807

Cause: Preterm gestation (e.g., fetus did not yet "flip"); congenital (e.g., associated with torticollis (J Pediatr Surg 2000:1091)) or uterine (e.g., bicornuate) anomalies

Epidem: ~3% of deliveries

Si: Leopold's maneuvers to ascertain fetal lie and locate feet; vaginal exam for same reason. Buttocks presentation with feet about the head is *frank breech*, buttocks presentation with feet near bottom is *complete breech*, and leg presentation is *footling breech*

Crs: If breech lie is known, external version may have been performed prior to onset of labor—this is attempted after 37 weeks gestation in hospital birthing units

Cmplc: Entrapment of the fetal head, spinal cord injury, brachial plexus injury, asphyxia, intracranial hemorrhage—with consequent lower Apgar scores and orthopedic or internal organ trauma—also possible

Lab: U/S if possible to define fetal lie

ED Rx:

- OB and anesthesia available for delivery if possible, and may prefer to perform C-section (Obstet Gynecol 1987:965). Should be alerted even for precipitous delivery

- *If delivery is imminent*, let the buttocks and trunk deliver to the midabdominal region, with the fetal back facing anterior. A frank breech may need help with leg delivery; put a finger in the popliteal area behind the fetal knee, fully flex the hip so that the knee delivers followed by the leg and foot. For complete and footling breech, attempt to deliver the legs first—gently direct the feet out. Gently feed out the umbilical cord to have some extra length, wrap the body in a blanket, and when the scapula are seen, sweep your finger across the chest to deliver the arms one at a time—try to hook the volar aspect of the elbow to facilitate arm delivery. Then gently lift so that fetal midscapular region is aiming for mother's superior pubic symphysis region—this gentle lifting should be performed in conjunction with an assistant. While angling the body as above, use one hand and place one finger on the maxilla of the fetal face. Avoid hyperextension of the neck, and use fundal pressure as well to help deliver the head

• Pitfalls: 1) be prepared for a neonatal recovery; 2) perform an elective episiotomy if this delivery has to occur in the ED; 3) the head may get trapped at the cervix, and if the cervix is going to tear, you may elect to perform Dursin's incisions to facilitate head delivery and then know where the lacerations are which are directed away from the urethra. If the cervix closest to the urethra is 12 o'clock, the incisions are made at 2 o'clock, 6 o'clock, and 10 o'clock; and 4) call OB and anesthesia as soon as it appears that precipitous breech delivery is occurring

LIMB PRESENTATION

Cause: Seen with vertex, breech, and transverse lie presentations
Si: Hand or leg presenting
Crs: Hand and head presentation OK if vertex precedes the limb during delivery
Cmplc: Leg as with breech (footling breech); transverse lie at risk for umbilical cord prolapse
Lab: U/S if possible to delineate anatomy
ED Rx:
   • To hospital birthing center if possible, OB and anesthesia consults
   • Hand presentations preceding the vertex and transverse lie presentations necessitate C-section and labor does not proceed precipitously
   • Precipitous footling breech presentations as above

PROLAPSED CORD

Lancet 1966:1443
Cause: No fetal body part applied to cervix allowing umbilical cord to extrude with rupture of membranes
Epidem: Incidence of 0.1–0.6%; more common with breech presentation, polyhydramnios, transverse lie. ~47% due to obstetrical intervention (Am J Perinatol 1999:479) without increased neonatal morbidity/mortality in these patients
Sx: Rupture of membranes
Si: Umbilical cord felt in vaginal vault—check for pulse

Crs: Poor perinatal outcome even with emergent C-section
(J Reprod Med 1998:129)
Cmplc: Fetal anoxia
Lab: None
ED Rx:
- Trendelenburg
- IV access, O_2
- Place hand in vagina and hold fetal presenting part from compressing the cord between the fetus and the cervix
- Immediate OB consult

SHOULDER DYSTOCIA

Asia Oceania J Obstet Gynaecol 1994:195; Obstet Gynecol Clin North Am 1995:247

Cause: Large fetus/small pelvis but macrosomia with subsequent shoulder dystocia is not predictable (Surg Gynecol Obstet 1992:515)
Epidem: Not uncommon
Pathophys: As above
Sx: "Turtle head"—the fetal head partially emerges and then retracts with relaxation without any progress being made
Si: As above
Crs: Varies
Cmplc: Fetal injury such as fracture or brachial plexus injury; fetal death
Lab: None specific
ED Rx:
- IV fluid, O_2
- Episiotomy
- Legs up and out—McRobert's maneuver is the most effective maneuver (Am J Obstet Gynecol 1997:656)
- Fundal pressure, push towards spine with hand just above symphysis pubis
- Wood's screw maneuver, or try to push anterior shoulder from behind symphysis pubis by rotating the shoulder either way
- Deliver posterior shoulder first; fracture clavicle

- Zavenelli's maneuver—push fetal head back into vagina and hold it while C-section performed; 92% successful (Obstet Gynecol 1999:312)

14.8 PREECLAMPSIA AND ECLAMPSIA (TOXEMIA)

Clin Obstet Gynecol 1984:836

Cause: Unknown, some association with gestational diabetes mellitus (Diabetes 1991:79; J Reprod Med 1998:372) and/or lupus anticoagulant (N Engl J Med 1985:1322)

Epidem: Incidence 1.5% of private OB patients, whereas 12% of teaching hospital patients; 20% of urban poor, and ~5% in primips who represent 85% of all patients with PIH/eclampsia; 25% of patients with chronic hypertension. This is the second most common cause of maternal deaths—pulmonary embolus is first. Risk for development increases as pregnancy progresses

Pathophys: Preeclampsia is hypertension in pregnancy associated with edema and/or proteinuria. If this progresses to seizures and/or coma, then the patient has developed eclampsia. Those with isolated hypertension (excluding proteinuria as well) in pregnancy probably have a mild form of the preeclampsia spectrum (Clin Exp Hypertens [A] 1989:1565). Sympathetic vasoconstriction that abates with delivery—this is in contrast to the normal pregnancy reduction in peripheral vascular resistance mediated by an increased resistance to angiotensin; somehow this effect is lost via a trophoblast-dependent process with platelet dysfunction—hyperaggregation? CNS changes associated with reversible brain edema and leukoencephalopathy

Sx: Rapid weight gain; edema; headache; visual changes; epigastric abdominal pain

Si: Hypertension starting after 20 weeks' gestation—before this probably due to chronic hypertension—look for systolic >140 or diastolic >90, with diastolic >110 foreboding eclampsia; edema; proteinuria; hyperreflexia; papilledema if eclampsia—funduscopic exam somewhat controversial if suspecting eclampsia since light stimulation may induce seizures

Crs: All symptoms disappear by 72 hours postpartum in 95% of people. If signs and symptoms occur in first trimester, consider mole or trophoblastic tumor

Cmplc:

- Preeclampsia can be severe and these cases are associated with a 1% maternal and 10% prenatal infant mortality—without treatment, 25–50% of those who are severe will evolve to eclampsia
- Eclampsia (toxemia) includes seizures, and may be predicted by the same criteria for preeclampsia, as well as renal failure, CHF, CNS bleed; DIC; Sheehan's syndrome; fetal distress or demise; hepatic hemorrhage and rupture; HELLP—*H*emolysis, *E*levated *L*iver profile, *L*ow *P*latelets—syndrome; newborn neutropenias which are transient in 50% but also associated with sepsis

Diff Dx: Transient hypertension of pregnancy; chronic hypertension in pregnancy; pheochromocytoma

Lab: CBC with diff, look for thrombocytopenia (Am J Perinatol 1989:32); metabolic profile; liver function tests (Am J Perinatol 1988:146); uric acid; consider Mg level; consider Ca level; U/A; consider 24-hour urine for Ca—looking for hypocalciuria; consider DIC profile

ED Rx:

Eclampsia

- Stabilize, protect airway, O_2, IV access
- $MgSO_4$ 4-g IV bolus, then 2 g per hour drip; may use IM option of 10-g loading, then 5 g q 4 hours (J Reprod Med 1979:107). $MgSO_4$ superior to phenytoin (N Engl J Med 1995:201)
- Immediate OB consult; definitive treatment is delivery

Preeclampsia

- OB consult for all decisions on treatment and outpatient options
- May use hydralazine 5–10 mg IV, or labetalol 10–20 mg IV to acutely treat hypertension; nifedipine 10 mg sl not advocated here
- Outpatient hypertension treatment may use α-methyldopa (Aldomet), hydralazine, propranolol, or clonidine. Not ACE inhibitors—teratogenic
- Outpatient prevention may include low-dose aspirin (Obstet Gynecol 1990:742)—data is equivocal
- Treatment of hypertension does convey some benefit to the mother, not much to the fetus. Definitive treatment is delivery

OBSTETRICS

15 Ophthalmology

15.1 ACUTE GLAUCOMA (ANGLE CLOSURE)

Aust N Z J Ophthalmol 1999:358

Cause: Genetic predisposition, hyperopia (farsightedness); after LASIK procedure (J Cataract Refract Surg 2000:620); intranasal cocaine (J Laryngol Otol 1999:250)

Epidem: ~0.2% of population; especially in middle-aged and elderly (>50 years of age)

Pathophys: Smaller eye with shallow anterior chamber that impedes the normal aqueous humor flow, trapping the fluid posteriorly. Pressure then builds, compressing the optic nerve

Sx: Rainbow halos; eye pain that is sudden and bilateral; headache; nausea and vomiting; scotomas in nasal fields; precipitated by mydriatics, antacids, anesthesia, and darkness

Si: Red eye, especially circumcorneal; partially dilated fixed pupil; corneal edema with blistering and haziness; visual field defects (Graefes Arch Clin Exp Ophthalmol 1999:908); corneal pressure >30 mm Hg—pressures >18 mm Hg have a 65% sensitivity and specificity

Crs: Tonometry of 20–30 will have 3.5% go on to glaucoma in 5 years

Cmplc: Blindness; other eye affected within 5–10 years in 40–80%, and use of pilocarpine does not confer protection

Lab: Tonometry *Note*: Anesthetic drops used to facilitate tonometry will not take the discomfort away

ED Rx:
- Ophtho consult, with consideration of pilocarpine 1–2% drops q 5–10 minutes until relieved and systemic carbonic anhydrase inhibitor (acetazolamide 1 g IV or 0.5 g po immediately) to lower pressure
- Definitive Rx is surgical laser iridotomy (Eye 1999:613) or laser iridoplasty if within 48 hours (Eye 1999:26)

15.2 CONJUNCTIVITIS

Am J Ophthalmol 1991:2S

Cause: Bacterial 50–80% of the time, mostly pneumococcus in colder climates, consider *Staphylococcus*, *Corynebacterium*, *Haemophilus* (including Koch-Weeks bacillus), *Chlamydia* in warmer climates (Arch Ophthalmol 1966:639); viral 20% of the time—especially adenovirus; allergic, such as giant papillary conjunctivitis, which is associated with soft contact lens use, trauma, and foreign body but is truly allergic (Acta Ophthalmol Scand Suppl 1999:17)

Epidem: Second most common reason for red eye; if exclude foreign body, is 95% of the reason for a red eye

Pathophys: Obvious—inflammation of conjunctiva

Sx: Sand feeling in eye; discharge from eye(s)

Si: Conjunctival injection; PERRLA and with normal vision; allergic types with preponderance of itching

Crs: Usually clears in 3–4 days, rarely protracted unless secondary problem (foreign body), or if allergic but treating for infectious

Cmplc: Protracted course

Diff Dx: Conjunctivitis associated with paraneoplastic syndrome or inflammatory skin disease—cicatrizing conjunctivitis (Am J Ophthalmol 2000:98); hemorrhagic conjunctivitis with enterovirus 70 (Am J Epidemiol 1975:533)

Lab: None, although consider viral and bacterial cultures for atypical or severe cases

ED Rx:

- Recommend fluorescein with Wood's lamp exam for all red eyes with pain looking for corneal abrasion, also consider iritis
- *Infectious conjunctivitis*: try sulfacetamide 10%; Tm/S (Polytrim) drops are bacteriocidal rather than bacteriostatic and sting less than sulfa but cost 10× as much; neomycin/polymyxin qid; erythromycin eye ointment; gentamicin eye drops; tobramycin eye drops; not chloramphenicol which can lead to aplastic anemia, although just as efficacious (J Antimicrob Chemother 1989:261)
- *Allergic conjunctivitis* (Drugs 1992:154; Med Lett Drugs Ther 2000;42:39): consider topical ketorolac (Acular) 0.5% 1 drop qid; or topical antihistamine levocabastine (Livostin) 0.05% 1 drop qid; or mast cell stabilizers such as cromolyn (Crolom) 4% 1–2 drops OU qid; or lodoxamide (Alomide) 0.1% 1–2 drops qid; or

mast cell stabilizer/H$_1$ antihistamine olopatadine (Patanol) 0.1% 1–2 drops OU bid

15.3 CORNEAL ABRASION/FOREIGN BODY

Optom Clin 1991:119

Cause: Trauma; extended wear contact lens (Optom Clin 1991:123)

Epidem: Most common reason for red eye

Pathophys: Direct trauma or rubbing causing trauma to cornea or abrasion

Sx: Teary, red eye

Si: Usually unilateral conjunctival injection, check under upper and lower eye lids for foreign body. Metallic foreign bodies with more injection

Crs: Unremarkable if foreign body removed and timely intervention

Cmplc: Corneal ulcer, with *Pseudomonas* reported after patching (Clao J 1987:161); conjunctivitis

Diff Dx: Occult globe rupture if significant trauma

Lab: None

ED Rx:
- Topical anesthetic—this usually alleviates all the discomfort; if patient still uncomfortable, rethink this working diagnosis. If foreign body known to be under lid, may withhold topical anesthetic so that removal can be confirmed by patient's response to FB removal
- Fluorescein with Wood's lamp/slit lamp exam; may have to rinse excess fluorescein to see small abrasions

Foreign Body
- Remove foreign body with soft, cotton applicator which is moistened—touch and lift, do not rub; 25-G needle; or eye spud—remove rust ring if present with drill if available. This is a taught skill. Once removed, follow corneal abrasion instructions

Corneal Abrasion
- Antibiotic eye ointment (such as erythromycin) tid for 3 days
- Topical ketorolac 0.5% ophtho solution 4 times a day for 5 days (Ophthalmology 1997:1353) or diclofenac 0.1% eye drops 1 drop every 6 hours for 36 hours (Eye 1997:79; Ann Emerg Med 2000:131) for pain relief

- Consider mydriatic eye drops, such as 2.5% phenylephrine/1% tropicamide (Ophthalmology 1995:1936)
- Patching is equivocal (Ophthalmology 1995:1936). May provide some comfort
- Ophtho consult (may be next day) if unable to remove foreign body completely, or if not completely better in 3 days
- Home with narcotic pain meds—manipulation of eye will have significant discomfort
- Avoid contact lens use, although topical diclofenac with soft lens use (J Refract Corneal Surg 1994:640) and a bandage lens (Br J Ophthalmol 1987:285) both tried, but not advocated here as an emergency department procedure secondary to potentiating possible keratitis or ulcer

15.4 HERPETIC KERATITIS

Optom Clin 1991:45

Cause: Usually herpes simplex, but consider herpes zoster, adenovirus, and other viruses

Epidem: Excluding foreign bodies, 1% of the reason for a red eye

Pathophys: Inflammation of cornea

Sx: Photophobia; foreign body sensation

Si: Corneal ulcer; PERRLA; check under lids

Crs: Usually associated with iritis—look for ciliary flush

Cmplc: Chronic ulcers; persistent viral presence (Arch Ophthalmol 1993:522); hypopyon (white cells in anterior chamber); long-term corneal opacity to some degree (Acta Ophthalmol 1970:214)

Diff Dx: Overnight contact lens use giving infectious keratitis (Br J Ophthalmol 1998:1272); ultraviolet light exposure (Optom Vis Sci 1994:125), and UV eye drops no help (Ophthalmic Res 1998:286); exanthems; bacterial (Acad Emerg Med 1994:391, 412); chronic topical anesthetic use; bacterial and fungal keratitis after corneal transplant (Ophthalmology 1988:1450)

Lab: Consider bacterial and viral culture; perhaps PCR for HSV DNA (Can J Ophthalmol 2000:134)

ED Rx:
- Topical anesthetics will not fully relieve the discomfort
- Fluorescein with slit lamp exam may show dendrites—consistent with herpetic keratitis
- Do not patch nor instill steroids
- Immediate ophtho consult for consideration of the following: trifluridine (Viroptic) 1 drop 1% solution q 2 hours as first line; second line is ARA A; topical/oral acyclovir (Ophthalmologica 1997:29); antibacterials; cycloplegics to relax ciliary spasm such as 1% atropine bid or 5% homatropine tid

15.5 IRITIS

Postgrad Med 1989:117

Cause: Idiopathic by far the most common; iatrogenic (many causes, e.g., IV cidofovir (Arch Ophthalmol 1997:733)); autoimmune diseases (Ann Ophthalmol 1978:147) (Behçet's syndrome, RA, SLE, ankylosing spondylitis, Reiter's syndrome, Sjögren's syndrome (Arthritis Rheum 1992:560), ulcerative colitis (Gastroenterology 1967:78), Wegener's granulomatosis; tuberculosis; syphilis; histoplasmosis; sarcoid; coccidioidomycosis; toxoplasmosis; perhaps autoantibody viral related; herpes simplex; herpes zoster; CMV; Candida; hypermature cataract; trauma; intraocular tumor (Cancer 1979:1511); Whipple's disease bacterium; Hansen's disease; intranasal drug use such as cocaine (Ann Emerg Med 1991:192)

Epidem: Excluding foreign body, 2% of the reason for a red eye

Pathophys: A form of uveitis

Sx: Pain; photophobia; tearing without exudate

Si: Tenderness; visual blurring; turbid aqueous humor; low pressure; miosis—constricted pupil with pain on direct and consensual pupillary response to light (Lancet 1981:1254); circumcorneal injection—ciliary flush; have the patient accommodate with their own finger—a specific (97%) yet not sensitive (74%) test (Br Med J (Clin Res Ed) 1987:812). Do slit lamp exam with fluorescein to look for other causes; check under lids

Crs: Variable depending on etiology

Cmplc: Refractory course; rare renal-ocular syndrome with interstitial nephritis (Am J Med 1984:189)

Diff Dx: Acute angle closure glaucoma, keratitis, foreign body

Lab: None

ED Rx:
- Ophtho consult immediately—will consider topical steroids and cycloplegics
- Future role of prostaglandin synthetase inhibitors, including NSAIDs (Arch Ophthalmol 1980:1106; Fortschr Ophthalmol 1987:353)

15.6 RUPTURED GLOBE

Int Ophthalmol Clin 1995:71

Cause: Usually traumatic

Epidem: Uncommon; usually a male in third or fourth decade of life; ETOH a risk with leisure time activities (Ophthalmologica 1999:380)

Pathophys: Usually ruptures at site of muscular insertion if not readily apparent on exam

Sx: Eye pain; visual loss

Si: Complete hyphema; protrusion of globe contents; loss of usual globe contours; perform a careful eye exam without instilling any medicines into eye

Crs: Visual recovery is usually scant

Cmplc: Vision loss

Diff Dx: Foreign body in anterior chamber (Ophthalmic Surg 1985:586)

Lab: Facial/head CT (AJNR Am J Neuroradiol 1995:936)

Rx:
- Metallic or plastic eye shield
- Keep head of bed elevated
- NPO
- Consider broadspectrum IV antibiotics, and update tetanus as in any trauma if needed
- Immediate ophthalmology consult

OPHTHALMOLOGY

15.7 SUDDEN VISION LOSS (TRAUMATIC)

Acad Emerg Med 1996:1056; Neurol Clin 1998:323

Cause: Trauma to the optic nerve—laceration, contusion, compression; retinal detachment; retinal hemorrhage. Trauma to the globe or lens (see 15.6)

Epidem: Uncommon, but must be able to recognize

Pathophys: Optic nerve compression, retinal detachment, and retinal hemorrhage can be reversible if limited involvement. Optic nerve laceration and contusion usually with irreversible vision loss

Sx: Pain; loss of vision; retinal detachments may simulate flashing lights

Si: Trauma to the globe either penetrating or blunt; look for abnormality to the retina and vitreous humor

Crs: As above

Cmplc: Vision loss

Diff Dx: Atraumatic causes (much more common): orbital (see 10.5) or sinus (see 17.11) infection (Laryngoscope 1984:1050); CVA (see 13.2)—e.g., amaurosis fugax; migraine (see 13.9); hypertensive crisis (see 2.5); cerebral blindness; ischemic optic neuropathy, central retinal artery or vein occlusion (J Neurol Neurosurg Psychiatry 1993:234); optic neuritis; uveitis; ectopia lentis; toxins such as methanol or quinine (Ann Emerg Med 1987:98); acute cataract formation; rheumatologic disorders such as giant cell arteritis (Semin Ophthalmol 1999:109) or SLE

Lab: Facial/head CT; MRI if available

ED Rx:
- Update tetanus if needed
- NPO
- IV pain control if needed
- Immediate ophthalmology consult for consideration of emergency orbital decompression (Otolaryngol Head Neck Surg 1981:252)
- Minor retinal detachments and minor retinal hemorrhages may have next day follow-up after discussion with ophthalmologist

16 Orthopedics

16.1 BURSITIS/TENDONITIS

Med Sci Sports Exerc 1998:1183

Cause: Inflammation of bursa or tendons; may be infectious in etiology—especially olecranon and prepatellar areas (see 16.5)

Epidem: Common

Pathophys: Overuse or acute stress phenomenon; multifocal bursitis may be associated with homozygous homocystinuria (J Inherit Metab Dis 1999:185)

Sx: Pain of specific joint; remember referred pain such as neck to any location in upper extremity, back to hip, hip to knee, etc.

Si: Pain with palpation in bursitis; pain with range of motion in tendonitis—have patient hold specific position in opposition to your force to isolate specific area; Finkelstein's test in de Quervain's tendonitis

Crs: Acute with resolution within 2 weeks, or chronic if more protracted

Cmplc: Chronic pain

Diff Dx: Arthritis; ligamentous sprain; rarely due to sea urchin spines, which do not resolve until spines removed (Joint Bone Spine 2000:94)

Lab: Consider plain radiographs if suspicious for significant fracture. Consider needle aspiration if nonprosthetic joint to ascertain etiology

ED Rx:
- Inject with anesthetic agent (lidocaine, bupivacaine) and steroids—pro study of anserine bursitis (South Med J 2000:207), equivocal for shoulder tendonitis (Scand J Rheumatol 1985:76) and perhaps negative for Achilles tendonitis (Clin J Sport Med 1996:245); tendonitis (such as de Quervain's) does not have to have injection into tendon sheath to be effective

- Splinting of shoulder or elbow (tennis elbow) for example—if using sling, be sure to have daily shoulder movements to avoid adhesive capsulitis. Heel cup for plantar fasciitis or Achilles tendonitis (Br J Sports Med 1981:117)
- Ice for 24 hours
- Acetaminophen and NSAIDs about equal efficacy in traumatic situations (Curr Opin Rheumatol 2000:150), NSAIDs better in inflammatory realms (RA, gout, etc.); IM ketorolac as efficacious as po ibuprofen (Acad Emerg Med 1998:118; Ann Emerg Med 1995:117)
- Dimethyl sulfoxide of no help (Med Sci Sports Exerc 1981:215)

16.2 DISLOCATIONS

Cause: Usually traumatic, although those with joint laxity due to connective tissue disorder may need minimal trauma. Less force needed for recurrent injuries. In peds, remember to consider child abuse. Consider complication of seizure

Epidem: Variable

Pathophys: If fracture of joint surface, may go on to arthritis

Sx: Pain; deformity

Si: Tenderness; decreased to no range of motion of affected joint; deformity—palpate location of dislocated part; check distal neurovascular status

Crs: Reduction curative, coincident fracture may prolong rehabilitation

Cmplc: Fracture, neurovascular damage

Lab: Plain radiographs—2 pictures 90° from each other. The Y-view in shoulder dislocations is key. Postreduction views are standard, yet necessity in some areas (shoulder (Ann Emerg Med 1996:399)) has been questioned

ED Rx:
- IV access for pain control
- Local block such as digital, radial nerve, or median nerve if feasible
- Ortho consult for all dislocations with neurologic or vascular compromise
- Conscious sedation with midazolam should be considered for large joints such as ankle, elbow, shoulder, etc.

- Steady and gradual traction over 2–5 minutes is more effective than more force attempted quickly
- Get postreduction films

Specific examples:

Ankle

Obvious deformity should be reduced if possible to prevent skin tearing/breakdown. Most of these have coincident fractures. Most fracture fragments will move during reduction; patient should be well sedated so that there is minimal muscle tension during the maneuver to avoid injury to the articular cartilage

Digit

Digital block, being sure to infiltrate the dorsal surface on the hand and the plantar surface on the foot to get a complete block. Reduction should first have outward traction in the direction of the long axis of the dislocated phalanx. With your other hand, move the base of the dislocated bone towards its natural position. Then move the long axis of the phalanx to its natural neutral position, so that the digit is now normally aligned

Elbow

Five types of elbow dislocations. Peds: nursemaid elbow dislocations are pediatric dislocations of the radial head, and these are uncommon in adults. To reduce a pediatric nursemaid elbow, place your thumb over the radial head, extend the elbow and supinate the forearm, and then flex the forearm. A pop may be felt/heard. Adult: the elbow may dislocate posteriorly (most common), anteriorly, laterally, or medially, or the radius and ulna may diverge laterally and medially, respectively. Reduction may be accomplished with conscious sedation, having an assistant anchor the humerus, distract the elbow, and guide the proximal forearm bones around the humeral condyles. Bring the elbow into flexion once the olecranon/radius is felt to reseat, and apply posterior splint with elbow at 90° flexion. Ligamentous injury is common (Clin Orthop 1987:221), but conservative treatment is usually adequate (Clin Orthop 1987:165)

Hip

Done with ortho; posterior dislocations are more common

Knee

A true ortho emergency; the popliteal artery is at large risk with a knee dislocation. Reduction should be done with ortho involved; splint in position of comfort. Consider arteriogram

Patella

Lateral more common than medial. Completely extend knee, which may reduce patella. If not, keep the knee extended while attempting the following. Put thumbs at medial edge if medial dislocation and lateral edge if lateral dislocation, and gently push towards anatomic alignment; may need to lift leading edge with fingers just a little

Shoulder

Med Sci Sports Exerc 1984:444; Am J Emerg Med 1999:288)

May dislocate anterior, inferior, or posterior. Associated compression fracture of the humeral head is called a Hill-Sachs deformity. Some general reduction principles: 1) the patient needs to be relaxed; 2) distract the humerus so that the humeral head can slip past the glenoid rim; 3) sometimes guiding the humeral head directly is needed as distraction is being applied; 4) 3 cc of 2% lidocaine in the affected shoulder joint can bring about significant relief (sterile prep and injection); and 5) bring the arm to the patient's side, elbow 90° of flexion, and immobilize in this position once reduction completed

• Anterior dislocation (Am J Emerg Med 1991:180): methods include. 1) Weight (aka Stimson or Wait)—patient prone with 10 lb of weight wrapped to freely hanging arm, reduction accomplished over time—this is a good wilderness rescue technique. One variation is with patient sitting in chair with arm draped over backrest and hanging straight down (Injury 1992:479). 2) Hippocratic variation: patient supine and anchored with one sheet wrapped around affected axilla for countertraction and reducer grasps elbow, which is flexed to 90° with forearm pointing to ceiling. Distract the humerus—original method was with physician's heel in patient's axilla as countertraction, but can either put other sheet around you and tie off to patient's elbow and lean back, or just hold elbow in antecubital fossa firmly. Walk the humerus into abduction, and gently externally and internally rotate. 3) Scapular rotation (Ann Emerg Med 1992:1349): patient prone (supine if necessary (Ann Emerg Med 1996:92)), weights in hand, rotate the inferior scapular pole medially and superiorly until reduced. 4) External rotation (Jacep 1979:528): patient is supine, humerus is completely adducted, elbow at 90° with forearm pointing to ceiling, slowly and gently externally rotate the shoulder. 5) Walk (Milch) (J Trauma 1992:801): patient supine, bring the arm from adduction with 90°

elbow flexion to full abduction with external rotation while gently walking it to this position. 6) The backstroke: begin with patient supine, arm in adduction with elbow at 0°, gently walk the arm to 180° of forward flexion, as if doing a swimming backstroke

• Inferior dislocation (Instr Course Lect 1985:232): significant trauma. Patient is supine; place the sheet over the shoulder for countertraction; the arm vector for reduction is approximately 180° abduction. May truly be irreducible with closed technique

• Posterior dislocation: patient supine; vector for reduction is the long axis of humerus with arm adducted

16.3 FRACTURE MANAGEMENT

Emerg Med Clin North Am 2000:85, vi

Cause: Usually traumatic, possibly due to child abuse in children, or osteogenesis imperfecta as underlying cause in children with multiple fractures and low-intensity trauma, pathologic fractures in people with either neoplastic or other chronic diseases such as TB in which the bone is abnormal, and more common in the elderly or in those with impaired mobility due to osteoporosis; a difficult diagnosis is that of stress fractures where repetitive forces may cause X-ray–negative fractures. Be sure to screen the whole patient in the setting of multisytem trauma, and look for syncope or other comorbid illnesses in the elderly or those with chronic diseases

Epidem: Common

Pathophys: Bony anatomy core knowledge includes bony landmarks (e.g., the trochanteric area in the hip is the basis for our hip fracture descriptions) and remembering that pediatric bones will a have growth plate (physis)—with regard to the physis, the segment at the end of the bone with the joint cartilage is called the epiphysis, and the segment towards the major portion of the bone mass is called the metaphysis. Transverse or oblique fractures usually due to uniform load without rotation, whereas spiral fractures associated with a rotational force to the bone. Children may have fractures involving the physis that are called Salter fractures:

- Salter I is a fracture through the complete physis and may not show on initial X-ray
- Salter II is the physis with a portion of the metaphysis
- Salter III is a portion of the epiphysis and physis
- Salter IV is an oblique fracture through the physis so that the fracture segment has both metaphysis and epiphysis
- Salter V is a compression injury of the physis and may not show on initial X-ray

When *describing fractures*, we need to be specific in the following areas:
- Bone involved
- Displacement of bones from their usual anatomic location
- Angulation from their normal anatomic angle
- Look for secondary dislocation
- Assess overlying skin tension
- Assess peripheral vascular and neurologic function

Specific Considerations

OTTAWA ANKLE RULES

Jama 1993:1127 (see Figure 16.1)

Patients aged 18 years or older (may be applicable to older children (Acad Emerg Med 1999:1005)) may have ankle or foot radiographs based on some basic triage criteria (100% sensitive for significant fracture) which are the following:
- Injury is 10 days old or less
- Not a reassessment

OTTAWA KNEE RULE

Ann Emerg Med 1995:405

Patients 18 years or older should have plain X-rays of the knee for acute knee injury for any of the following (95% sensitivity and specificity for significant fracture (Jama 1996:611)):
- Age ≥55 years old
- Tenderness at head of fibula
- Isolated patella tenderness
- Inability to flex knee to 90°
- Inability to bear weight for 4 steps immediately and in the ED

Sx: History of trauma; pain, usually with pinpoint location to affected bone; obvious deformity. Referred pain—knee pain in hip fractures is common (Ann Emerg Med 1997:418)

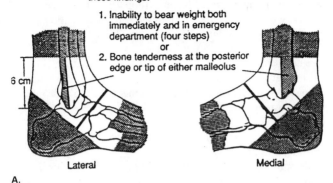

An ankle x-ray series is only necessary if there is pain near the malleoli and any of these findings:

1. Inability to bear weight both immediately and in emergency department (four steps)
   or
2. Bone tenderness at the posterior edge or tip of either malleolus

6 cm

Lateral   Medial

A.

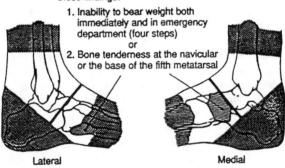

A foot x-ray series is only necessary if there is pain in the midfoot and any of these findings:

1. Inability to bear weight both immediately and in emergency department (four steps)
   or
2. Bone tenderness at the navicular or the base of the fifth metatarsal

Lateral   Medial

B.

Figure 16.1. A. Refined clinical decision rule for ankle radiographic series in ankle injury patients. **B.** Refined clinical decision rule for foot radiographic series in ankle injury patients. (Reproduced with permission from Stiell IG, et al., Decision rules for the use of radiography in acute ankle injuries. Jama 1993;269:1130.)

Si: Tenderness; edema; ecchymoses; angulation; crepitus; tendon or ligamentous instability about specific joint; perhaps auscultatory percussion in hip fractures (Clin Orthop 1977:9)—place stethoscope over the pubic symphysis, percuss over the patella one at a time, and an ipsilateral fracture should have decreased sound conduction

Crs: Extremely variable depending on what type of fracture, the cause, and patient's overall health. Osteoporotic fractures may not be amenable to reduction or repair, and therapy should be tailored towards osteoporosis treatment (including exercise (Br J Sports Med 1999:378))

Cmplc: Non-union; open fracture (skin not intact); vascular or neurologic compromise

Diff Dx: Rupture of ligaments with or without avulsion injury; tendon rupture (elbow (Orthop Clin North Am 1999:95))

Lab:
- Potential need for CBC with diff, PT/PTT, metabolic profile, type and screen, EKG if patient needs operative repair and has age-related anesthesia concerns
- X-ray: plain radiographs (facial (AJR Am J Roentgenol 1983:587)), and children may need comparison views from the contralateral side, although utility of comparison views controversial (Ann Emerg Med 1992:895); with CT if unable to adequately assess if true fracture (such as femoral head cortical fracture (AJR Am J Roentgenol 1990:93)) and would be operative repair (as seen in some hip fractures) or if need further detail delineation (facial fractures), or if vertebral body fracture and assessing for retropulsion or posterior element involvement. Simple mandibular views as good as pantomographic for mandibular fractures (Acad Emerg Med 2000:141). Special rib films are not clinically indicated, but chest films are helpful to look for associated injuries with complaint of traumatic rib pain (AJR Am J Roentgenol 1982:91). Algorithms for CT dependent on area in question; e.g., Le Fort facial fractures use coronal CT, whereas zygoma with axial (AJNR Am J Neuroradiol 1991:861); give the radiologist clinical info

ED Rx:
- Immediate pain control, consider IV access or appropriate block—do block only after distal neurovascular exam is completed
- NPO
- Splint, with traction splint (Hare, Sager) for femur fractures

- Ice
- If possible, reduce to anatomic alignment fractures causing vascular compromise, and get postreduction films
- Any fracture with neurologic or vascular compromise needs immediate ortho referral
- Open fractures need IV ABX (cefazolin), update Td if needed, and ortho referral
- Fractures that involve articular surfaces (<24°) need urgent ortho follow-up
- If no fracture, treatment of contusion/sprain/strain based on clinical grounds with splint, immobilization, ice, elevation, NSAIDs, and/or po narcotics; 2–4 week f/u

Specific Considerations

Fractures of weight-bearing joints/bones need to be assessed carefully; approach these with the consideration that ortho should be immediately involved in all of these:

- *Toe digits*: reduce if angulated, ortho referral if joint space involved or unable to reduce; Rx with buddy tape and/or cast boot
- *Foot* (Semin Roentgenol 1994:152; Radiol Clin North Am 1997:655): look carefully for tarsal-metatarsal dislocations (Lisfranc's (Clin Orthop 1963:116; Radiology 1976:79)), a transverse fracture of the fifth metatarsal (Jones Fracture (J Bone Joint Surg [Am] 1978:776)), and for calcaneal fractures—these necessitate immediate ortho referral. Other fractures will be referred based on extent of injury and may need further studies or perhaps second radiographic opinion to decide on extent of injury such as fifth metatarsal avulsion fractures. If no immediate referral, splint/cast boot and 1–2 week follow-up
- *Ankle* (Curr Opin Pediatr 2000:52): ankle fractures are classified on which malleoli (lateral—fibula, medial—tibia, posterior—tibia) are involved and whether or not the mortise is intact. Most significant is the lateral malleolus; a lone lateral malleolus fracture may have an abnormal mortise view with ankle instability because the deltoid (tibial-calcaneal) ligament is ruptured on the medial side—although isolated anterior talofibular sprain with inversion ankle injury is very common (Foot Ankle Int 2000:138). All unstable ankle fractures need ortho referral, whereas chip fractures are managed as moderate to severe sprains as long as no clinical or radiographic instability exists. Ankle taping helps with proprioception (Med Sci Sports Exerc 2000:10)

ORTHOPEDICS

- *Tibia*: tibia fractures need to be non-weight-bearing for Rx, and proximal tibia metaphysis fractures may have an arterial injury as well, especially with valgus angulation. Tibial shaft fractures associated with ligamentous injury to the ipsilateral knee (J Bone Joint Surg [Am] 1989:1392). Ortho referral/outpatient follow-up based on degree of injury/patient discomfort
- *Fibula*: if they do not involve the ankle joint, they usually do very well. Individual preference as far as splinting and outpatient follow-up
- *Knee* (Emerg Med Clin North Am 2000:67, v): look carefully for tibial plateau fractures and intercondylar eminence fractures (tibia), the latter being the attachment of the anterior cruciate ligament. Patellar fractures and tibial tubercle fractures can sometimes be difficult to judge, as normal variants may show separate osseous bodies in these locations. The knee can suffer significant ligamentous and internal derangement without bony fracture, and those with traumatic hemarthroses or ligamentous instability should have ortho referral (Injury 1984:96). Remember to assess for vascular compromise if displaced fracture or dislocation of the knee. The aforementioned fractures and all epiphyseal fractures also need ortho referral
- *Femur*: the femoral shaft fracture may lead to local hemorrhage with a hematoma collection of ~1 L not being unusual—use a traction splint (Injury 1973:35) (e.g., Hare, Sager) to stabilize femur. Hip fractures (J Trauma 1970:51; Am J Orthop 1999:497) include femoral head, femoral neck, intertrochanteric fractures, and subtrochanteric fractures—these are sometimes difficult to diagnose; look carefully at the trabeculation pattern—it should be uninterrupted. Also look carefully for wedge-shaped defects in the head of the femur and consider AVN. In adolescents, consider slipped capital femoral epiphysis (SCFE); correlation noted in those that are obese (Clin Orthop 1996:8). Ortho referral for all of these, and those with femoral neck fractures do better if operation within 12 hours (Injury 1992:83). Prevent hip fractures with fall prevention, treatment of bony disease, and hip protectors (Am J Orthop 1998:407)
- *Pelvis* (Emerg Med Clin North Am 2000:1, v): the ring usually breaks in two spots; search for the second when seeing the first—diastasis of the pubic symphysis may be the second fracture location. Hemorrhage, bladder rupture, and urethral injury are

potential major complications of pelvic fractures. Look for associated fractures in the hip; if blood is seen at the urethral opening, do a urethrogram to document an intact urethra before placing a urinary catheter. Ortho referral for anything more than ramus (not including the acetabulum!), coccyx, or pubic symphysis fractures with no other problems, although general surgery or interventional radiology may need to be involved for unstable patients as well (Am Surg 1998:862). Geriatric patients have problems with this fracture secondary to other comorbid problems (Am J Emerg Med 1997:576). X-rays not necessary in neurologically and hemodynamically intact adults with blunt trauma, negative physical exam, and no anemia (J Trauma 1995:722)

- *Vertebral body*: traumatic vertebral fractures, those with retropulsion of the body fragments (Neurosurgery 1979:250) and those with rotational fracture-dislocation (J Bone Joint Surg [Am] 1970:1115) or posterior element involvement, should have CT imaging (J Bone Joint Surg [Am] 1978:1108) to look at the spinal canal, although those with single-level and minimal anterior compression would probably do OK with just plain films. BAFL (big air, fractured lumbar) is a term coined with regard to those who snowboard and have minimal and single-level anterior compression fractures. Transverse fracture through a vertebral body is a Chance fracture, and is associated with seatbelt use (Am J Roentgenol Radium Ther Nucl Med 1971:844). The cervical spine has special issues (see 26.2). Neurosurgical referral

- *Rib*: rib fractures should be used as markers for associated injuries: 1) look for associated pneumo- or hemothorax on chest films; 2) high rib fractures (1–3) may be associated with great vessel injury and look for widened mediastinum, pleural effusions, or associated history and physical to decide on further testing, e.g., CT, TEE, aortogram (Ann Thorac Surg 1983:450); 3) low rib (9–12) fractures may have associated local organ injury, e.g., diaphragm, kidneys, liver, or spleen; 4) multiple rib fractures in a row have a higher likelihood of underlying lung injury (flail chest is three or more adjacent ribs fractured each in two or more locations and moving counter to the rest of the chest wall); 5) three or more rib fractures in general associated with a higher likelihood of other significant injuries (J Trauma 1990:689). If secondary injuries, appropriate referral. Rib belts do convey some comfort (Am J Emerg Med

1990:277). For those with severe pain, intercostal, interpleural (J Emerg Med 1994:441), or epidural block may be used

- *Clavicle*: "A clavicle fracture will heal as long as both ends are in the same room" (Anon). If no complications from the fracture (underlying vessel injury rare (J Trauma 2000:316)), then primary care outpatient follow-up after sling and swathe. Figure 8 immobilization is controversial
- *Scapula*: most significant as marker of significant trauma; look for associated injuries. Glenoid, coracoid, and acromion fractures with ortho referral; others may sling if no other associated problems and outpatient ortho follow-up
- *Shoulder*: this implies the humeral head (anatomic neck) and be sure to exclude coincident dislocation (J Trauma 1999:318). Most of these fractures are treated with shoulder immobilization (via spica splint or prepackaged tool), but those with rotation of the humeral head may necessitate immediate surgical intervention. Both anatomic neck and surgical neck fractures are at risk for AVN to the head of the humerus, especially if rotation of the humeral head has occurred—those with rotation or displacement need immediate ortho referral; otherwise 1–2-day follow-up OK
- *Humerus*: humeral shaft fractures are usually managed nonoperatively despite how significant the X-rays may look. Radial nerve palsy may occur in 10–20% of people, and most of those resolve without operative intervention. Due to the fact that a radial nerve injury may occur with manipulation/splinting, ortho consult for all of these even for splinting
- *Elbow* (Emerg Med Clin North Am 1999:843, vi): we usually speak of intercondylar fractures in adults and supracondylar fractures in children as being significant here. Radial head fractures may occur, and are usually treated with a posterior splint plus a sling and 1-week ortho follow-up. In an adult, a simple nondisplaced condylar fracture can be posterior splinted with 1-week follow-up, but any displacement or rotation of the condyles necessitates immediate ortho referral. In children, a supracondylar fracture may go on to a myriad of problems (neurologic (Orthop Clin North Am 1999:91), vascular (Int Angiol 1995:307), non-union, etc.) so get ortho involved early for even nondisplaced fractures. If a posterior fat pad or billowing anterior fat pad is seen (Injury 1978:297), treat as an occult elbow fracture if none is obvious

- *Radius/ulna*: a partnership (Emerg Med Clin North Am 1992:133). If you see an isolated fracture of either bone, look carefully at the complete length of its partner. Look carefully at the radial styloid and radial-ulnar joint on the radiographs to be sure fractures or disruptions have not occurred here—minimal injuries here can have significant consequences and necessitate urgent ortho referral. Any radius/ulna fracture with more than ~10° of angulation or greater than 25% displacement needs ortho consult. Specifics: Monteggia's fracture is an isolated proximal ulna fracture with a radial head dislocation; a Galeazzi fracture is a distal radius fracture with a distal radial-ulna joint dislocation; a Colles fracture is a distal radial metaphysis fracture/ulna styloid fracture with dorsal angulation of the fractured segment; a Smith fracture is a distal radial metaphysis fracture with volar angulation. A risk factor for distal radius/ulna fracture is being left-handed, or being naturally left-handed but forced to be right-handed (Am J Epidemiol 1994:361)
- *Carpal bones* (Emerg Med Clin North Am 1993:703): proximal row radial to ulna is scaphoid, lunate, triquetrum, and pisiform over triquetrum, with the second row radius to ulna as trapezium, trapezoid, capitate, and hamate. All fractures here may be difficult to diagnose on plain radiographs, and the most important fractures are to the lunate and scaphoid. The scaphoid crosses both rows, which makes it more susceptible to injury. To the radial side of the scaphoid is a triangular soft tissue density that is disrupted if the scaphoid is fractured (variable reliability). Both of these fractures can go on to AVN (AVN of lunate is Kienböck's disease), so thumb spica splint if clinically suspected with ortho follow-up in 3–7 days. Some advocate slight extension when splinting for scaphoid fractures (J Bone Joint Surg Br 1999:91). Fractures of the pisiform and hook of the hamate may sometimes be diagnosed with a reverse oblique X-ray, where the wrist is angled toward supination (J Emerg Med 1998:445). Wrist guards do help prevent these and distal forearm fractures (Ann Emerg Med 1997:766)
- *Metacarpals* (Occup Med 1998:549): most important to assess the cascade (rotational alignment) if fracture noted in the shaft or neck; have the patient bring the fingers to the palm with the nail beds showing. Trade names: fifth metacarpal neck fracture known as boxer's fracture and thumb metacarpal fracture involving the metacarpal-carpal joint is a Bennett fracture—a Bennett fracture needs immediate ortho referral. Most metacarpal fractures can be

treated in a radial or ulnar gutter splint with 1–2-week follow-up. Immediate ortho referral for fractures that are cleanly transverse (these have a predisposition to rotate), if the shafts are rotated more than 15° of angulation of second or third metacarpals, or more than 30° of angulation of fourth or fifth metacarpals

• *Hand digits*: articular surface fractures should be reduced and referred urgently to ortho; shaft fractures that are transverse or comminuted require a radial or ulnar gutter splint. Trade names: chip fracture of distal phalanx at the extensor tendon insertion is a mallet finger—splint this joint (DIP) in extension for 2–3 months and refer for ortho follow-up

• *Mandibular*: mandibular fractures are common, and the decision for admission versus outpatient follow-up (next day) has to do with whether the patients can protect their airway and the amount of displacement. To clinically diagnose, look for facial asymmetry and malocclusion, and have patient bite on a tongue depressor placed over the molars (one side at a time) (Am J Emerg Med 1998:304); if patient can oppose you twisting the tongue depressor so that it breaks, then most likely not a fracture; if cannot oppose, a fracture more likely. More than 25% displacement, or if the airway appears to be at risk (inability to swallow or control the tongue), then the patient should be admitted. Remove loose teeth from fracture site unless essential for splinting, clear liquids only, next day follow-up if discharged from ED

• *Facial bones* (Plast Reconstr Surg 1979:26): these are fractures of the zygoma, orbital floor, maxilla, mandible, and nasal bones (in descending order (J Trauma 1989:388)), and others (cribiform plate, pterygoids, etc.). Look for cranial nerve deficits and facial asymmetry for keys to correct diagnoses. Maxilla fractures carry the Le Fort classification (Plast Reconstr Surg 1980:54), and other midface variations also occur (Int J Oral Surg 1980:92); maxillofacial surgeons should be consulted when suspected—the upper dental plate will move independent of the rest of the head. Orbital floor fractures may show entrapment of an intraocular muscle clinically, and look for secondary globe trauma—ophtho consult, but they usually advocate delayed repair for isolated orbital floor fractures. The zygoma may show a fracture line, but always compare the contralateral side and look for cheek flattening of affected side. Nasal fractures if isolated and closed do not need X-rays, but the diagnosis of open fracture can be made with having the patient gently blow out their nose while occluding both nares—if air escapes through an open wound, this is an open fracture. Epistaxis is seen in zygoma fractures, nasal bone fractures, and cribiform plate fractures—put bloody nasal discharge on gauze and see if halo of clear fluid encompasses the spot of blood; if so, this is a CSF leak, and consult neurosurgery. No correlation of facial fractures with closed head injury (if closed head injury not clinically suspected) except for those in car accidents—they have a 1.5 increased risk for closed head injury (Ann Emerg Med 1988:6). Conversely, facial fractures do not help prevent injuries to the brain (Arch Surg 1999:14)

16.4 GOUT/PSEUDOGOUT

Curr Opin Rheumatol 1999:1; Am J Med 1967:322; Radiology 1977:1

Cause:
- *Gout* is hyperuricemia due to two possible reasons—either a transferase deficiency (possibly genetic with sporadic penetrance), or increased tissue breakdown (Arthritis Rheum 1965:765) and/or decreased renal tubular excretion of urate. White blood cells may ingest the crystals, but the main problem is then deposition of uric acid in joints and other tissues
- *Pseudogout* is calcium pyrophosphate crystal deposition

Epidem:
- *Gout* due to a transferase deficiency is seen 20:1 male:female, with males affected in fourth decade of life, females postmenopausal. The secondary type is seen in those with leukemia (especially if treated), polycythemia, hemolytic anemia, starvation, diuretic Rx, lead ingestion (N Engl J Med 1981:520), and alcoholics due to increased urate production and perhaps decreased excretion
- *Pseudogout* has an increased incidence in neuropathic joints, hemochromatosis, hypothyroidism, hypomagnesemia, hyperparathyroidism, gout, RA, and osteoarthritis

Pathophys:
- *Gout* depends on uric acid physiology. Uric acid is normally 100% filtered, 100% resorbed, and 100% excreted in distal tubule. This may be competitively inhibited by lactate, ETOH, and ketone bodies; perhaps increase in uric acid production correlating with

hypertriglyceridemia (Metabolism 1989:698). Podagra comes from traumatically increased synovial fluid from which water is resorbed at night faster than urate, leading to a gouty attack
• *Pseudogout* occurs with polyingestion of crystals resulting in enzyme release in the joint and subsequent inflammation

Sx:
• *Gout*: family history (50%); podagra (84%)—inflammation of first MCP joint of big toe; low-dose ASA (<4 g) precipitates or worsens
• *Gout* or *pseudogout*: other painful arthritides

Si:
• *Gout*: podagra; tophi of ear > elbow > finger > foot
• *Pseudogout*: arthritis of knee > MCP > wrist > shoulder

Crs: Acute gouty attacks last 1–14 days, symptom free between attacks but with increasing frequency over the years; without treatment permanent damage ensues

Cmplc: *Gout*: osteoarthritis; no increase in *pseudogout*; renal stones, but the nephropathy is only associated with lead-related gout

Diff Dx:
• *Gout*: sarcoid arthritis that also improves with colchicine; Reiter's syndrome; septic arthritis; RA; pseudogout: osteoarthritis; Lesch-Nyhan syndrome—choreoathetosis, dystonic spasticity, self-mutilation
• *Pseudogout*: calcium oxalate deposition in renal failure, septic arthritis (Jama 1979:1768)

Lab:
• *Gout*: hyperuricemia nonspecific and is seen in idiopathic without gout, hemolysis, leukemia, diuretics, psoriasis, Fanconi syndrome, chronic beryllium disease, Down syndrome (and never get gout), starvation, lead poisoning, and alcoholism. False hypouricemia seen with ASA, allopurinol, and X-ray dyes; false hyperuricemia with methyldopa and L-dopa. Perhaps serum creatinine to assess renal function before initiating colchicine (J Rheumatol 1991:264) and hypophosphatemia secondary to impaired renal tubular phosphate transport (Nephron 1992:142)
1) *Joint fluid* with long thin urate crystals, some inside WBCs, negatively birefringent
2) *X-ray* with soft tissue swelling, possible erosions
3) *24-hour urine* for uric acid ≥1 g

- *Pseudogout*: with joint fluid showing rhomboid and positively birefringent crystals; may be small enough to require oil immersion lens. X-ray with semilunar calcifications of joint cartilages

ED Rx:

Gout

- Colchicine 0.6 mg po q 1 hour up to 7 mg, or IV dosing of 1 mg q 12 hours (J Clin Pharmacol J New Drugs 1969:410; Jama 1987:1920)
- ACTH 80 IU IM/IV then 40 mg 12 hours later, especially if symptoms >1 week

Gout and Pseudogout

- Indomethacin 50 mg po tid or qid, then rapid 1-week taper
- Intra-articular or systemic steroids

Gout Prevention

- Colchicine 1–2 mg po qd (Arthritis Rheum 1974:609)
- Probenecid 1–3 grams po qd divided, start with 0.5 g—prevents resorption and good if 24-hour urine with urate <600 mg
- Sulfinpyrazone 800 mg po divided—same conditions for use as probenecid
- Allopurinol 200–400 mg po qd if 24-hour urine with urate >600 mg, or renal disease and if failure of probenecid (Am J Hosp Pharm 1989:1813)—decrease dose to 100 mg qd in anuria to prevent rash/fever/hepatitis syndrome, or tophi; can precipitate attack

16.5 SEPTIC ARTHRITIS

J Am Geriatr Soc 1985:170; Rheum Dis Clin North Am 1997:239; J Rheumatol 1999:663

Cause: Immunosuppression, chronic joint disease, overlying skin disease or artificial joint as template for *Staphylococcus* or other gram-positive bacteria to infect, although gram-negatives and anaerobes seen in those with joint replacements or if elderly

Epidem: ~30% incidence in those >60 years of age; 1–2% risk in those with joint prosthesis; decreased *Haemophilus influenza* type B infection with vaccination (J Bone Joint Surg Br 1998:471)

Pathophys: Either direct introduction through skin or hematogenous spread of offending organisms to joint space

Sx: Painful joint; fevers; chills

Si: Red hot joint with palpable effusion

Crs: Sepsis if unrecognized/untreated

Cmplc: Septic shock; may occur in the setting of gout or pseudogout (J Rheumatol 1983:503)

Diff Dx: Hip and children: transient synovitis (Ann Emerg Med 1992:1418)—physical exam and laboratory evaluation rarely helpful and consider diagnostic aspiration by ortho consult. Rarely *Mycobacterium marinum* (J Cutan Med Surg 1999:218)

Lab:

- CBC with diff; ESR; blood cultures; tap bursa for Gram's stain and culture
- *Joint fluid* with low viscosity, poor mucin clot, usually 80–200 K WBCs/mm^3 but 95% with >20 K, >75% of WBCs are polys, low glucose, positive Gram's stain and culture—consider anaerobic cultures, especially if monoarticular or history of puncture wound (Ann Emerg Med 1981:315)
- *X-ray* (AJR Am J Roentgenol 1995:399): consider radiographs for osteomyelitis/erosion evaluation, perhaps U/S of hip in children if effusion is suspected; bone scan if plain films equivocal

ED Rx:

Bursitis

J R Soc Med 1999:516

- Keep open, consider drain
- Antibiotics such as cephalexin, dicloxacillin, or erythromycin—IV antibiotics such as cefazolin considered if lymphangitis; IV antibiotics advised if systemic response to infection
- Pain control: acetaminophen, NSAIDs, narcotics
- Next day follow-up, ortho consult/admission if lymphangitis or worse clinical picture

Arthritis

- Aspirate joint—ortho referral for aspiration if joint is prosthetic
- Irrigate joint if septic; consider ortho referral so that done in OR
- IV antibiotics: cefazolin (Ancef); consider antipseudomonal coverage if diabetes mellitus or sickle cell history—such as ciprofloxacin (J Infect Dis 1985:291)
- Perhaps NSAIDs of some benefit if due to *S. aureus* (J Orthop Res 1997:919)
- Consult ortho/medicine for admission, early mobilization for hand joints (Ann Plast Surg 1999:623, discussion, 628)

17 Otolaryngology

17.1 BAROTRAUMA

Am Fam Physician 1992:1777

Cause: Direct blows to the external ear with pressure wave damage to the middle ear (Tm); closed space bomb explosion (Am J Otol 1993:92); rapid changes in atmospheric pressure as seen in nonpressurized aircraft, scuba diving (Ear Nose Throat J 1999:181, 184, 186, passim), or hyperbaric (dive) chambers (Undersea Hyperb Med 1999:243)

Epidem: Common in scuba divers, with pulmonary barotrauma seen in those with lung cysts or end-expiratory flow limitation (Thorax 1998:S20)

Pathophys: Rapid changes in pressure can cause systemic effects from higher to lower pressure gas phase shifts. Association with closed space bomb explosion conveys significant injury possibilities for patient. Middle ear perforation benign in scuba diving, but inner ear perforation can lead to inner ear dysfunction problems such as hearing loss, dizziness, tinnitus, and vertigo

Sx: Ear pain, sinus pain, chest pain, difficulty breathing, abdominal pain

Si: Tm perforation is both sensitive and specific for barotrauma—unless Valsalva or other pressure-equalizing phenomenon has occurred, including myringotomy tubes (Stein, M.; 4/6/88). Hypesthesia in the infraorbital area on ipsilateral maxillary barotrauma (Undersea Hyperb Med 1999:257). Also look for subcutaneous emphysema, subconjunctival hemorrhage, absence of breath sounds over usual lung fields, lack of bowel sounds with peritoneal signs—perforation

Crs: Extremely variable, with full spectrum of simple Tm perforation to multiple organ breaches—lung, bowel, skin

Cmplc: Deafness, respiratory failure, peritonitis

Diff Dx: Perforated Tm from acute otitis media

Lab: None for isolated ear trauma; CBC with diff, BMP and U/A to guide fluid therapy in scuba accidents; multisystem trauma evaluation for bomb explosions

ED Rx:

Isolated Tm Rupture

• Oral pain meds, NSAIDs, and narcotics

• Antibiotic ear drops, either cortisporin otic suspension (not solution) or gentamicin ophthalmologic drops, for example

• Follow-up with primary physician in 2 weeks; perforation needs to be followed until closed. Perhaps patching/Hyaluronan by ENT (Acta Otolaryngol Suppl 1987:88)

• No scuba diving, surface diving, or swimming deeper than 3 feet in water—use earplugs when swimming until healed

Scuba Accident

• O_2

• IV fluid, resuscitation guided by hematocrit and urine specific gravity

• Refer to hyperbaric chamber

Bomb or Other Environmental Explosion

Toxicology 1997:17

• Trauma resuscitation, with trauma/general surgery consult

17.2 EPIGLOTTITIS

Jama 1974:671; Pediatr Emerg Care 1989:16; Am J Emerg Med 1996:421

Cause: *Haemophilus influenzae* type B usually in adults, rarer now in the immunized child; staphylococcus, *S. pneumoniae*, rarely other type streptococcus. Rarely due to thermal injury (Pediatrics 1988:441)

Epidem: Now more common in adults with HIB vaccine in peds; mortality rate 1.2% (Laryngoscope 1998:64)

Pathophys: Obstruction of upper airway by edematous epiglottis

Sx: Extremely sore throat (95%), more than the dysphagia (94%), plus respiratory distress over 6–24 hrs—mainly in peds

Si: Epiglottis or other supraglottic structures inflamed and edematous by direct or indirect laryngoscopy, need to sit erect (21%), muffled voice (54%), fever (50%), drooling (40%), stridor (15%) (Am J Dis Child 1988:679); pharynx is often normal (50%)

Crs: Variable

Cmplc: Sudden and unpredictable airway obstruction, 7% mortality without prophylactic airway (vs. recognition of event?); decreases to 1% with airway placed

Crs: Lingual cellulitis; lingual abscess (Am J Emerg Med 1998:414)

Lab:
- CBC with diff; blood culture
- X-ray: soft tissue lateral neck looking for abnormal soft tissue swellings with or without air/fluid levels; look for swollen epiglottis (thumb sign) with loss of air in the vallecula (Ann Emerg Med 1997:1)

ED Rx:
- Do not startle children, perhaps blowby O_2
- Unknown value of racemic epi nebulizer (Anesth Analg 1975:622)
- IV access in adults
- ABX with IV cefuroxime or ceftriaxone (J Paediatr Child Health 1992:220) (second- or third-generation cephalosporin)
- Equivocal, but advocate for use of IV steroids (methylprednisolone or dexamethasone) (J Pediatr Surg 1979:247)
- Early airway in OR is controversial, even in peds

17.3 EPISTAXIS

Cause: Bleeding from nares may be due to trauma externally such as nasal fracture, direct mucosal trauma, foreign body in nares, sinusitis, cocaine use, hypertension, thrombocytopenia, carotid artery aneurysm, or bleeding disorder

Epidem: Common, most resolve with conservative treatment (Otolaryngol Head Neck Surg 1993:60); 5% are posterior bleeds, and these are associated with previous epistaxis and hypertension (Ann Emerg Med 1995:592). Medical issues/habits associated with persistent bleeds are hypertension, aspirin use, and alcohol abuse (Arch Otolaryngol Head Neck Surg 1988:862)

Pathophys: Exposed vessel bleeds are those that usually come to medical attention, those with extensive mucosal involvement, or hematologic/bleeding disorders

Sx: Blood from nares

Si: Look for blood running down pharynx with patient head neutral, with noted blood suggestive of posterior bleed—if head has been rested back, then blood in posterior pharynx will not help distinguish anterior from posterior bleeds; check the septum for perforation; multiple petechiae or ecchymoses to implicate systemic process; coincident hemotympanum (J Emerg Med 1988:387)

Crs: ENT consult for repetitive, uncontrollable, or briskly flowing anterior bleeds, and all posterior bleeds

Cmplc: Anemia, hypoxia, bleeds elsewhere if systemic problem, sinusitis if packing or other obstructive method used as treatment

Lab: If elderly, with multiple medical problems, significant bleed, or anticipating admission, consider ordering CBC with diff; PT/PTT; and/or type and screen (J Laryngol Otol 1999:1086; 2000:38)

ED Rx:

All Bleeds
- Pinch nose below bridge
- Head forward slightly (neck flexed)
- Ice over nose
- Trial of oxymetazoline HCl 0.05% (Afrin) nasal spray; most will resolve with this and pressure alone (Ann Otol Rhinol Laryngol 1995:704)
- Address hypertension if needed, with either acute treatment or follow-up with primary physician for treatment; hypertension is a ubiquitous problem in those with spontaneous bleeds (Ann Emerg Med 2000:126)

Brisk Bleeds
- Soak cotton ball with cocaine 4% or oxymetazoline HCl 0.05% (Afrin) nasal spray, and place in naris that is bleeding—if bleeding stems, this is an anterior bleed. Then pinch nose for 10 minutes
- If bleeding does not stem, follow posterior bleed instructions

Anterior Bleeds
- Pack with Vaseline gauze, Merocel pack, Gelfoam, or Surgicell—packing goes smoother if viscous lidocaine instead of Surgilube is used to facilitate insertion
- Trial of cautery if able to get clear site; may use silver nitrate
- Trial of microfibrillar collagen (J Otolaryngol 1980:468), if able to get clear site. Hold pressure for 3 mintues once collagen placed over site
- Use nasal drops as needed to keep packing moist and to stem bleeds

- Pack out in 1–2 days, 3 days at the most
- Keep in cool environment. Avoid bending and straining. Hold nose if sneezing and expel force through the mouth

Posterior Bleeds
- Posterior pack, with viscous lidocaine for insertion
- Inflate distal balloon first, then proximal balloon—do only 1/2 the amount of balloon capacity, and add more if needed (J Oral Maxillofac Surg 1982:317)
- Foley catheter may be used if posterior pack is not available (Surg Neurol 1979:115); perhaps umbilical cord clamp at external nares to secure position (J Otolaryngol 1996:46)
- O_2
- Antibiotic prophylaxis for sinusitis, such as cefazolin
- ENT consult for admit

Thrombocytopenia
- Transfuse platelets if <50 K and symptomatic (epistaxis counts)

17.4 FOREIGN BODIES (NASAL, AURAL, PHARYNGEAL)

Cause: Usually volitional, rare bug

Epidem: Usually children 2–4 years of age

Sx: Pain, decreased hearing if aural; purulent nasal discharge if nasal

Si: Noted foreign bodies (FBs), ubiquitous malodor with nasal FBs (Jama 1979:1496)

Crs: To OR with ENT if unable to remove

Cmplc: Pharyngeal FBs may be aspirated; aural FBs may cause a perforation; batteries cause tissue destruction (Jama 1986:1470)

Lab: Suspected pharyngeal FB should have radiographs if not visible on exam—soft tissue neck, CXR if necessary, and AXR if necessary

ED Rx:
Nasal
Am J Emerg Med 1997:54
- Have patient occlude contralateral naris while closing mouth and forcing air out of occluded side
- Variation: have mom/dad give puff of air in child's mouth while holding unaffected naris closed, or use Ambu-bag (Practitioner 1973:242; Am J Emerg Med 1996:57)

- Try to grasp with smooth forceps—4% cocaine preprocedure may help
- Crazy Glue on small stick (cotton swab) and touch object—wait a few minutes and then remove
- No. 5 or 6 French balloon catheter lubricated with 2 or 4% lidocaine, snaked past the FB, inflated, and withdrawn (Ann Emerg Med 1980:37)

Aural

- Mineral oil or lidocaine instilled to "kill" potential bug is not advocated—may have unrecognized Tm perforation, and sterile saline works just as well
- Try smooth forceps delivery
- Locate object with otoscope, sit right on top of it with ear speculum (disposable), open magnifying end and place wood stick (cotton swab) with Crazy Glue inside of speculum and "marry" object to stick and speculum, wait a minute, and remove
- Flushing may work—stop if any pain, and do not try if noted Tm perforation
- Dark room/light usually does not work for insects—cannot turn around

Pharyngeal, Visualized

- If easy to reach and patient cooperative, remove object
- If infant, turn infant head down, extend neck, and finger sweep to remove visualized object

Pharyngeal, Nonvisualized (with X-ray)

- If object not found, may be radiolucent or abrasion in pharynx from FB—if symptoms still present next day, follow-up with ENT if no airway compromise
- If FB in skeletal muscle (top 1/3) esophagus or higher, ENT consult to remove. If lower, see 6.2

17.5 OTITIS EXTERNA

Br Med J 1980:1616; Emerg Med Clin North Am 1995:445
Cause: Allergic; seborrheic; infectious (J Otolaryngol 1984:289); bacterial (*Staphylococcus*, *Pseudomonas*) most common, fungal—aka otomycosis (*Aspergillus niger*)—if chronic, viral is rare (herpes simplex, zoster)

Epidem: Bacterial is most common. Bacterial/fungal—swimmer's ear. More common in those with allergies or prolonged water exposure, not with local trauma (J Laryngol Otol 1993:898)

Pathophys: Bacterial—local furunculosis that becomes more diffuse

Sx:

- *Allergic*: 1+ pain, 3+ itching
- *Seborrheic*: 1+ pain, 1+ itching
- *Bacterial*: 3+ pain, especially with movement of pinna
- *Fungal*: 1+ pain, 3+ itching
- *Viral*: 1+ pain with herpes simplex; 3+ pain with herpes zoster

Si:

- *Allergic*: acute with weeping small vesicles; chronic with fissures and scales
- *Bacterial*: Pain with pressure on tragus and pinna traction; erythema and edema (stenosis) of external ear canal
- *Seborrheic*: Greasy scales; dandruff
- *Fungal*: Looks like wet newspaper; black discharge is diagnostic
- *Viral*: Vessels in ear may rupture, or form hemorrhagic bullae

Crs: Variable

Cmplc: Bacterial may go on to malignant otitis externa, a severe form of perichondritis, now only a problem in pts with resistant organisms or diminished resistance, e.g., in patients with diabetes, cancer, AIDS, etc.

Diff Dx: Mastoiditis

Lab: Consider culture of drainage, especially if chronic

ED Rx:

All Types
- Avoid water in ear
- Topical Auralgan for pain

Allergic
- Antihistamines; topical steroids

Seborrheic
- Keep hair away from ears; topical steroids

Bacterial/Fungal
- Remove wax/debris usually by speculum/irrigation—relatively painless
- Domeboro's solution, boric acid 4% (J Laryngol Otol 1987:533), or 9:1 alcohol:vinegar solution drops to acidify area which prevents *Pseudomonas* growth; use wick if stenosis (no stenosis and wick will fall right out) either from commercial source or roll a piece of

tissue paper—helps delivery of therapy (Eye Ear Nose Throat Mon 1974:458)

- Topical antibiotics and steroids (Cortisporin or Cipro) drops qid (Ear Nose Throat J 1978:198), or ofloxacin (Floxin) drops bid; if Tm perforation, use Cortisporin otic suspension or antibiotic eye drops (gentamicin ophthalmologic solution (Curr Med Res Opin 1993:182)) to avoid damaging the ossicles
- Glycerin with nonaqueous acetic acid to decrease swelling by hydroscopic action (Vosol) or with steroid (Vosol HC) are both effective (Curr Ther Res Clin Exp 1974:431)
- Systemic antibiotics, e.g., penicillin, dicloxacillin, cephalothin, or ciprofloxacin especially if *P. aeruginosa* and if sensitive; malignant external OM, Rx with ceftazidime (Ann Otol Rhinol Laryngol 1989:721; Rev Infect Dis 1990:173) or fluoroquinolones (Cmaj 1994:669; Am J Otolaryngol 1988:102)

Viral

- Analgesia; occasionally local antibiotics; ? acyclovir

17.6 OTITIS MEDIA

Br Med J 1980:1616; Emerg Med Clin North Am 1995:445

Cause: Three types
- *Acute (AOM)*: 70% are bacterial—pneumococcus up to 50%, *Moraxella (Branhamella) catarrhalis* up to 30%, *H. influenzae* up to 25% but lower in immunized children, and other streptococci. Viral ~30%
- *Chronic*: above plus staphylococcus, *Proteus*, *Pseudomonas*
- *Serous*: fluid secretion without organism, usually, although 1/3 may have organisms

Epidem: Some viral infections predispose, e.g., RSV, influenza, adenovirus. Childcare outside home and parental smoking also increase risk of acquiring; breast feeding is protective, and pacifier use appears equivocal (Clin Infect Dis 1996:1079). Serous OM often follows infectious resolution

Pathophys: Rhinitis and sinusitis spread along eustachian tube. Pharyngeal closure of eustachian tube may cause ear pain with normal ear exam—eustachian tube dysfunction

Sx: Pain, decreased hearing, sense of fullness or water sloshing

Si: No pain with manipulation of external ear; bulging or retracted Tm with loss of normal landmarks (light reflex), with erythema (erythema is the least helpful sign), and fluid visualized if able to see through the Tm. Lack of Tm movement with pneumatic otoscopy (Pediatr Infect Dis J 2000:256)

Crs: AOM usually begins clearing in 48 hours, but fluid may persist for 2–3 weeks. Serous OM lasts for months and may have associated hearing loss

Cmplc: All rare:
- Ossicle necrosis, especially of incus
- Chronic otitis with granulomas and polyps
- Mastoiditis
- Meningitis and encephalitis
- Lateral sinus thrombosis
- Facial nerve paralysis in chronic OM; Rx with surgical decompression
- Labyrinthitis
- Chronic serous OM
- Hearing acuity decreases if chronic, but no diminished verbal/intellectual abilities with delayed tubes

Lab: None if >28 days of life, and if not septic. Acute phase reactants (ESR, CRP) not helpful in differentiating AOM from other acute invasive bacterial processes (Am J Dis Child 1992:1037). Tympanometry or acoustic otoscopy helpful if diagnosis in question (Ann Emerg Med 1989:396)

ED Rx:

AOM
- ABX (Pediatr Infect Dis J 1994:1054), although current pediatric prescription practice probably not justified (many reasons— diagnostic criteria, strength of study data, placebo controlled studies lacking) (Br J Gen Pract 1998:1861): po with amoxicillin 40–80 mg/kg/day divided tid is first line (Jama 1991:2249); amoxicillin clavulanate (Augmentin); Tm/S (8/40 kg/24 hours) bid; erythromycin + sulfa (Pediazole); cefaclor, etc. Treatment length has varied from 2–10 days for po meds (Br Med J (Clin Res Ed) 1985:1243)
- If no po possible, ceftriaxone 50 mg/kg up to 1 g IM with lidocaine—single dose Rx (Pediatrics 1993:23)
- Advocate ibuprofen 10 mg/kg q 6–8 hours for pain (Fundam Clin Pharmacol 1996:387), although no difference between acetaminophen 15 mg/kg q 4 hours

- Topical Auralgan may be helpful (Arch Pediatr Adolesc Med 1997:675)
- Decongestants and antihistamines of no help (Ann Emerg Med 1983:13), and may actually worsen with analogous dry sinus syndrome—fluid not able to drain from ear
- Have peds <4 years of age recheck with primary care in 4 weeks

Serous OM
- ABX may help (Arch Otolaryngol Head Neck Surg 1997:695); may try for 2-week course but many will clear spontaneously
- Steroids × 7–14 days
- Recheck with primary care in 4 weeks

Chronic OM
- *Pseudomonas* coverage—flouroquinolones if >15 years of age
- ENT follow-up in 1 week or less

17.7 PAROTITIS/PAROTID DUCT STONE

Arch Otolaryngol Head Neck Surg 1992:469

Cause: Mechanical (stone), Stensen duct abnormalities, infectious (e.g., mumps, TB), drugs (anticholinergics), irradiation

Epidem: Bacterial parotitis is bilateral ~20% of the time and not uncommon postoperatively. *S. pneumoniae* and *H. influenzae* common in chronic cases (Pediatr Infect Dis J 1997:386)

Pathophys: Inability to effectively drain the gland allows bacteria to flourish if due to calculi or duct problem; the gland itself is primarily inflamed if due to systemic infectious or irradiation cause; drugs may cause parotitis secondary to causing ineffective drainage or cause direct inflammation of the salivary tissue. Chronic inflammation perhaps secondary to local release of kallikrein

Sx: Painful neck/face

Si: Tenderness, fluctuance, and erythema over parotid; oral inspection may show drainage from Stensen's duct

Crs: Weeks to clear, longer in the elderly

Cmplc: Abscess, osteomyelitis, facial nerve palsy (Arch Otolaryngol Head Neck Surg 1989:240), sepsis

Diff Dx: Enlarged parotid may not be an acute infection; consider the following:

- Chronic infection: cat-scratch disease, atypical mycobacterial disease, actinomycoses, and TB
- Enlargement without infection: alcoholism, malnutrition, celiac disease, DM, uremia, cirrhosis, cystic fibrosis, hypothyroidism, heavy metal poisoning, or drugs (e.g., phenothiazines)

Lab: Gram's stain and culture of drainage; consider CBC with diff and blood cultures if febrile; other labwork based on patient's history and clinical exam

ED Rx:
- If parotid not draining, attempt to milk the gland—IV access with parenteral narcotics will probably be needed. Milk the gland by having one hand massaging the parotid, the other hand with one finger intra-oral below the duct and gently massaging it along its anterior/posterior course
- Antibiotics to cover for penicillinase-resistant *Staphylococcus* until cultures are known, such as nafcillin or ampicillin/sulbactam IV; or dicloxacillin or amoxicillin/clavulanate po
- IV hydration and hold possibly offending meds if necessary
- If unable to drain or to D/C to home, ENT consult for admission and further evaluation. Parotidectomy considered only if chronic and after failure of all conservative therapies (J Otolaryngol 1996:305)
- If home, po antibiotics, pain meds, warm compresses, order to suck on a lemon or lemon candy tid, and 1-week follow-up with primary physician
- Perhaps aprotinin (kallikrein inhibitor) for chronic cases (Arch Otorhinolaryngol 1985:321)

17.8 PERITONSILLAR ABSCESS (QUINSY)

J Otolaryngol 1990:226; Arch Otolaryngol Head Neck Surg 1993:521; Laryngoscope 1995:1

Cause: Group A, β-hemolytic *Streptococcus pyogenes* (J Otolaryngol 1998:206); rarely group C or D that is an extension from pharyngitis; *Peptostreptococcus*; *Fusobacterium*; with anaerobes in 75% of cases

Epidem: Most common deep head and neck abscess

Pathophys: This may set up a tonsillar vein phlebitis, rarely progressing to PE

Sx: Sore throat; difficulty swallowing; drooling

Si: Asymmetric tonsillar pillars, dysphonia, dysphagia, trismus

Crs: Most will drain spontaneously

Cmplc: Recurrent infection and abscess formation

Lab: Throat culture. X-ray: Soft tissue lateral neck series if extending down into neck and looking for air/fluid level

Diff Dx: Peritonsillar cellulitis—may exactly mimic peritonsillar abscess (Arch Emerg Med 1990:212), except at 1-day follow-up after parenteral antibiotics, trismus as measured from incisor to incisor is better in patients with cellulitis (Laryngoscope 1988:780); unfortunately, no threshold value exists. Infectious mononucleosis—rare to have secondary abscess

ED Rx:

If Airway Appears at Risk

- IV for pain control (narcotics), antibiotic (ceftriaxone 2 g, or clindamycin), and steroids (dexamethasone 12 mg in adult or higher (Otolaryngol Head Neck Surg 1983:593)), and ENT consult with patient in ED

If Airway Is Patent

- Treat as outpatient with PCN, cephalexin, second-generation cephalosporin (Arch Otolaryngol 1982:655), or clindamycin; or perhaps IV ceftriaxone with next day follow-up
- Steroid taper (prednisone 60 mg taper or dexamethasone 8 mg taper)
- Oral narcotics
- Salt water gargle
- ENT consult in ED for needle aspiration (Otolaryngol Head Neck Surg 1981:910), outpatient treatment still feasible
- Call ENT to arrange 1-day F/U; interval tonsillectomy in those with history of tonsillitis (Ear Nose Throat J 2000:206)

17.9 STREPTOCOCCAL PHARYNGITIS

Cause: Group A, β-hemolytic *Streptococcus pyogenes*; rarely group C or D

Epidem: Respiratory droplets; foodborne; carrier state in 15% of the population

Pathophys: Possibly due to some breach in the mucosa or increased bacterial load or relative immune state nadir—all theoretical. Treatment to prevent ARF (Pediatrics 1995:758), and perhaps to shorten clinical course and infectious potential

Sx: Sore throat; abdominal pain (although not predictive of strep pharyngitis (J Fam Pract 1998:159))

Si: Fever; pharyngeal edema, erythema or exudates; soft-palate or widespread petechiae (Am J Dis Child 1969:156); anterior cervical adenopathy; normal abdominal exam

Crs: 10 days without Rx

Cmplc: Acute glomerulonephritis; acute rheumatic fever—currently <1/10,000 without Rx, and <1/100,000 with Rx in adults, not seen in peds <3 years of age; peritonsillar abscess—see 17.8

Diff Dx: Chlamydia—TWAR; viral—e.g., EBV (mono), rhinovirus, adenovirus, parainfluenza virus, RSV, coxsackie; mycoplasma; non-Group A strep; periodic fever, such as familial mediterranean fever (FMF) or periodic fever, aphthous stomatitis, pharyngitis, and adenopathy (PFAPA) syndrome (J Pediatr 1999:98); *Legionella*; gonorrhea; diphtheria

Lab:
- Controversial—treatment is geared toward preventing acute rheumatic fever, and cultures and rapid strep tests are 90% sensitive at best. Treating everyone based on clinical grounds *may* miss more, but there is probably just as reasonable a chance that in the group of 10% that the culture misses would be the 1/10,000 person who goes on to acute rheumatic fever. Alternatively, culture those who you do not believe need treatment (they should at least have pharyngeal erythema) and empirically treat all others (J Fam Pract 1975:173)
- Rapid strep vs. culture: Most labs "back up" their rapid strep with cultures—this is because the latex agglutination tests have ~87% positive predictive value and 96% negative predictive value (J Fam Pract 1986:245). Some believe that teleologically a 2-day wait

period was helpful in bolstering the patients immune response, and this still prevented ARF. Since it appears to make no difference, if you must order a test on every patient—order just one. The idea that the marginal cost incurred by ordering both tests is offset by preventing 17 cases of rheumatic fever (Pediatrics 1990:246) is flawed, unless you do not provide patient follow-up for cultures that you order

- Thoughtful ordering: those who are immunosuppressed; septic; have an abscess, glomerulonephritis, or recurrent strep throat; a large group outbreak; or if considering parenteral antibiotics, then a quantitative culture (Lancet 1976:62) would be helpful. May also help to culture a patient if considering treating a family

ED Rx:

- PCN (Pediatrics 1996:955) or macrolide (Am J Med 1991:23S) or first-generation cephalosporin or clindamycin (warn patients about diarrhea with clindamycin, since predisposition to go onto C. diff colitis)
- PCN G benzathine and procaine (Bicillin C-R, or Bicillin C-R 900/300) IM × 1 (Jama 1976:1112)
- Perhaps steroids if severe, such as single dose dexamethasone 10 mg IM for ages 12–65 years (Ann Emerg Med 1993:212); helps pain in 24 hours
- Abbreviated or simple daily dosing for antibiotics that are usually tid or qid has not been shown to be effective (Antimicrob Agents Chemother 1996:1005)
- ENT referral outpatient if >3 episodes/year over several years for consideration of tonsillectomy/adenoidectomy—this decreases recurrence

17.10 RETROPHARYNGEAL ABSCESS

J Laryngol Otol 1997:546

Cause: Direct trauma (e.g., candy cane that was not well masticated before swallowing, fishbone (Ann Otol Rhinol Laryngol 1990:927)); extension from pharyngitis or other head/neck infection

Epidem: Usually Group A, β-hemolytic strep in peds; staph, strep, *Klebsiella, Neisseria,* and other gram-negatives and anaerobes in adults

Pathophys: Inoculation into fascial space that is contiguous with mediastinum

Sx:
- *Peds*: Airway obstruction
- *Adults*: Painful to swallow

Si:
- *Peds*: Drooling, stridor, dysphonia, dysphagia, meningismus, cervical adenopathy
- *Adults*: None, or as with peds (J Emerg Med 1996:147)

Crs: More serious in peds and older adults

Cmplc: Mediastinitis, empyema (Thorax 1994:1179), airway obstruction, jugular vein thrombosis, sepsis

Diff Dx: Retropharyngeal perforation—may be managed as outpatient in healthy adolescent or young adult with amoxicillin/clavulanate and steroids and next day follow-up; epiglottitis; pharyngeal foreign body; retropharyngeal hemorrhage (Jama 1973:427); meningitis in peds

Lab:
- Blood tests if septic—CBC with diff; blood culture
- X-ray: Soft tissue lateral neck, look for swelling in the prevertebral space, or air, or air/fluid level (J Otolaryngol 1999:134)—infants may have air here that disappears with inspiration and is thus a normal variant (Pediatr Radiol 1993:186); CXR if respiratory symptoms or abnormal lung sounds; CT of neck if simply prevertebral edema without air

ED Rx:
- IV access
- ABX—ampicillin/sulbactam, clindamycin and aminoglycoside, ceftriaxone with metronidazole, for example
- ENT consult for admission

17.11 SINUSITIS

Emerg Med Clin North Am 1999:153, ix

Cause: Viral, *Pneumococcus*, *H. influenzae*, strep, staph, *Moraxella catarrhalis*, sometimes anaerobes, chronic may be fungal

Epidem: Occurs at any age >2 years; anywhere from 0.5–5% of URIs complicated by acute sinusitis (Pediatr Infect Dis 1985:S51)

Pathophys: Edema around sinus ostia blocks drainage; all sinuses drain to medial meatus (ostial meatal complex—OMC) except posterior ethmoidals to superior meatus, sphenoid to sphenoethmoid recess (posterior to the concha), and nasolacrimal duct to inferior meatus

Sx: Fever; headache; maxillary toothache; purulent nasal discharge; outpatient trial of decongestant without relief

Si: Rhinitis (90%); postnasal discharge; dental caries (10%); purulent material on middle turbinate; sinus tenderness with palpation or percussion; loss of sinus transillumination (for frontals—light below and pointing upwards from medial supraorbital rim; for maxillaries—light at medial inferior orbital rim and pointing downwards while looking in mouth); infraorbital nerve hypesthesia in maxillary sinusitis; noting sinus fluid is sensitive but not specific for acute bacterial sinusitis

Crs: May be chronic

Cmplc: Meningitis/intracranial sepsis (J Laryngol Otol 1995:1061); lateral sinus thrombosis; osteomyelitis

Lab:
- None unless septic—cultures and plain radiographs are nonspecific
- *If septic*: CBC with diff, blood cultures, and other evaluation based on history and physical exam
- X-ray: radiographic imaging may show fluid or not, with a lack of fluid not excluding bacterial sinusitis, and a fluid level possibly denoting viral, allergic, or fungal sinusitis, or trauma. If diagnostic dilemma, CT is the better test (Acad Emerg Med 1994:235)

ED Rx:

If Septic (Usually Seen in Frontal or Ethmoidal Sinusitis)
- O$_2$, IV access for fluid resuscitation and antibiotics
- ABX: ceftriaxone 2 g IV; or ampicillin/sulbactam 3 g IV; or cefuroxime 1.5 g IV
- ENT consult for admission

- Local nasal decongestants like epinephrine drops 0.5–2% or phenylephrine 0.25% in saline qid for 4–5 days
- Amoxicillin (40–80 mg/kg/day divided tid to max 1500 mg/day) first line in peds and adults except with ethmoidal and sphenoidal when need penicillinase-resistant penicillin like amoxicillin/clavulanate (Augmentin), erthromycin/sulfa (Pediazole), Tm/S (Bactrim), cefaclor (Ceclor), cefuroxime (Ceftin)—short courses appropriate in healthy patients, e.g., 3 days of Tm/S as effective as 10 days
- Outpatient follow-up in 1–2 weeks with primary care doctor if first evaluation, with ENT if becoming a chronic problem

17.12 VERTIGO

Ann Otol Rhinol Laryngol 1968:193; Emerg Med Clin North Am 1987:211

Cause: Perhaps viral (labyrinthitis); positional vertigo (Brain 1972:369)—either positional nystagmus which persists or benign paroxysmal positional vertigo (BPPV); cerebellar insult (hemorrhage)—see 13.2; or other central causes

Epidem: BPV idiopathic in half its cases (inner ear stones?), but may have etiologies such as head trauma or viral labyrinthitis; female:male 2:1; most commonly posterior semicircular canal (Neurology 1987:371)

Pathophys:

Arch Otorhinolaryngol 1984:23

Stability conferred via 3 mechanisms: vision, proprioception, and semicircular canals (for rotational stability). We need 2 out of 3 of these intact to avoid vertigo, unless inaccurate input from one site, such as lesion along the vestibular tract including the semicircular canals, the eighth cranial nerve, or eighth cranial nerve lesion. A lesion may be stones not settling correctly in the semicircular canals. As far as the specifics for the induction of vertigo, this is all conjecture

Sx: Room spinning, nausea

Si: Horizontal nystagmus with otherwise normal neurologic exam including hearing; BPPV may be elicited with Hall-Pike (head-hanging) maneuver—move patient from sitting to supine with one ear down and symptoms/nystagmus occur after ~15 seconds and pass in 2 minutes, and then repeat with the other ear down

Crs: Labyrinthitis and BPPV may have chronic course

Cmplc: Misdiagnosis

Diff Dx:

- Meniere's disease—with tinnitus and decreased hearing; use salt, caffeine and ETOH restriction; may try antihistamines, antivertigo meds as listed below, diuretics such as thiazides and benzodiazepines for symptoms; refer to ENT as outpatient
- Cerebellar-pontine angle tumor—diagnosed with auditory evoked potentials
- Inner ear hemorrhage—acute with hearing loss
- Temporal bone fracture—usually with trauma history and severe hearing loss
- Seizure

Lab: None, but head CT without contrast if suspect cerebellar hemorrhage or skull fracture or other acute CNS event, head MRI if suspect CNS neoplasm (Clin Imaging 1998:309)

ED Rx:

Labyrinthitis and BPPV

- IV benzodiazepines (diazepam or lorazepam) of equivocal efficacy (J Otolaryngol 1980:472), but relax patient
- Meclizine (Antivert, Bonine) 25–50 mg po q 6 hours (Arch Neurol 1972:129)
- Dimenhydrinate (Dramamine) po or scopolamine (Transderm) patch
- Outpatient primary care follow-up

Labyrinthitis

- Consider steroid taper if presenting within first 24 hours

BPPV

- Canalith repositioning procedure (Epley's maneuvers) (Otolaryngol Head Neck Surg 1992:399; Am J Otol 2000:230)
- Homeopathy effective, specifically Vertigoheel (Heel, Inc.) (Arch Otolaryngol Head Neck Surg 1998:879)

18 Pediatrics/Pediatric Surgery

18.1 BRONCHIOLITIS/RSV

Pediatrics 1999:1334

Cause: Respiratory syncytial virus

Epidem: Peak incidence in November–April. Major issue in immunocompromised, premature infants, and cardiopulmonary disease in peds <2 years of age (Jama 1999:1440)

Pathophys: Bronchial infection/reactivity

Sx: Respiratory distress

Si: Tachypnea with wheezing

Crs: Fever associated with more severe clinical course (Arch Dis Child 1999:231). Lifelong increased chronic course of airway hyperreactivity in children if bronchiolitis after 1 year of age (Am J Respir Crit Care Med 2000:1501), but this is not found if disease affects one only as an infant (<12 months of age) (J Pediatr 1999:8)

Cmplc: Respiratory failure

Diff Dx: Adenovirus; parainfluenza virus; foreign body; pneumonia; cystic fibrosis if recurrent

Lab: Nasal wash RSV; capillary blood gas, pulse oximetry, and CXR if significant distress

ED Rx:
- Isolation—prevent nosocomial spread
- O_2
- IV fluids if in extremis
- Nebulized racemic epinephrine (1 mg in 2.0 cc NS) in extremis (J Pediatr 1993:145)
- Albuterol neb 2.5 mg/Rx, or 10 mg/hr continuous

- Consider steroids (controversial)—parenteral, oral, or inhaled—pro, parenteral study (Pediatrics 2000:E44) and con, budesonide inhaled study (Arch Dis Child 1999:343) and fluticasone inhaled study (Eur Respir J 2000:388)
- Nitric oxide data is equivocal (Intensive Care Med 1999:81)
- Peds consult for admit if not responding or unstable, may need intubation +/– aerosolized ribavirin as inpatient—con (Am J Respir Crit Care Med 1999:829)
- Next day follow-up with peds if well enough to go home, consider home albuterol nebs (q 3–4 hours). Outpatient follow-up may include RSV immune globulin (q 1 month in high-risk infants)

18.2 CERVICAL ADENITIS/ CAT-SCRATCH DISEASE

Pediatr Infect Dis J 1997:163; 1985:S23

Cause: *Bartonella* (*Rochalimaea*) *henselae* and *quintana*, a small pleomorphic gram-negative, probably rickettsial organism. Sometimes *Afipia felis* (J Clin Microbiol 1998:2499)

Cervical adenitis itself is usually a self-limited viral (adenovirus, enterovirus, CMV, Epstein-Barr, herpes simplex) disease which resolves quickly, but can be caused by staph, strep, and anaerobes (Clin Pediatr (Phila) 1980:693); less likely anaerobes, atypical organisms, cat-scratch disease, and toxoplasmosis

Epidem: From young cats, infected for a few weeks; transmit via bites, scratches, and fleas, thus common name is a misnomer. 80% of cases in patients under age 21

Pathophys: 7–14 day incubation. *Bartonella* sp. also found in bacillary angiomatosis and bartonellosis (Int J Dermatol 1997:405)

Sx: Bite or scratch from kitten (90% positive); papule at site of scratch

Si: Fever; signs of scratch or bite with papule noted; adenopathy with 40% of nodes suppurative; potentially many ocular findings including Parinaud's oculoglandular syndrome (infection of eye surface and regional lymphadenopathy) (Curr Opin Ophthalmol 1999:209)

Crs: Usually self-limited, even with complications

Cmplc:
- Encephalopathy (J Pediatr 1999:635); encephalitis (10%); osteolytic bone lesions; conjunctivitis; purpura; mesenteric adenitis
- *Immunocompromised pts*: disseminated disease; bacillary angiomatosis—looks somewhat like Kaposi's sarcoma; peliosis hepatitis—sometimes seen in the immunocompetent

Diff Dx: Rare—TB and other mycobacterium (Clin Pediatr (Phila) 1997:403); *Haemophilus influenzae*; syphilis; fungal; *Yersinia pestis*

Lab: CBC with diff showing mild eosinophilia; ESR; liver function tests if systemically ill; obtain CSF if neuro changes and look for increased protein; *R. henselae* titer of >1:64 is 84% sensitive and 96% specific. PCR may be needed (Hum Pathol 1997:820)

ED Rx:
Mild Disease (Only Papule at Site)
- No treatment, outpatient follow-up in 2–3 days with primary physician

Moderate/Severe Disease
- Ciprofloxacin 500 mg po bid; perhaps azithromycin 500 mg day 1 followed by 250 mg days 2–5, or 10 mg/kg day 1 in peds followed by 5 mg/kg days 2–5 (Pediatr Infect Dis J 1998:447)
- Peds—Tm/S
- Erythromycin 500 mg po qid for disseminated forms; second line is doxycycline 100 mg po bid
- May also consider gentamicin, ceftriaxone, cefotaxime, or amikacin
- Primary care consult for admission if moderate or severe disease

18.3 CHILD ABUSE

Hosp Community Psychiatry 1992:111; J Med Assoc Ga 2000:5

Cause: Potentially anyone—parents, caregivers, strangers

Epidem: Linked to parental unemployment/poverty, especially fathers (Child Abuse Negl 1998:79). Adolescent mothers at higher risk than older counterparts, especially if they had been abused (Child Abuse Negl 2000:701). False allegations or misinterpretation uncommon (2.5%) (Child Abuse Negl 2000:149)

Pathophys: Abuse or neglect in the physical, sexual, or emotional (verbal) realm

Sx: Sleep disorders; nightmares; inappropriate sexual play; school and developmental problems; phobias; depression

Si: Delay in seeking treatment. Recurrent injury; patterned bruises; fractures; head injuries; retinal hemorrhages; facial and oral injuries (Child Abuse Negl 2000:521). Injuries inappropriate for age, not consistent with history, and to different body planes

Crs: Potentially fatal

Cmplc: Failure to thrive; may impact all aspects of life, including long-term neurobehavioral problems (J Child Psychol Psychiatry 2000:97)

Lab: Consider radiographic bone survey if evidence of trauma (J Am Acad Orthop Surg 2000:10); forensic photos

ED Rx:
- Peds consult for admission
- Department of Health/Human Services referral

18.4 CROUP

Pediatr Pulmonol 1997:370; Pediatr Clin North Am 1999:1167

Cause: Parainfluenza virus, and others

Epidem: 3/100 under age 6 years; 1.3% must be hospitalized; adult croup does exist (Chest 1996:1659)

Pathophys: Two forms, and both occur mainly at night with child in recumbent position—whether this is due to fluid shifts with consequent edema or meridian causality is unknown
- *Acute laryngotracheitis*—follows 2–3 days of URI
- *Spasmodic croup*—no antecedent illness; acts like hypersensitivity syndrome

Sx: Barky cough

Si: Cough like a seal bark; tachypnea; hoarseness or other voice change; inspiratory stridor; accessory respiratory muscle use; cyanosis when severe

Crs: Most self-limited, protracted course with herpes simplex (Acta Paediatr 1996:118); increased risk of asthma in school-aged children with recurrent croup, with an even higher risk if family history of asthma (~37%) (Acta Paediatr 1996:1295)

Cmplc: Hypoxia

Diff Dx: Aspirated foreign body; epiglottitis; bacterial tracheitis—such as diphtheria; congenital anomaly—such as vascular ring

Lab: None. X-ray: May be done to exclude other causes of airway obstruction, look for tracheal edema (steeple sign) (Radiol Clin North Am 1998:175)

ED Rx:
- Most patients improved at ED secondary to cool night air and upright posture
- Mist tent, or humidified O_2
- Racemic epinephrine 0.25–1 cc of 2.25% solution neb (Pediatr Emerg Care 1996:156), although L-epinephrine 1:1000 5 cc neb (cheaper and more available) perhaps as efficacious (Pediatrics 1992:302). Observation time post epinephrine is debatable (Ann Emerg Med 1995:331)
- Heliox 70/30 may be helpful in mild to moderately ill children (Acad Emerg Med 1998:1130)
- Steroids (Bmj 1999:595)—dexamethasone 0.6 mg/kg po (Jama 1998:1629) or IM (Acta Paediatr Scand 1988:99); or prednisone 2 mg/kg po; or methylprednisolone 2 mg/kg IV; or nebulized budesonide (Pulmicort) 2 mg in 4 cc neb (Br J Gen Pract 2000:135)
- Outpatient follow-up next day with primary physician if home, with trial of steam from shower or cool night air if recurrent. If severe, peds/primary care consult for admission

18.5 HIRSCHSPRUNG'S DISEASE

Dig Dis 1994:106; Crit Rev Clin Lab Sci 1999:225

Cause: Unknown, probably many types of Hirschsprung's disease with complicated genetic inheritance (Proc Natl Acad Sci U S A 2000:268)

Epidem: Usually in infants with male:female 1:4

Pathophys: Aganglionic segment of colon, variable in length from a few cm in rectum to all rectum and descending colon. No neurons in this segment resulting in constant contractions and no relaxation—eventually with intestinal obstruction; seen as acute in infants, chronic in children and teenagers

Sx: Abdominal pain; chronic constipation

Si: Distended and tender abdomen

Si: Distended and rigid abdomen; possibly palpable mass in right upper quadrant; look for rectal prolapse; guaiac positive stools

Crs: Variable, more emergent course of action needed the younger the child; look for the triad of intermittent abdominal pain, vomiting, and palpable right upper quadrant mass, with gross or occult blood also significant (J Pediatr 1998:836)

Cmplc: Dehydration; intestinal ischemia; peritonitis

Diff Dx: Appendicitis; foreign body obstruction—ileocecal valve region; hernia; gastroenteritis; infectious colitis; Meckel's diverticulum, although this is usually painless

Lab:
- CBC with diff; metabolic profile; consider type and screen
- X-ray: 3-view abd series should show intestinal dilatation with air/fluid levels (Pediatr Emerg Care 1992:325); barium enema is both diagnostic and many times curative if no evidence of perforation; perhaps U/S for low-risk patients (J Pediatr 1992:182)

ED Rx:
- IV access for fluids, pain and nausea control
- Peds/surgical consult, with expectation to do barium enema or air pressure enema reduction (J Pediatr Surg 1986:1201) if no signs of perforation or shock

18.8 KAWASAKI DISEASE

J Pediatr 1991:680; Arch Dis Child 1991:185

Cause: Unknown

Epidem: Incidence of ~5/100,000/year; commonly presents as fever of unknown origin

Pathophys: A mucocutaneous lymph node disease, with the immune response precipitating a vasculitis (Immunodefic Rev 1989:261)

Sx: Prolonged fever; variety of rashes

Si: Fever in peds 1–8 years of age; nonpitting edema; cervical lymphadenopathy; desquamation of skin on palms, perineum, trunk, and lips; nonexudative conjunctivitis; "strawberry" tongue

Crs: Difficult diagnosis in those <6 months of age, consider echo of heart looking for coronary aneurysms in those with prolonged fever (J Pediatr 1986:759)

Cmplc: 25% get coronary aneurysms later, which may cause an MI if thrombosed (Intern Med 1992:774); cardiac conduction system may become infiltrated/scarred (Am Heart J 1978:744); polyserositis which includes cardiac tamponade

Diff Dx: Infantile periarteritis nodosa; adenovirus; measles; scarlet fever; RMSF; leptospirosis; EBV; JRA

Lab:
- CBC with diff (look for anemia); ESR; metabolic profile; blood cultures; CK-MB and troponin I for myocarditis (Pediatr Cardiol 1999:184); rapid direct fluorescent antigen test for adenovirus (Arch Pediatr Adolesc Med 2000:453); EKG—none of these overwhelmingly specific
- X-ray: CXR

ED Rx:
- Peds/primary care consult for admission
- IgG 2 g/kg IV over 10 hours to prevent complications (N Engl J Med 1991:1633; Pediatr Int 1999:1)
- ASA 100 mg/kg, with more free salicylate available compared to normals (J Pediatr 1991:456)
- IV streptokinase (3500 IU/kg over 30 minutes, followed by 1000 IU/kg/24 hours) for acute MI (Cathet Cardiovasc Diagn 1995:139)
- Consider methylprednisolone 30 mg/kg/day × 3 days if impending cardiac tamponade (Intensive Care Med 1999:1137)

18.9 PYLORIC STENOSIS

J Paediatr Child Health 1993:372

Cause: Possibly genetic/sex-linked

Epidem: Males > females; 50% of affected mother's children will have, 10% of affected father's offspring will have; 1/100–1/600 births

Pathophys: Concentric muscular hypertrophy of pyloric smooth muscle, in which nitric oxide synthetase deficiency precipitates the disease

Sx: Well and gaining weight for first 3–5 weeks of life, and then nonbilious projectile vomiting

Si: Palpable "olive" in right upper quadrant 70% of the time; since we routinely image patients, our clinical diagnosis skills are declining (Bmj 1993:553)

Crs: Benign with surgical repair

Cmplc: Dehydration

Diff Dx: All uncommon—annular pancreas; duodenal atresia; addisonian crisis due to congenital adrenal hypoplasia; antral diaphragm; eosinophilic gastroenteritis (J Pediatr Gastroenterol Nutr 1987:543)

Lab:
- Metabolic profile shows a hypochloremic, hypokalemic metabolic alkalosis—this metabolic derangement is becoming more uncommon (J Pediatr Surg 1983:394; Am J Emerg Med 1999:67)
- X-ray: Upper GI barium study vs. abdominal U/S—increased use of radiologic diagnostic testing has not led to a significant change in management (Bmj 1993:553), although is the standard for current diagnosis and perhaps allows earlier diagnosis if patients present earlier (Pediatrics 1997:E9)

ED Rx:
- IVF rehydration if needed
- Surgery consult

18.10 SIDS

Emerg Med Clin North Am 1983:27; Acad Emerg Med 1995:926; 1995:996; 1995:1077

Cause: Unknown, but some cases due to unrecognized abuse

Epidem: 1.4 deaths/1000 live births in U.S.; familial tendency; increased incidence by sleeping prone, use of deformable mattress, swaddling, warm room, URIs, and exposure to passive cigarette smoke; associated with primary *Pneumocystis carinii* infection (Clin Infect Dis 1999:1489); no association with DPT immunizations.

Pathophys: Hypothesized that several sleep apneas (>15 seconds) precede fatal event

Sx: Deceased

Si: Deceased

Crs: Medical Examiner case

Diff Dx: Trauma; smothering asphyxia; other types of abuse

Lab: None; near SIDS requires full physiologic evaluation including Hgb F level (look for elevation) (N Engl J Med 1987:1122;

Med Hypotheses 2000:987), and EKG showing no shortening of
QT with rate increase

ED Rx:
- Resuscitative efforts while looking for other treatable causes
- Counseling to parents and report to Medical Examiner
- Prophylactic measures of supine or side position; firm bedding; and
  apnea monitor have been equivocal in efficacy

19 Plastic Surgery

19.1 BITES (HUMAN AND ANIMAL)

Curr Clin Top Infect Dis 1999:99; N Engl J Med 1999:138

Cause: Human or domestic or wild animal bite, or awakening in a room/tent with a bat as additional occupant (Wis Med J 1996:242)

Epidem: *Pastuerella multocida* is in >50% of animal bite and cat-scratch infections; polymicrobial infections in human and mammalian bite wounds (N Engl J Med 1999:85); higher risk in animal control officers (Am J Public Health 1984:255)

Pathophys: Inoculation of bacteria—cat bites frequently become infected because of deep inoculation; possible rabies virus in unvaccinated or wild animal saliva; see 1.3 for envenomations

Sx: Obvious wound; no obvious wound for bat bite Rx

Si: Wound—note tenderness, erythema pattern, adenopathy, depth, and discharge; evaluate distal neurovascular status, check for tendon injury

Crs: Varies with potential need for rabies prophylaxis

Cmplc: Cellulitis, lymphangitis, tenosynovitis, or osteomyelitis (Arch Emerg Med 1992:299); rabies; sepsis—infections more common in those who are immunosuppressed such as those with diabetes mellitus

Lab:
- Uncomplicated bites without specific lab evaluation; consider CBC with diff, ESR, wound Gram's stain and culture for those with more significant infections. For assailant in human bites, obtain HIV, hep B, and hep C if possible
- X-ray: consider for osteomyelitis, look for periosteal reaction—not seen acutely

ED Rx:
- Clean wound, soap and water as good as anything else
- Update/initiate tetanus if needed, see 10.10
- Treat for rabies if mammalian bite from unvaccinated animal such as dog, cat, bat, fox, raccoon, or skunk with no quarantine ability of attacking animal, or if awaken with bat in the same room, see 10.7. Not usually seen in mice, squirrels, or other rodents, nor in rabbits
- For envenomations, see 1.3
- Do not close wounds if possible, although those on the head and neck may be closed if repaired within 12 hours (Ear Nose Throat J 1998:216). If closing on other areas of the body, consider placing a drain and do not use tissue adhesives for any bite wound closures. Debride all devitalized tissue, surgical consult if this extends beyond the myofascial plane or into tendons, ligaments, joint spaces, or bone
- Splint and elevate the injured area
- Consider oral prophylactic antibiotics for human bites (Plast Reconstr Surg 1975:538), especially to any part of the hand, and all animal bites (Arch Emerg Med 1989:251). Human bites—dicloxacillin, erythromycin, cefuroxime (Ceftin), or amoxicillin/clavulanate (Augmentin) for 3–5 days. Animal bites—amoxicillin/clavulanate (Augmentin) as first choice; penicillin, tetracycline, dicloxacillin, erythromycin, and first- or second-generation cephalosporin as second line
- If antibiotics for treatment of minor infection such as cellulitis or minimal lymphangitis (no adenopathy) in an otherwise healthy person, first dose IV such as ampicillin/sulbactam, home with amoxicillin/clavulanate, and next day follow-up—probably in the ED
- If antibiotics for all other infections, IV antibiotic as above, and ortho/plastic/general surgery consult (one of these) for admission

PLASTIC SURGERY

19.2 TOPICAL AND LOCAL ANESTHESIA

Selection and site of appropriate anesthesia is important for surgical procedures. All infiltration should be done through the cleanest field possible, and nerve blocks should have sterile prep performed

Lidocaine: An aminoamide, maximum subcutaneous infusion is 2.5–3 mg/kg (N Engl J Med 1979:418). Thus, goal of 1% solution (1 g/100 cc) is ~0.45 cc/kg, or 30 cc in the 70-kg person. Gives ~2 hours of local anesthesia. Iontophoresis effective (J Dermatol Surg Oncol 1994:579), yet not an ED modality

The role of epinephrine: Added to local anesthetic solutions such as lidocaine, its vasoconstrictive properties are such that duration of anesthesia and control of hemostasis are enhanced (Anesthesiology 1989:757), and may use a larger amount of anesthesia since it is absorbed into circulation slower and over more time. Do not use epinephrine in nerve blocks, or locally into digits, tip of the nose, on to the ear, or penis

The role of NaHCO$_3$: Along with warming injected solution (hand-rub filled syringe or 40°C heater) and injecting slowly, buffering is thought to decrease the pain of injecting (J Dermatol Surg Oncol 1990:842). The solution of lidocaine:bicarb is 10:1. May keep up to 2 weeks with refrigeration at 0–4°C (J Dermatol Surg Oncol 1991:411)

The role of benzyl alcohol 0.9%: Allows to increase amount of fluid injected if epinephrine is not an option, or if lidocaine allergy. Works better than diphenhydramine (Ann Emerg Med 1998:650)

The role of diphenhydramine 0.5% (Benadryl): Allows to increase amount of fluid injected for local anesthesia if epinephrine is not an option or in lieu of lidocaine; diphenhydramine is a weak anesthetic (Ann Emerg Med 1994:1328). Combined with lidocaine, the solution is prepared 1:1

Bupivacaine (Marcaine): Long-acting (8–12 hours) anesthetic available in 0.25% or 0.5% solution, has a lower safety profile than lidocaine, and do not use with epinephrine or bicarb. No need to combine with lidocaine for faster onset of action (Ann Emerg Med 1996:490)

TAC:

Ann Emerg Med 1980:568

Solution of 0.5% tetracaine/0.5% adrenaline/11.8% cocaine applied topically to face or scalp for 20 minutes to facilitate anesthesia in children. Avoid to tip of nose, directly onto ear, or on mucous membranes. No advantage over LET (see next), and LET avoids any issues physicians may have with using cocaine. Evidence of effect is with observed blanching to surrounding tissues; may need to boost anesthesia in some with 1% lidocaine locally injected

LET:

Ann Emerg Med 1995:203

Solution of 4% lidocaine/0.1% epinephrine/0.5% tetracaine used in the same circumstances as with TAC, same onset of action, same parameters

4% viscous lidocaine: For use in injured skin where TAC or LET cannot be used; takes 30–60 minutes for onset of action, and most children will need additional 1% lidocaine supplementation, but allows you to infiltrate with much less pain

EMLA:

J Dermatol Surg Oncol 1994:579

Solution of lidocaine and prilocaine for use over intact skin, such as prior to IV access. For elective situations since requires 60 minutes for onset, and use occlusive dressing such as Opsite or Tagaderm when applied to facilitate action

Local infiltration: 25–30 gauge needle for injecting, do the proximal edge first since this will facilitate pain control for the distal edge. Injecting through the wound is less painful than going through the skin, but beware of debris. Inject slowly; lidocaine has onset in 5–10 minutes, and bupivacaine 10–15 minutes

NERVE BLOCKS

Postgrad Med 1999:69, 77

Digital finger block: Injections are just distal to the MCP. The neurovascular bundle runs on both the radial and ulnar sides of the phalanx, with some dorsal nerves also crossing the proximal phalanx. Begin on either the radial or ulnar side of the proximal phalanx and you will be blocking the web area—raise a wheal using a 25–27 gauge needle, and then go deeper towards the bone, inject here, and then aim to the volar aspect and inject a little more (total 1–1.5 cc). Keep the needle in but skew the aim (almost completely withdraw to re-aim) so that your needle is now across the extensor (dorsal) surface, and put 1 cc or less through here. Now block the web area on the other side of the finger exactly the same way as the first side. Total infiltration solution volume should be 3–4 cc, and remember not to use any epinephrine

Digital toe block: Same approach as with the digital finger block, but it is important to get the plantar aspect of the toes. Begin on either the medial or lateral side of the proximal phalanx and you will be blocking the web area—raise a wheal using a 25–27 gauge needle, and then go deeper towards the bone, inject here, and then aim to the plantar aspect and inject a little more (total 1 cc). Now place the needle more toward the plantar aspect but within your anesthetized area, and put 1 cc of fluid across the plantar aspect. Now block the web area on the other side of the toe exactly as done on the first side. Total maximum solution volume should be 3 cc, and remember not to use epinephrine. The hallux may need 0.5–1 cc injected across its dorsal surface, so that a ring-like area of anesthesia has been performed. Total maximum solution volume for the hallux is 4 cc

Metacarpal block: This is performed dorsally and just proximal to the MCP joint, and can accommodate more fluid than a digital block—it is not to be used for the thumb. Anesthetize the skin using a 25–27 gauge needle. Introduce the needle just ulnar and radial to the metacarpal in question, and position it so that the tip is just deep (in a volar sense) to the metacarpal. Inject while withdrawing the needle, placing ~3 cc in this space. Inject both sides—this is not a palmar approach

Radial nerve block: Block the superficial branch of the radial nerve when anesthetizing the thumb. The anesthetized area will resemble a half-circle. Infiltrate the dorsum of the hand just below the skin beginning at the proximal "snuff box" area and end at the proximal second metacarpal using a 25–27 gauge needle. The convexity of the half-circle should be away from the thumb

Median nerve block: Useful when working on the palmar aspect of the index or middle finger, and when working on the thumb. Imagine a line that is an extension of the radial side of the middle finger and extends to the wrist. Two tendons are palpable at the wrist on either side of this line—the palmaris longus to the ulnar side and the flexor carpi radialis to the radial side. The median nerve is deep to the flexor retinaculum between these two tendons (~2 cm deep) and can be anesthetized with a 25–27 gauge needle

Ulnar nerve block: Useful when working on the little finger or the ulnar side of the hand. On the volar aspect of the wrist, the last large tendon toward the ulnar side is that of the flexor carpi ulnaris. At the distal end of this palpable tendon off to its medial aspect runs the ulnar nerve. It is just deep to the tendon, ~1 cm deep and can be anesthetized with a 25–27 gauge needle

Auricular block: When working on the ear, it is preferable not to inject directly into the skin of the ear. Just before the skin reflects onto the ear, anesthetize this area both anteriorly and posteriorly using a 25–27 gauge needle. The external canal may also have some vagal branches that will require local anesthesia

Dental blocks:

Gen Dent 1982:414

Most common is the inferior alveolar nerve block. This nerve enters the mandible on the medial aspect (at approximately its midpoint in the anterior/posterior axis) of the body of the mandible (just in front of the tonsillar pillars)—it is about a finger's breadth superior to the top of the lower teeth. If you place your needle a finger's breadth above the lower row of teeth anteriorly at the body of the mandible, and then aim posteriorly while keeping parallel to the teeth, you can gauge the depth by having your noninjecting hand on the posterior and anterior aspects of the mandible. Inject about 1 cc

19.3 WOUND MANAGEMENT

This is a review of key points, and not a substitute for proper training and practice. Adjunctive materials are available (J Emerg Med 1998:651)

All wounds: Examine for foreign body (X-ray if necessary), and check for involvement of tendons, joint spaces, ligaments, or bone. Check distal neurovascular function; it is not uncommon to have a small area of skin anesthesia distal to a laceration. Remember tetanus

Puncture wounds: Special wounds in the sense that an inoculum of bacteria may be deposited and then quickly sealed over. Although potentially more serious, overall incidence of secondary infection is only ~6% (J Accid Emerg Med 1996:274). All these wounds should be cleaned and left open, and perhaps soaking 3 times a day in warm water. If the wound is completely sealed, conservative treatment with surface cleaning and non-weight-bearing for 24 hours and 1–2 day follow-up is OK (J Emerg Med 1995:291); providing a crosshatch so that drainage can occur may be appropriate in those not deemed reliable. Foot wounds are high-risk for *Pseudomonas aeruginosa*, especially if nail through sole of shoe (ABX of choice is ciprofloxacin in those >15 years of age (Clin Infect Dis 1995:194)) (Jama 1968:262). Dirty wounds or wounds in high-risk patients (congenital heart disease, diabetes mellitus, HIV, etc.) should have prophylactic antibiotics (first-generation cephalosporin such as cephalexin), and perhaps consideration of having polymicrobial infections in those with diabetes mellitus (J Foot Ankle Surg 1994:91)

Irrigation: Irrigate with copious amounts of sterile saline, and wounds that are heavily contaminated or need significant debridement should be treated in the OR. If you elect to use antibacterial skin prep agents such as iodophor or chlorhexidine, avoid getting these into the open wound, as these will destroy the healthy tissue in the wound

Repair: Debride all devitalized tissue. Make edges smooth leaving an elliptical opening if possible, and undermine tissue to reduce tension if necessary. Stiches do not need to be water tight, and if too tight, may lead to skin necrosis. If a myofascial layer has been violated, it is not necessary to repair this, and it actually may be necessary to extend the defect to avoid a compartment syndrome as in the anterior tibial region. All facial and nail bed injuries need repair, and tendon and joint capsule repair should be done by an orthopedic surgeon (OK to repair extensor tendons if trained to do so). Deep or heavily contaminated wounds may need a drain for 2–3 days to prevent abscess formation. Remember to close deep layers so that a potential space is not left (>3 cm depth is considered necessitating a deep closure). The palmar aspect of the hand has a high propensity for infection (Arch Emerg Med 1987:211), and the palm itself should not be explored in the emergency department. Most body areas need to be repaired within 12 hours of injury but the face can be delayed for 24 hours—this can be modified with surgical debridement and if this needs to occur, should be done by a surgeon

- Staples (Ann Emerg Med 1989:1122): the fastest way to close a wound, thus useful for hemostasis control. Helpful in large or multiple lacerations from a trauma. Also used primarily in locations where scar formation is not an issue, such as the scalp
- Sutures: better cosmesis; the basics of absorbable stitches deep and nonabsorbable or absorbable with subcuticular closure at the skin are important to remember. Do not make stitches tight, and it is OK to run the stitch in incision injuries rather than place repeated simple stitches (J Trauma 2000:495). Use mattress stitches to evert the edges of wound and help evenly distribute wound tension. Facial injuries require 5–0 or 6–0 stitches, hands/digits 4–0 or 5–0, and 3–0 or 4–0 for the trunk and extremities. Be sure to repair the nail bed/matrix, and place nail back in place or surrogate (aluminum foil) to preserve nail fold
- Wound closure tape: a tape that can hold minimally tense wounds that have good hemostasis. Use tincture of benzoin on either side of the wound to help secure this tape. Best are Steri-strip, Nichi-strip, and Curi-strip (J Emerg Med 1987:451)
- Tissue adhesive: for wounds with no tension, controlled bleeding, not a bite, and not over an extensor surface
- Watchful waiting: it is not necessary to manipulate all wounds; puncture wounds, bites, and heavily contaminated wounds would do better with cleaning, no closure, and 1–2 day follow-up. Small scalp wounds that are not bleeding can also just be observed. If the scalp injury is from a relatively clean source, manipulating the wound with cleaning or repair is often not necessary, and it can be left to heal on its own. Infection of scalp wounds is rare unless retained foreign body

20 Procedures

20.1 AIRWAY MANAGEMENT

The first step in every assessment is to evaluate for a secure airway.
The following information is intended as a refresher, and does not
substitute for hands-on training with an appropriate instructor.
Always first open an airway with a chin lift or jaw thrust. Any
techniques that violate the skin should have sterile prep and drape
performed. The cricothyroid membrane is bound by the inferior
border of the thyroid cartilage above and the cricoid below

Note: Peds do well with bag-valve mask (BVM) out of hospital
compared with ET for medical or trauma in urban environment
(Jama 2000:783)

Oral pharyngeal airway (OPA): This curved plastic airway may be the
first step in an oral airway adjunct. This is sized by having one
end resting on the tip of the nose and the other end resting at the
angle of the jaw. Insert with the concavity upwards, and then
rotate 180° when it is halfway in. The final position is with the
flange at the lips. This lifts the tongue from the back of the throat,
and is not for use in a conscious person. Adult size is 5–6, with
smaller numbers for smaller sizes

Nasal pharyngeal airway/nasal trumpet (NPA): This is sized as with the
OPA; the lubricated tip goes through a naris, and the flange rests
at the external naris when done. Many people have asymmetric
naris passages—if it does not work on one side, try the other. Size
8–9 in adult (internal diameter in millimeters); may be used on
the conscious patient, but should not be used in those with
maxillofacial trauma

Laryngeal mask airway (LMA): An anesthesia device which has limited
application in emergency medicine, but may be useful for those
in C-spine immobilization (Anaesthesia 1999:793) or when an
endotracheal tube cannot be introduced successfully. The distal tip

of this device sits in the posterior pharynx and is then inflated to "occlude" the esophageal opening; air vents just proximal to this area direct air towards the larynx. Not as secure as an endotracheal tube, and some people intubate through this device with an endotracheal tube, sometimes using fiberoptic assistance (Paediatr Anaesth 2000:53)—the intubating laryngeal mask airway is of equivocal usefulness (Anaesth Intensive Care 1998:387; Anaesthesia 1996:389)

Orotracheal intubation: This tube is placed through the mouth and into the trachea. Peds tubes are uncuffed and can be sized using the patient's little finger, or consulting a Breslow tape. Adult tubes are typically in the 7–8 range (internal diameter in millimeters) and have an inflatable cuff. "Cricoid" pressure from an assistant helps (BURP—manipulate the thyroid cartilage in a *b*ack or posterior, *u*p, and *r*ightward *p*ressure), and this is commonly known as the Sellick maneuver (Anaesthesist 1998:45). Confirmation of placement with checking for breath sounds over anterior lung fields and lack of sounds over stomach; CXR is confirmatory. Not uncommon to have right mainstem intubation, and simply withdraw the tube 2–4 cm

Nasotracheal intubation: This can be done in a conscious adult patient, and the same caveats with NPA with regard to facial trauma. The patient must have spontaneous respirations, because listening and feeling for breath sounds at the end of the tube is the mechanism for guiding the tube into the trachea (J Emerg Med 1999:791). Lubricate the tip of the tube, insert through largest naris passage, and follow the breath sounds, with gentle back and forth rotation of the tube to facilitate placement. Application of oxymetazoline HCl 0.05% (Afrin) nasal spray prior to procedure may decrease nasal bleeding. Advancing during early inspiration is the timing most important to pass through the vocal cords. May be facilitated with digital intubation guidance (J Emerg Med 1989:275)

Digital intubation: A deeply comatose patient with obscure landmarks may be digitally intubated (J Emerg Med 1984:317). Place two fingers of your nondominant hand past the tongue and behind the epiglottis. Pass the tube down along the hand and use the two fingers at the epiglottis to guide the tube into the trachea. Not uncommon to have left mainstem intubation (Am J Emerg Med 1994:466). Beck airway airflow monitor (BAAM) may be helpful with these type of intubations; produces a whistle noise that intensifies with placement into trachea (Prehospital Disaster Med 1993:357)

Rapid sequence intubation:
Ann Emerg Med 1993:1008

A protocol for allowing paralysis of a patient who is difficult to intubate, secondary to jaw clenching such as seen in those with head injury. Different protocols exist with all meds IV, with succinylcholine and vecuronium being two examples. Use of this sequence necessitates knowledge of these drugs, and learning about preanesthesia. Typically, pain and amnestic modulation can occur with fentanyl (2–5 µg/kg) and midazolam (0.1 mg/kg), although consider substituting ketamine (2 mg/kg) for midazolam in those with status asthmaticus. Premedicate with meds of choice, including lidocaine 1 mg/kg to blunt reflex ICP increase from initiating gag reflex with laryngoscope blade—this can be blunted with lidocaine directly on posterior tongue, as well. Wait 3–5 minutes, and then give your muscle relaxants. Succinylcholine is 1.5 mg/kg, and should be used with caution in those with massive muscle trauma or other reasons for hyperkalemia, in those with increased intraocular pressure, and in those with brain tumors giving an increased ICP—may be used as sole paralytic agent (Ann Emerg Med 1992:929). Vecuronium is an example of a nondepolarizing agent, and these agents usually require a priming dose given with the premedications for quick action. For example, the dose for vecuronium is 0.1 mg/kg, but give 10% of this with the premedications. Once the muscle relaxant has been given, the Sellick maneuver must be employed and held until the airway is controlled to avoid regurgitation (BURP—*b*ackward, *u*pward, *r*ightward *p*ressure). As well as the usual monitors for heart rate, blood pressure, and O_2 saturation, also consider end-tidal CO_2 monitor. Working with the hospital anesthesia department can help provide protocols for individual EDs

Gum elastic bougie: A 2–3-foot length of Teflon that facilitates intubation in those with anatomy that makes it difficult to visualize the vocal cords (Anaesthesia 1992:878), or if patient with C-spine immobilization (Anaesthesia 1993:630). This performs better than using a stylet (Anaesthesia 1996:935). The end of this Teflon rod has a slight bend to it, and snaking this past the epiglottitis and toward the larynx should place this rod within the trachea—moving the rod back and forth and feeling slight bumps (tracheal rings) is a positive sign, whereas complete smoothness probably denotes esophageal intubation. Leave the rod in place, and pass an endotracheal tube over this. Passage of the ET tube over the bougie is facilitated by leaving the laryngoscope in place and rotating the bougie so that the bevel is facing posteriorly once it is sitting in the trachea (Anaesthesia 1990:774)

Retrograde intubation: A-time consuming technique (Crit Care Med 1986:589) (not for the apneic patient) that relies on identification of the cricothyroid membrane, passing a needle through this membrane followed by a J-wire through the needle and the J-wire passed into the oral cavity. Put the J-wire into the distal side port of the ET tube and then out through the proximal opening (i.e., opening of ET tube out of body) (Anesth Analg 1974:1013). Keep the J-wire taut at this point. Pass the tube until it can no longer go forward, cut the wire where it enters the neck, pull the wire, and pass the tube into its final position

Translaryngeal insufflation: Demand valve or oxygen wall units that can deliver 50 psi of pressure may be used in this set-up. The cricothyroid membrane should be punctured with a 14-gauge needle, and the plastic catheter advanced towards the carina after removal of the needle. Insufflate for 1–2 seconds, and allow chest relaxation for 4–5 seconds. The plastic catheter commonly bends and occludes

Cricothyrotomy: This is a rapid surgical airway when less invasive techniques have not been successful. Identify the cricothyroid membrane, make a vertical 4-cm incision centered on the membrane, and make a horizontal incision through the membrane itself. Pass a hemostat or dilator (such as the Trousseau (J Emerg Med 1999:433)) through the membrane, and then a No. 4 Shiley tracheostomy tube or a No. 5 ET tube. Be sure that the tube is not positioned in the anterior mediastinum. Sew this in place. Placement with a guidewire following the Seldinger technique is also available with similar operator profiles (time needed and complications of procedure) (J Emerg Med 1999:957; Anesthesiology 2000:687)

Esophageal detector devices: A device used to ensure correct tube placement (nonesophageal). Two examples are the esophageal detector device (Tube Check®), or the "turkey baster," and the end-tidal CO_2 detector. The bulb is squeezed and then placed on the end of the ET tube—if it quickly inflates, then it is a tracheal intubation. If it slowly reinflates, then it is a presumed esophageal intubation. The CO_2 monitor is placed in-line with the BVM, and is situated between the ET tube and the BVM. The litmus paper inside the plastic housing turns yellow with CO_2 and this is good; turns purple without CO_2 and this is bad

Fiberoptic devices: Passage of an ET tube can be facilitated with a bronchoscope, or a fiberoptic laryngoscope if it is the only device available (Lab Anim 2000:199). Place the tube over the scope to begin with, advance the scope into the larynx/trachea, and then advance the tube. This may be particularly useful in burn patients with evidence of facial burns. Also may be preferable in those with C-spine immobilization (Anesthesiology 1999:1253). If abnormalities are noted, early elective intubation is usually advocated, and this can be quickly done if the tube is in position. A fiberoptic stylet is also available, which functions similar to a gum elastic bougie with an eyepiece (Anesth Analg 1999:526)

20.2 CONSCIOUS SEDATION

Curr Opin Pediatr 1995:309; N Engl J Med 2000:938

Many situations abound in medicine where patients feel uncomfortable or cannot tolerate procedures that need to be done. For example, suture repair in pediatrics, I + D of abscess (Arch Otolaryngol Head Neck Surg 1999:1197), chest tube placement, central line placement, foreign body removal, lumbar puncture, or perhaps CT or MRI exam. We can use large doses of medications and combine analgesics and sedatives to provide pain control, anxiolysis, and amnesia. When we impair a patient's reflexes and mentation, then we have induced conscious sedation

A variety of medications are available to help in these situations, and learning to use them should be done with direct preceptorship. Intravenous dosing is more effective for titrating to effect

When using these drugs as conscious sedation, one is doing more than simple pain control or anxiolysis. Continuous cardiac monitoring, O_2 saturations, and blood pressures should be employed (Ann Emerg Med 1992:551); end-tidal CO_2 monitoring via divided nasal cannula

may herald respiratory depression earlier than other measures
(Pediatr Emerg Care 1997:189)

- The opiates for pain control include MSO_4 at 0.05–0.1 mg/kg, fentanyl at 1–3 µg/kg, and meperidine at 1–2 mg/kg. These work best IV, but morphine and meperidine may be given IM, and fentanyl has a lollipop (Ann Emerg Med 1994:1059)
- The benzodiazepines include midazolam at 0.05–0.07 mg/kg IM, which may be helpful with ketamine IM; midazolam 0.01–0.03 mg/kg IV (Ann Emerg Med 1993:201) or perhaps up to 0.1 mg/kg IV; and lorazepam at 0.01–0.02 mg/kg IV
- The barbiturates include thiopental at 3–5 mg/kg IV and 25 mg/kg pr, and IV use is an effective induction agent for RSI. Methohexital at 25 mg/kg pr is also useful (AJR Am J Roentgenol 1993:577)

Other sedatives include choral hydrate, ketamine, nitrous oxide, etomidate, and propofol

- Chloral hydrate is 25–50 mg/kg either po or pr, and has found a niche in radiology studies (AJR Am J Roentgenol 1995:905)
- Ketamine is 1–2 mg/kg IV and 3–5 mg/kg IM (Acad Emerg Med 1999:21). Medication of choice for RSI in asthma, and may be of some use combining with midazolam 0.05–0.07 mg/kg IM and atropine 0.02 mg/kg IM to prevent emergence reactions and hypersalivation, respectively. Midazolam pro and con (Ann Emerg Med 2000:229). All three (ketamine, midazolam, atropine) can be combined in the same syringe for IM use in peds, and no IV is necessary using this protocol (Ann Emerg Med 1998:688)
- Nitrous oxide is a 50% nitrous oxide/50% oxygen mixture that is a "self-use" system (Acad Emerg Med 1998:112), and remember that nitrous oxide causes bowel edema. Efficacy is equivocal (Pediatr Dent 2000:125)
- Etomidate is an imidazole that is useful for conscious sedation at 0.1 mg/kg (ACEP Annual Meeting, Burton, 10/98), and for induction at 0.3 mg/kg IV (J Emerg Med 2000:13; Pediatr Emerg Care 2000:18)
- Propofol is 0.5–2 mg/kg IV bolus, followed by 25–125 µg/kg/min infusion. This may be useful for RSI and then to ICU patients, not yet for conscious sedation (Acad Emerg Med 1999:975)
- Reversal of medications may "wake" patients faster, but does not shorten time to discharge postprocedure (e.g., flumazenil for benzodiazepines (Acad Emerg Med 1997:944))—advocate for letting patients "lighten" on their own

20.3 INTRAOSSEUS TECHNIQUE

J Crit Illn 1993:539

An effective access technique in children less than 5 years of age,
but also effective if significant osteoporosis or nonuse of lower
extremity. The site of insertion is the flat anterior portion of the
proximal tibia. Clean with iodine, local lidocaine anesthesia if
available, and place needle by puncturing skin and then screwing
into place. Angle of insertion is perpendicular to the long axis of
the tibia. When "pop" is felt, aspirate marrow to confirm placement,
and secure in place by screwing plate to skin surface (IO needle)
and/or taping into place. In an IO needle, the center tap is removed
by unscrewing the top of the needle, and the IV line is placed into
the exposed receptacle

20.4 PEDIATRIC BLADDER CATHETERIZATION

Suprapubic tap is less efficient than urethral catheterization, with no
benefit as far as risk (Ann Emerg Med 1994:225). Additionally,
suprapubic tap less likely to succeed if bladder is not full. Thus,
the suprapubic tap is not advocated

20.5 VENTRICULAR SHUNT MANAGEMENT

Malfunction or secondary infection is possible with indwelling shunts,
and ventriculoperitoneal shunts are the most common today
Malfunction is most common with proximal occlusion, and
secondarily distal occlusion. The bladder(s) of the shunt can be
palpated subcutaneously over the skull. If one-bladder system,
inability to easily compress it is consistent with distal obstruction,
and slow filling (>2 seconds) is consistent with proximal obstruction.
If two bladders, compress the proximal one first, and inability to
easily compress the second bladder is consistent with distal

obstruction; after releasing the distal bladder, lack of quick filling of the proximal bladder is consistent with proximal obstruction. Head CT may show ventricular enlargement

Infection can occur at any site along the catheter, and may present as an acute abdomen or meningitis/encephalitis. If considering either of these conditions, neurosurgical consult is mandatory

21 Psychiatric/Substance Abuse

21.1 CHEMICAL AND PHYSICAL RESTRAINT

This section encompasses the issue of how to best help a violent and aggressive patient. The procedures surrounding chemical and physical restraint should provide a safe environment for the patient and the staff (HEC Forum 1998:244)

- Initial physical restraints may include wrist and ankle restraints to a stretcher/bed (J Nurs Adm 1998:19). If the patient does not respond to this immobilization, it may be necessary to secure the chest and pelvis, and be sure that the gurney is anchored to the floor. If the patient is spitting or biting, a mask may need to be positioned, and someone should be available at all times to remove the mask if a patent airway becomes an issue

- Chemical restraints are medications used to modify and subdue a patient's behavior so that the patient is not a danger to him/herself or staff, and so that a medical evaluation can occur. Some options are haloperidol (Haldol), droperidol (Inapsine) (Ann Emerg Med 1992:407), diphenhydramine (Benadryl), lorazepam (Ativan), or perphenazine (Trilafon) (Curr Ther Res Clin Exp 1972:478)

- Once chemical restraints begin to work, physical restraints can be modified and eventually eliminated. Frequent reassessment and treatment of underlying medical issues may help release patients from physical restraints in a timely manner

21.2 DELIRIUM

Am J Psychiatry 1999:1; Geriatrics 1999:28, 36, 39; Dement Geriatr Cogn Disord 1999:310

Cause: Drugs (intoxication discussed in 21.3); intracranial lesion or process, such as encephalitis, meningitis, amyloid, or primary neoplasm or metastatic disease; systemic diseases such as infections (syphilis) or autoimmune phenomenona; ETOH or sedative withdrawal; drug abuse, e.g., ecstasy (J Psychoactive Drugs 1999:167); metabolic such as hyperammonemia, sodium disorders, hypoglycemia, etc.; seizures

Epidem: High incidence in elderly, with 15% developing this after general surgery; higher rate noted in those with dementia

Pathophys: Dependent on process, but overall leading to CNS dysfunction (Dement Geriatr Cogn Disord 1999:330). Increased serum anticholinergic activity in the elderly (J Gerontol A Biol Sci Med Sci 1999:M12) and elevated serotonergic activity in general (Dement Geriatr Cogn Disord 1999:339)

Sx: Hallucinations, often visual but also auditory

Si: Acute onset and fluctuating course; transient global disorder of cognition and attention. Inattention; loss of attention span is most prominent deficit; test by serial 7's; serial digits up to 7, such as phone numbers; spell "world" backward; disorganized thinking or altered level of consciousness; may also "sundown"—exacerbated at night (Dement Geriatr Cogn Disord 1999:353)

Crs: Variable depending on underlying illnesses and cause. Prognosis/course may be guided by the Delirium Rating Scale (Psychosomatics 1999:193), which is a tool applied over time (e.g., 24 hours)

Cmplc: Inherent with cause

Diff Dx: Psychoses are not global; consider total global amnesia in patient who recovers in 1 day

Lab: Directed by exam and past medical history. Consider metabolic (Chapter 11), intoxication (see 21.3 and 25.1), infectious disease (Chapter 10), and CNS (Chapter 13) work-up

ED Rx:
- Consider 1-to-1 staffing to watch patient
- Consider medication to help calm patient, such as haloperidol, droperidol, or a benzodiazepine; use low doses in the elderly; such Rx may change the exam
- Medical evaluation as above, with medicine consult for admission

21.3 INTOXICATION

Cause: Ingestion, inhalation, injection, or dermal absorption of substance which alters brain function (J Emerg Med 1999:679)

Epidem: Unknown, but drug intoxication linked to trauma (Jama 1997:1769)

Pathophys: Per substrate

Sx: Hallucinations, often visual but also auditory (may be seen in withdrawal, too)

Si: Variable, from acute onset to fluctuating course; transient global disorder of cognition and attention. Inattention, loss of attention span is most prominent deficit; disorganized thinking or altered level of consciousness anywhere from agitation to coma

Crs: Variable depending on underlying illnesses and cause

Cmplc: Inherent with cause

Diff Dx: If febrile, consider CNS infection (meningitis, encephalitis) or NMS; hypoglycemia; head trauma or other CNS pathology

Lab:
- Rectal temperature with hypothermia thermometer if low; CBC with diff; glucoscan; metabolic profile with calcium and magnesium levels; liver profile; acetaminophen level; salicylate level; ETOH level, especially in all trauma patients (J Trauma 1999:1131, discussion, 1135); measured vs. calculated osmoles; methanol, ethylene glycol, or isopropyl alcohol level if suspicion by history or if metabolic acidosis without other cause; serum levels of specific drugs based on history, clinical exam, metabolic abnormalities, EKG, or positive indicator found on urine drug screen if necessary (Br J Clin Pharmacol 1999:278)
- U/A; urine toxic drug screen; Wood's lamp evaluation of urine to assess for ethylene glycol
- X-ray: Consider head CT without contrast to check for bleed

ED Rx:

- Airway, intubate if necessary
- Staffing with 1-to-1 watch if needed
- IV access, with fluid resuscitation if needed
- Consider D50, naloxone; give thiamine 100 mg IV
- Physical/chemical restraint as needed

Alcohol

- Ethanol withdrawal may be treated with IV lorazepam 2 mg, or other benzodiazepine or chlordiazepoxide (Librium) orally if able. Treat tremors, hypertension, and tachycardia to avoid delirium tremens. Seizure treatment as in 13.11. No effect on clearance with IV NS (J Emerg Med 1999:1) or coffee
- Methanol intoxication (Med Toxicol 1986:309) may lead to blindness (Arch Ophthalmol 1999:286) and other complications with ingestions as low as 15 cc of a 40% solution. Treatment is with IV NaHCO₃ to maintain normal pH and ETOH (Am J Kidney Dis 1987:441) to maintain level >100 mg/dL. Institute Rx if methanol suspected, do not wait for the serum level to return (intoxication usually with level >20 mg/dL). IV ETOH is 10% ETOH in D₅W—bolus 10 cc/kg, then 1.6 cc/kg/hr infusion. Also give folate 50 mg IV q 4 hours. Hemodialysis for those with CNS dysfunction, visual complaints, or methanol level >50 mg/dL. Do not withhold ETOH Rx pending dialysis. 4-Methylpyrazole (Fomepizole) (J Toxicol Clin Toxicol 1999:777; Intensive Care Med 1999:528) and N-acetylcysteine (Drug Alcohol Depend 1999:61) may be of some use
- Isopropranolol intoxication should be treated with supportive therapy, consider IV NaHCO₃ if acidosis with hypotension, and dialysis for patients who are hemodynamically unstable, have significant CNS or respiratory depression, or if serum level is >400 mg/dL

Cocaine

- Use IV benzodiazepines to treat tremors, anxiety, and vasospasm. Vasospasm of coronary arteries and intracerebral arteries may cause acute coronary syndrome and acute stroke syndrome, respectively
- Treat hyperthermia with cool mist and cooling blanket, usually no benefit with acetaminophen, avoid ASA
- Seizure treatment in 13.11, use phenobarbital before dilantin in these cases

- Acute coronary syndrome Rx should be ASA, TNG, benzodiazepines, and MSO_4. Avoid β-blockers (α activity would then be unopposed) and thrombolytics may be useful although probably vasospastic and possible secondary thrombotic etiology
- HTN crisis with IV benzodiazepines and nitroprusside—not labetalol
- Mules (cocaine transporters who have swallowed packaged condoms) who have no signs of toxicity should be given oral charcoal and Golytely. If symptomatic, general surgery referral for package removal—not endoscopy

Narcotics
- Reversible with naloxone 0.1 mg/kg, up to 2 mg IV. Use higher doses in those with propoxyphene (Darvon) and pentazocine (Talwin) intoxication
- Short half-life of naloxone may necessitate repeated dosing or drip—0.4 mg/hour titrated to effect

21.4 MEDICAL SCREENING EXAM

Acad Emerg Med 1997:124

This is a term applied to those who come to the ED with psychiatric issues but first need a medical evaluation. Even those patients with an emotional or stressful nidus accounting for increased psychiatric lability or somatization may have a significant medical condition that needs attention

If a patient has had a medical evaluation previously, and no presenting symptoms have changed, further laboratory evaluation may not be necessary in the setting of a stable physical exam. If a patient has not been previously evaluated, or has an abnormal exam, then further medical evaluation may be necessary

Intoxicants can also lead to coping or behavioral problems, and these may need to be screened as well. Indiscriminate and universal toxicology screening is not supported by the literature (Am J Emerg Med 1984:331; J Emerg Med 2000:173). On the other hand, those with intentional overdose or any ingestion with suicidal overtones should be screened for both salicyclates and acetaminophen (Am J Emerg Med 1996:443) (see 21.2). Occult infections, metabolic abnormalities, or CNS lesions are more common in the elderly presenting for the first time for psychiatric evaluation. The value of random thyroid function testing (TSH) is equivocal in the young, and more helpful in the elderly

The most important part of the exam is the mental status and neurologic exam. In psychiatric cases that are not clear-cut, disposition can be difficult. No historical data (suicidality, homicidality, hallucinations) in a patient's evaluation or screening tool exists that helps us decide who needs emergent hospitalization, and who will be benefit from other types of disposition

22 Pulmonary

22.1 ASPIRATED FOREIGN BODY

Ann Surg 1972:720

Cause: Usually accidental, may be anything that can be inhaled, such as small pieces of toys, coins, candy and peanuts

Epidem: Common in infants

Pathophys: Inhalation of object in mouth or nose with lodging in larynx or bronchopulmonary tree

Sx: Dyspnea; stridor; hemoptysis

Si: Wheezing; tachypnea; decreased lung sounds in one lobe

Crs: Benign if not obstructing entire airway/lung, and able to be retrieved with a bronchoscope

Cmplc: Asphyxia; pneumothorax; pneumonia; pulmonary edema (Pediatr Emerg Care 1986:235)

Diff Dx: Asthma, croup, pneumonia

Lab: X-Ray—CXR with expiratory film if radiolucent foreign body to look for area that does not symmetrically compress. If unable to locate foreign body, do lateral neck X-ray and abdominal X-ray to locate (Radiol Clin North Am 1998:175)

ED Rx:
- O_2, keep patient calm
- IV access
- ENT or pulmonary consult immediately if in trachea, mainstem bronchus, or beyond (Endoscopy 1977:216)
- If severe respiratory distress or impending respiratory failure, consider rapid sequence intubation. Look for FB in larynx, remove with Magill forceps, and intubate. If cannot locate the FB, intubate and try to push object down one mainstem to oxygenate and ventilate the contralateral lung

22.2 ASTHMA

Ann Intern Med 2000:219

Cause: Innumerable allergens, with genetic susceptibility—chromosome 5—, and is also found more often in those with atopic susceptibility

Epidem: ~5% of U.S. population and increasing; seen more in low-income groups; common in those exposed to first- and second-hand smoke

Pathophys: Airway inflammation with decreased airway lumen size, bronchial edema, and increased mucus production. Inflammatory airway secretions with eosinophils, but neutrophils predominate (Am J Respir Crit Care Med 2000:1185). Multiple types including allergic; exercise-induced; infectious—(25% of those with bronchiolitis go on to asthma, bronchiectasis, chronic bronchitis, and eventually some form of COPD); and emotional stress

Morning wheezing due to circadian decrease in epinephrine and steroids. ASA sensitivity is a direct action on kinin receptors by acetyl groups, may be genetic as well. Food sulfites precipitate, as does exposure to cigarette smoke

Sx: Dyspnea; wheezing; exercise or cold induction of symptoms; opiate or ASA exacerbation induction

Si: Wheezing, check with exertion or cough if lung exam is normal at rest; dyspnea; nasal polyps correlate with atopic type; cyanosis, papilledema, pulsus paradoxus are three late signs

Crs: Overall mortality has not increased

Cmplc: Status asthmaticus—respiratory arrest with respiratory acidosis as most common mode of death (not arrhythmia); multifocal atrial tachycardia associated with hypoxia, theophylline, and catechol Rx; allergic asthma in mother associated with premature labor and respiratory distress syndrome of the newborn. Minor complication of mild hypokalemia in those with β-agonist therapy (Pediatr Pulmonol 1999:27)

Diff Dx: Aspirated FB in the young and elderly; croup; CHF in the elderly and peds with heart disease; vocal cord dysfunction; conversion reaction; pulmonary emboli, rarely

Lab:
- If toxic or severe case—CBC with diff; ABG; blood cultures and sputum sample

- Peak flows poor predictor of severity in the ED (Am J Respir Crit Care Med 1996:889), length of speaking time just as useful (Am J Emerg Med 1998:572)
- X-ray: Chest film if severe, febrile, or not following classic asthma pathway

ED Rx:

Med Lett Drugs Ther 2000;42:19

- O_2
- Control airway, rapid sequence intubation if patient losing consciousness or in less than 1 word dyspnea and not responding—safer to do earlier rather than later; i.e., do not wait for pt to have cardiopulmonary arrest (Crit Care Med 1993:1727)
- β-agonists—nebulized albuterol (Proventil) at 0.1–0.15 mg/kg up to 5 mg/dose if >40 lb, may select as continuous at 10 mg/hour, all suspended in NS; terbutaline (Brethine) 1 cc in 2 cc of NS; or bitolterol (Tornalate)—all probably equally effective. Inhaler with spacer as effective as nebs if able to use effectively (J Pediatr 2000:497)
- Ipratropium (Atrovent) is not approved for acute asthma exacerbation but literature may support use of one-time dosing with albuterol at 0.5 cc in nebulized solution, definitely not a chronic Rx choice (Cochrane Database Syst Rev 2000)
- Steroids—hydrocortisone (100–300 mg q 6 hours), dexamethasone (4–8 mg q 8 hours), methylprednisolone (1–1.5 mg/kg IV q 12 hours), and prednisone (1–2 mg/kg qd) all equal at appropriate doses and give in ED; route of administration does not matter as far as onset of action or efficacy (6–8 hours or longer for onset of action). Outpatient treatment should include a short course of steroids, which may be extended depending on patient history (Cochrane Database Syst Rev 2000). Consider inhaled steroids such as triamcinolone or budesonide, and perhaps some benefit in combining oral and inhaled steroids (Jama 1999:2119)
- $MgSO_4$ 2 g IV or nebulized (3 cc isotonic) (Am J Med 2000:193) may help in severe cases (Cochrane Database Syst Rev 2000)
- Aminophylline may be considered in severe cases; load at 5.6 mg/kg over 20–30 minutes, then 0.5 mg/kg/hour, less in those with CHF, liver disease, pneumonia, or h/o cardiac dysrhythmia
- Consider Heliox 60–80% helium, probably better in sick patients, pro (Chest 1999:296) and con (Am J Emerg Med 2000:495)

- IVF important in severe cases, will need NaCl and KCl to reverse chloride depletion, be wary of pulmonary edema
- Antibiotics if bacterial focus or severe, consider macrolides (caution with theophylline), doxycycline, second- or third-generation cephalosporins, Tm/S
- NaHCO$_3$ probably not an ED intervention, treat acidosis with outline as above
- Internal medicine/primary care ED consult for those needing admission, outpatient follow-up with steroid taper for those with good response to Rx—peak flows ideally >80% predicted
- Salmeterol (Serevent), montelukast (Singulair), zafirlukast (Accolate), zileuton (Zyflo), cromolyn (Intal), nedocromil (Tilade), and the decision for outpatient theophylline (Slo-Bid, Theo-Dur) should be part of the outpatient physician's realm

22.3 COMMUNITY-ACQUIRED PNEUMONIA

Pediatr Infect Dis J 2000:251; Allergy Asthma Proc 2000:33; J Am Geriatr Soc 2000:82

Cause: By age

Pediatr Infect Dis J 2000:293

- *0–28 days*: *Escherichia coli*, group B streptococcus; less commonly *Staphylococcus aureus*, RSV, *Enterobacter* sp.
- *28 days to 5 years*: RSV, rhinovirus, *Streptococcus pneumoniae*, parainfluenza virus, adenovirus; less commonly *Chlamydia*
- *5 to 15 years*: *S. pneumoniae*, influenza A, adenovirus; less commonly *Mycoplasma*
- *Adults*: *S. pneumoniae*, *Haemophilus influenzae* (more common in smokers), atypicals (more common in young adults) including Mycoplasma and *Chlamydia*; less commonly aspiration (unless good history for such), *S. aureus*, gram-negatives, and *Legionella*

Epidem: Much more common in immunosuppressed individuals who constitute 60% of hospital admissions for pneumonia; worse prognosis in the elderly if elevated BUN, hypotensive, or respiratory rate >30 breaths/minute; incidence of 1.62/1000 population with males > females (Eur Respir J 2000:757). *Acinetobacter* in foundry workers (Ann Intern Med 1981:688)

sensitive and specific. The "blue bloater" is the pt with CHF, hypoxia, and hypercarbia. The "pink puffer" is the patient with weight loss, low Pco_2, moderate decrease in O_2 at rest, and possible left-sided CHF

Crs: Pink puffer has better prognosis than blue bloater because pulmonary hypertension is less

Cmplc: Polycythemia; pulmonary hypertension; peptic ulcer disease; acute respiratory failure; lithium worsens disease; treat hypophosphatemia—impairs diaphragmatic contractility

Lab:
- If severe distress or toxic—CBC with diff; metabolic profile including phosphate and magnesium; ABG
- X-ray: CXR—air trapping, large lung fields, and narrow mediastinum are common

ED Rx:
- O_2, keep SaO_2 at 90–92% if unsure about CO_2 retention
- Secure airway, intubate if necessary. Consider Bi-Pap with levels 10/4 if attempting to avoid intubation but patient still willing for intubation if this fails
- β-agonists—nebulized albuterol (Proventil) at 0.1–0.15 mg/kg up to 5 mg/dose if >40 lb, may select as continuous at 10 mg/hour, all suspended in NS; terbutaline (Brethine) 1 cc in 2 cc of NS; or bitolterol (Tornalate)—all probably equally effective (Am J Med 1983:697). Inhaler with spacer as effective as nebs if able to use effectively
- Ipratropium (Atrovent) 0.5 cc in first neb and then q 6 hours (Respiration 1998:354)
- Steroids—hydrocortisone (100–300 mg q 6 hours), dexamethasone (4–12 mg q 8 hours), methylprednisolone (1–1.5 mg/kg IV q 12 hours), and prednisone (1–2 mg/kg qd) all equal at appropriate doses; route of administration does not matter as far as onset of action or efficacy
- Third-generation cephalosporin (ceftriaxone, cefotaxime), Tm/S, fluoroquinolone, +/– macrolide will most likely help clear exacerbation sooner (Respir Med 1998:442)
- Aminophylline may be considered in severe cases, load at 5.6 mg/kg over 20–30 minutes, then 0.5 mg/kg/hour, less in those with CHF, liver disease, pneumonia, or h/o cardiac dysrhythmia
- Consider $MgSO_4$ 2 g IV in severe cases
- Internal medicine/primary care consult if requires hospitalization

- Outpatient: if able to clear quickly, home with appropriate inhalers with scheduled times, prednisone taper, antibiotics, and 1–2-day follow-up with primary physician

22.5 MASSIVE HEMOPTYSIS

Clin Chest Med 1994:147

Cause: Pulmonary vascular change (telangiectasia), TB (Radiology 1996:691), cancer, cystic fibrosis, trauma, massive PE, coagulation abnormalities

Epidem: <5% of those with hemoptysis with massive hemoptysis, but mortality in this small group ranges from 7–32%

Pathophys: Erosion into bronchopulmonary tree; self-limited cases usually from irritation

Sx: Coughing up blood

Si: Look in nares, oral cavity for other source; examine skin for petechiae or ecchymoses to consider systemic coagulopathy

Crs: Dependent on degree of bleeding; difficult to control true exsanguination

Cmplc: Asphyxia

Diff Dx: Minimal or limited usually—bronchitis; TB; mitral stenosis; nasopharyngeal, oral, or gastrointestinal source; bronchiectasis

Lab: Consider CBC with diff and PT/PTT if potential coagulopathy; get type and screen if pt exsanguinating. X-ray: CXR

ED Rx:
- O_2 if hypoxic, IV access, bed rest, and mild sedation for conservative treatment (Arch Intern Med 1983:287)
- Place in lateral decubitus position with affected side down
- Selective mainstem intubation of unaffected side if possible, especially in trauma (J Trauma 1987:1123); will probably need anesthesia consult
- Correct coagulopathy and replace blood if necessary
- Pulmonary consult for emergent bronchoscopy (Chest 1989:473) or perhaps embolization (Arch Surg 1998:862)

22.6 PNEUMOTHORAX

Cause: Trauma—either out of hospital (MVA, IV drug use) (Ann Emerg Med 1983:167) or iatrogenic (central lines, mechanical ventilation, emergency surgical airway) (Am J Emerg Med 1991:176; 1995:532; J Laryngol Otol 1994:69), bullous disease, postbiopsy via transthoracic or bronchoscopic approach (Thorax 1986:647)

Epidem: Spontaneous pneumothorax (SP) incidence changing from primarily a bleb nidus to those with AIDS and non-AIDS/nonbleb disease, which includes a host of diffuse interstitial lung diseases (Am J Surg 1992:528). No increase in risk of pneumothorax in those undergoing percutaneous pulmonary biopsies with history of COPD (Chest 1994:1705), but is related to depth and size (small) of lesion (Radiology 1996:371)

Pathophys: Violation of pleural space with air trapping and expansion

Sx: Dsypnea, chest pain

Si: Decreased breath sounds over lung field, with perhaps "crackling" or "bubbling" heard, which is louder than rales (Hamman's sign)—associated with both pneumothorax and pneumomediastinum (Chest 1992:1281); look for associated signs of subcutaneous emphysema in trauma; look for tracheal shift or hypotension to diagnose tension pneumothorax

Crs: Those with spontaneous etiology or bullous disease may need thoracic surgery

Cmplc: Tension pneumothorax—patient develops shock from pneumothorax with mediastinal shift to contralateral side as a feature. SP recurrence higher in those that are tall, with less recurrence with smoking cessation (Thorax 1997:805)

Diff Dx: Catamenial pneumothorax occurs in females; it is recurrent SP that occurs with menses (Pediatr Emerg Care 1997:390). Pneumothorax may be mistaken as Boerhaave's syndrome (J Accid Emerg Med 1999:235) or diaphragmatic hernia—congenital (Ann Emerg Med 1993:1221) or postsurgical

Lab: None for tension pneumothorax, otherwise CXR. Inspiration and expiration films increase yield of finding pneumothorax (Arch Emerg Med 1993:343). CT of chest in multisystem trauma will show occult pneumothoraces, which may need treatment if patient going on ventilator or to OR (AJR Am J Roentgenol 1984:987).

EKG changes may be noted that mimic acute MI (Ann Emerg Med 1985:164)

ED Rx:

Tension Pneumothorax
- Tap affected side going over the second rib in the midclavicular line, with over-the-needle catheter (14 G) be careful of withdrawing the needle completely because sometimes the catheter collapses, or use a 16 G Verres needle that automatically protrudes inner blunt tube when pleural cavity is entered (Crit Care Med 1978:378), or 16 F McSwain Dart, which has its plastic tip formed into a flange postinsertion to maintain patency (Ann Surg 1980:760)
- IV and O_2, conscious sedation if necessary
- Chest tube

Pneumothorax without Tension Physiology
- O_2 and IV access
- Conscious sedation with midazolam and MSO_4, for example
- Chest tube, 32 F for traumatic or those with fluid (hemothorax) component. May try simple aspiration (J Emerg Med 1986:437) although age >50 years, chronic lung disease, or >2.5 liters of aspirated air associated with failure of this therapy (J Accid Emerg Med 1998:317). Small tube with Heimlich valve an option in spontaneous or postprocedure pneumothoraces
- Post–needle biopsy of lung, having patient on affected side down or on the contralateral side has no influence on development of pneumothorax (Radiology 1999:59)

22.7 PULMONARY EMBOLUS

Chest 1998:499

Cause: Embolic clots to pulmonary arteries from systemic veins

Epidem: Associated with history of thromboembolic disease (Chest 1992:677); pregnancy, estrogen-containing birth control pills (Jama 1992:1689; Lancet 1996:983); hypercoagulable states from factor disorders or antiphospholipid syndromes; prolonged rest state. Equivocal association with occult malignancy (Arch Intern Med 1987:1907)

Pathophys: Thrombophlebitis causes thrombus, which breaks free and migrates to the lungs; it is possible to have small emboli chronically rather than one large one (one etiology for pulmonary hypertension). Calves and upper extremities are rarely the source; no signs or symptoms of DVT in 50% of pts

Sx: Dyspnea—sudden or chronic; pleuritic chest pain; hemoptysis; fever; syncope—seen in massive PE

Si: JVD; rales; wheezing; $P_2 > A_2$; BP cuff test for calf pain; cyanosis

Crs: Resolves over 10–30 days; 80% overall survival; 75% of deaths within the first 2 hours; DVT clinically resolves in 1/3 after 3 days of heparin

Cmplc: ARDS; chronic pulmonary hypertension

Diff Dx: Fat emboli—from bony fractures, 24–48-hour latency period, trial of methylprednisolone 1–1.5 mg/kg q 6 hours and other supportive care; amniotic fluid emboli in pregnancy

Lab:
- CBC with diff and PT/PTT if considering treatment with anticoagulants or thrombolytics; ABG may be of some value but cannot base further testing on Po_2 alone—$Po_2 <80$ mm Hg with 10% false negative, $Po_2 <90$ with 0% false negative; d-dimer equivocal with latex agglutination tests including SimplyRed—pro (J Nucl Med 1993:896) and con (Ann Emerg Med 2000:121)
- Noninvasive tests: duplex U/S if unsure if pt is high or low risk to help interpret the utility of pulmonary test (V/Q scan, helical CT) (Am J Emerg Med 1999:271); see 9.8
- X-ray: CXR to ascertain other reasons for hypoxia, look for pulmonary infarcts or newly elevated diaphragm—or perhaps future role in lieu of ventilation phase of V/Q scan (Thromb Haemost 2000:412). V/Q scan (87% sensitive, 97% specific) to look for multiple mismatched defects, helpful if normal or low probability with low index of suspicion, or high probability with high or moderate index of suspicion—otherwise not helpful (Jama 1990:2753). Helical CT to look for intraluminal clot in medium to large pulmonary arteries (Radiology 1997:447). Pulmonary angiography is the gold standard (not CT (Radiology 1997:453)), and should be used in cases where studies are persistently equivocal

ED Rx:
- O_2
- IV access
- Heparin 5000–10,000-unit IV bolus, large dose for larger thrombus/ emboli if considering clot consumption of heparin, then weight-based dosing per hour—OK in pregnancy. Low molecular weight

heparin effective (Fragmin (Thromb Haemost 1995:1432), tinzaparin (N Engl J Med 1997:663)); all low molecular weight heparins are not equivalent in action and efficacy

- Consider streptokinase to speed clearing with better PFTs and vein function; consider TPA if right heart failure with acute embolus (Lancet 1993:507)
- Medical consult for admission, with consideration of IVC umbrella, invasive radiology thrombolysis (rare) (Clin Cardiol 1999:661), or surgical embolectomy (rare)

23 Rheumatology

23.1 ACUTE RHEUMATIC FEVER (ARF)

Paediatrician 1981:158

Cause: Group A hemolytic (rarely nonhemolytic) streptococcus, with presence of M protein; post-strep, upper respiratory infection × 2–3 weeks, but bacteria must still be present

Epidem: Children peak incidence between 5–15 years of age (J Infect 1998:249); female:male 3:1; incidence of ~0.3/100,000 (Acta Med Scand 1988:587); see 17.9

Pathophys: Autoimmune theories with cross-reacting antibodies between group A strep and human tissues (such as T-cells (Clin Exp Immunol 1999:100)), but does not explain why only strep pharyngitis may go onto ARF

Jones criteria (Pediatr Ann 1999:9) for diagnosis—2 major, or 1 major + 2 minor, + positive ASO titer or culture or h/o scarlet fever. *Major criteria*: carditis; polyarthritis; erythema marginatum; subcutaneous nodules; chorea. *Minor criteria*: fever; arthralgias; distant h/o ARF; elevated WBC, ESR, or CRP; long PR interval or other EKG abnormalities. Members of the same family tend to have same major symptoms

Sx: Sore throat; fever; arthralgias—although transitory (Indian J Pediatr 1988:9)

Si: Erythema marginatum—associated with carditis; murmurs (valvular or nonvalvular) which are associated with pericarditis; subcutaneous nodules at bony prominences that are associated with carditis; pneumonitis; serositis; polyarthritis of large joints; Sydenham's chorea may follow other signs (or symptoms) by weeks or months

Crs: Less than 12 weeks in ~90%; ~95% of those with murmurs appear by 2 weeks of symptom onset

Cmplc: Chronic cardiac valve disease; mitral regurgitation with Jaccoud's arthritis (ulnar deviation which can voluntarily correct); transient glomerulonephritis

Diff Dx: Poststreptococcal reactive arthritis (J Intern Med 1999:261); familial Mediterranean fever (Clin Rheumatol 1999:446); septic arthritis; infective endocarditis; cat-scratch disease; rheumatoid arthritis; immune complex disease; Still's disease; pustular psoriasis; dermatomyositis; inflammatory bowel disease; sarcoidosis; SLE

Lab: CBC with diff; ESR; metabolic profile; U/A; throat culture if still inflamed; ASO titer or streptozyme test; consider anti-DNAase or antistreptodornase titer; EKG. X-ray: look for interstitial pneumonitis

ED Rx:
- PCN 25–50 mg/kg/day ÷ bid po for peds, 500 mg po bid for adults; PCN G benzathine and procaine (Bicillin C-R, or Bicillin C-R 900/300) IM × 1—this will be extended for years of prophylaxis in those with carditis
- ASA for all
- Steroids: for all with severe carditis or pneumonia; optional if sick without murmur; not needed for murmur alone
- Medicine consult for admit if ill, otherwise 1–2-day follow-up

23.2 BEHÇET'S SYNDROME

Curr Opin Rheumatol 1999:53; J R Coll Physicians Lond 2000:169

Cause: Genetic and viral hypotheses

Epidem: 27% of those affected with HLA B5 and B27; male:female 1.7:1 in eastern Mediterranean type

Pathophys: A vasculitis, onset in third decade of life. It is a multisystem disorder, and different classifications helpful for research, not as much in diagnosis (Ann Med Interne (Paris) 1999:477)

Sx: Oral ulcers; genital ulcers; eye pain

Si: Recurrent problems with the following—oral aphthous ulcers; genital ulcers with no preferred site, often painless in women; uveitis

Crs: Each attack lasts 1–4 weeks; unique pulmonary vasculitis is possible (Chest 1989:585); CNS disease has bad prognosis (Brain 1999:2183)

Cmplc: Blindness; cardiac problems; inflammatory arthritis; aseptic meningitis; thrombophlebitis; colitis; skin pustules

Lab: CBC with diff; ESR; viral and bacterial cultures of ulcers. Saline shot challenge—delayed hypersensitivity reaction is diagnostic

ED Rx:

Ann Med Interne (Paris) 1999:576; Cochrane Database Syst Rev 2000

- First line—ASA or indomethacin
- Second line—steroids
- Third line—azathioprine, cyclophosphamide, or chlorambucil
- Poor data—colchicine (Clin Exp Dermatol 1989:298)
- Oral ulcers—try mixture of 1:1:1:1 mylanta:benadryl:tetracycline:prednisolone elixir 5 cc swish and spit qid for 1 week. Thalidomide may be helpful
- Medicine consult for admit if CNS manifestations or same day ophtho consult for uveitis; otherwise outpatient medicine follow-up

23.3 TEMPORAL ARTERITIS

Semin Ophthalmol 1999:109; Br J Rheumatol 1996:1161

Cause: Autoimmune; giant cell arteritis

Epidem: 133/100,000; female:male ~2:1; usually in patients >60 years of age; occasionally associated with HLA DR4; associated with polymyalgia rheumatica (PMR) (Recenti Prog Med 1990:176; J Am Geriatr Soc 1992:515)

Pathophys: Arteritis of medium- and large-sized vessels. Sometimes with mild anemia and liver function abnormalities. Should spare the kidneys; equivocal association with thyroid disease (Rev Rhum Ed Fr 1993:493)

Sx:

Lancet 1967:638

Fever; headache; visual changes—e.g., diplopia or amaurosis fugax; scalp pain; sore throat; cough; claudication symptoms of leg, tongue, and jaw; weakness; joint stiffness; malaise; weight loss

Si: Fever; thickened temporal artery; retinal changes with ischemia or cherry red macular spot of retinal artery occlusion; synovitis; muscle tenderness

Crs: Most resolve with treatment over 1–2 years, some refractory cases. Arthritis of temporal arteritis not associated with progression to rheumatoid arthritis (unlike PMR) (Rheumatology (Oxford) 2000:283)

Cmplc: Blindness; cranial nerve deficits; MI; CVA; aortic aneurysms and dissections; psychosis; hypothyroidism

Diff Dx: Polymyalgia rheumatica—appears to be closely related to temporal arteritis; Takayasu's arteritis—arteritis of large vessels

Lab:

- CBC with diff, thrombocytosis with more significant disease (J Neuroophthalmol 2000:67); PT/PTT; ESR >80 mm/hr but significant cases will still be missed, and changing this to >30 mm/hr appears to be appropriately more sensitive (Clin Rheumatol 2000:73), degree of elevation inversely correlated with degree of anemia (Arch Ophthalmol 1987:965); metabolic profile with liver function tests; total CPK, consider aldolase—if myalgias; U/A; consider rheumatoid profile. Temporal artery biopsy is diagnostic
- X-ray: head CT or MRI to look for anatomic lesion of other cause if headache, visual disturbance, or cranial nerve deficits. CXR usually not helpful

ED Rx:

- If visual loss, give methylprednisolone (Solu-Medrol) 250 mg IV (Ophthalmology 1992:68; J Rheumatol 2000:1484) and medical consult for admission
- If no visual changes, begin prednisone 40–60 mg po qd × 12 weeks
- Arrange medicine follow-up, with temporal artery biopsy arranged through surgery—either directly arrange to have medicine assume this, or set up to have done within 1 week

24 Tools

24.1 ACLS GUIDELINES

Circulation 1998:1654; 2000:1129; Pediatrics 1998:E13
These guidelines are opinions, based on imperfect information. Best
   example, perhaps, is the study which shows that patients who receive
   ACLS medications do worse than those who do not (Ann Emerg
   Med 1998:544). This is because all people do better if their "code" is
   related to an arrhythmia treatable with electricity (Jama 1999:1175).
   Even success at early resuscitation still carries a poor ultimate
   prognosis (Resuscitation 1998:95). This is constantly updated, and
   please refer to the American Heart Association literature for the latest
   algorithms

24.2 APGAR SCORES

Developed by Patricia Apgar (Pediatr Dev Pathol 1999:292) to quickly
   stratify neonates and give a prognosis for the first minutes of life
   (Arch Intern Med 1999:125). Traditionally done at 1 and 5 minutes
   of life, has been extended to 10 minutes and other longer time
   intervals in an attempt to give further prognostic information (see
   Table 24.1). A persistently low score (3 or less) from 5 to 20 minutes
   of life is an indicator of increased neonatal morbidity/mortality
   (Arch Pediatr Adolesc Med 2000:294), with a finding of 3 or less
   at 5 minutes associated with cerebral palsy (Jama 1984:1843)

Table 24.1. Apgar Scores

Indicator	Score		
	0	1	2
A: appearance	Blue/cyanosis	Pink body/blue extremities (acrocyanosis)	Pink body
P: pulse	None	<100 bpm	>100 bpm
G: grimace (stroke sole)	None	Weak	Cry
A: activity	None	Weak flexor tone	Strong tone
R: respirations	None	Weak	Strong, crying

24.3 GLASGOW COMA SCALE

Lancet 1976:1031; Acta Neurochir 1976:45

The Glasgow Coma Scale was intended as a research tool with measurements originally 24 hours after injury to predict mortality and morbidity (see Table 24.2). Its primary usefulness has been its ease of use (Clin Neurol Neurosurg 1977:100), helping different practitioners communicate, and showing improvement or deterioration of a patient with repeat evaluations. Acute changes in this scale are now used to triage patients (J Emerg Med 1984:1). Its predictive value has not had rigorous evaluation (J Clin Epidemiol 1996:755), especially with regard to functional outcome (Am J Phys Med Rehabil 1996:364). Other tools (the APACHE scores (Intensive Care Med 1997:77), Acute Physiology Score, Reaction Level Scale, Simplified Acute Physiology Score, Therapeutic Intervention Scoring System, individual trauma scores such as the Maine Trauma Score) exist which may be better indicators and patient stratifiers in those with sepsis or trauma, but getting prognostic data on those with head injuries is still incomplete (J Trauma 1989:299). The APACHE II was found to be as predictive as the Glasgow Coma Scale in those with stroke (Stroke 1990:1280). The Baux Score, Edlich Burn Score, and Zawacki Score appear to be more prognostic in those with burns, and focus on size of burn and age of patient as bearing more weight prognostically (J Burn Care Rehabil 1991:560). As far as children, the Glasgow Coma Scale is as not as predictive in those with severe

Table 24.2. Glasgow Coma Scale

Indicator	Response	Score
Eyes	Open spontaneously	4
	Open to verbal stimuli	3
	Open to painful stimuli	2
	No movement	1
Verbal	Normally conversant/oriented	5
	Conversant/disoriented	4
	Inappropriate words	3
	Incomprehensible words (sounds)	2
	No response	1
Motor	Follows voice commands	6
	Correctly localizes painful stimuli	5
	Flexion-withdrawal to pain	4
	Decorticate posturing (flexion)	3
	Decerebrate posturing (extension)	2
	No response	1

traumatic injury (J Pediatr 1992:195), and mild abnormalities may be predictive of intracranial pathology (Neurosurgery 2000:1093). Other scales also exist for research methods, such as the Comprehensive Level of Consciousness Scale (J Neurosurg 1984:955). Add the best response from each category of eyes, verbal, and motor. This does not supplant a careful neurologic exam, and scores range from 3 (worst) to 15 (best)

25 Toxicology

25.1 ACETAMINOPHEN

Acad Emerg Med 1999:1115; Ann Intern Med 1999:52

Cause: Ingestion

Epidem: Most common reason for call to Poison Control

Pathophys: Causes liver failure secondary to metabolite which depletes reduced glutathione and perhaps secondary release of mitochondrial Ca^+. Stages will be covered below, and Stage I is within 24 hours, Stage II is 24–48 hours, Stage III is 72–96 hours, and Stage IV is 96 hours to 2 weeks

Sx: History of ingestion >10 g in adult in less than 24 hours, peds >140 mg/kg single dose
- *Stage I*: nausea, vomiting
- *Stage II*: abdominal pain, not urinating
- *Stage III*: laboratory abnormalities
- *Stage IV*: declaration of liver injury—either improving or failing

Si: None specific
- *Stage I*: clammy and pale skin
- *Stage II*: RUQ abdominal pain
- *Stage III*: laboratory abnormalities
- *Stage IV*: declaration of liver injury—either improving or failing

Crs: Most LFT abnormalities are transient, yet may be the harbinger of a fatal reaction

Cmplc: Co-ingestions (ETOH, anticonvulsants) can amplify toxic effects, or cause delayed symptoms and peak levels; nomogram not accurate in circumstances where co-ingested materials (cold remedies) alter uptake (Br J Clin Pharmacol 1999:278)

Lab: Acetaminophen level at 4, 8, and 12 hours gives prognostic data (Am J Health Syst Pharm 1999:1081, quiz 1091), (see Figure 25.1) and upon arrival to ED (Scand J Gastroenterol 1999:723) liver profile; salicylate level; ETOH level; CBC with diff; PT/PTT; urine

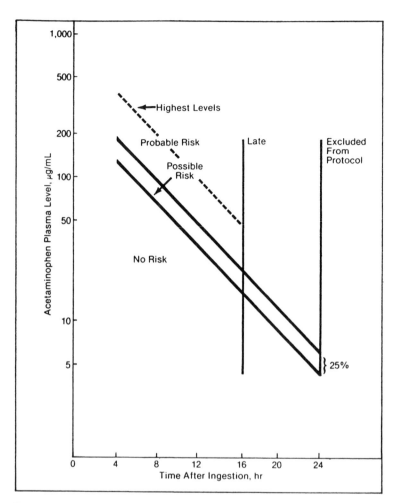

Figure 25.1. Study design nomogram. Possible risk is 25% below nomogram for multiclinic open-study purpose only. (Reproduced with permission from Rumack BH, et al., Acetaminophen overdose. Arch Intern Med 1981;141:382.)

toxic drug screen; EKG. Possible use of urine acetaminophen to R/O ingestion (J Toxicol Clin Toxicol 1999:769)

ED Rx:

- Acetylcysteine po 140 mg/kg load then 70 mg/kg q 4 hours for a total of 18 doses (Arch Intern Med 1981:380). IV as efficacious (J Toxicol Clin Toxicol 1999:759) and doses are the same of 3% solution infused over 1 hour (Crit Care Med 1998:40)

- Activated charcoal 1 mg/kg (J Toxicol Clin Toxicol 1999:753); do not use sorbitol as cathartic in these cases, but sodium sulfate instead if cathartic needed. No data that charcoal impedes absorption of acetylcysteine, but some advocate giving extra acetylcysteine in loading dose such as 150 mg/kg

- Studies have shown that hypothyroidism and cimetidine-induced delayed gastric emptying may have had a small beneficial effect in certain populations, but PTU and cimetidine are not advocated as ED Rx

25.2 ANTIDEPRESSANTS

Jama 1987:521; Pediatr Emerg Care 1998:293

Cause: Tricyclic antidepressants (TCAs) will be discussed here; MAO inhibitors and SSRIs discussed in 13.1. St. John's wort is a weak MAO inhibitor. Cyclobenzaprine (Flexeril) is similar to TCAs

Epidem: Most common intentional OD which causes death, since narrow therapeutic window

Pathophys: The mortal effect of TCAs has to do with Na-channel blockade in the myocardium. Sodium channel blockade causes decreased ionotropic action, conduction defects (heart block, widening QRS, ectopic beats), and resulting hypotension (Am J Emerg Med 1988:439). The anticholinergic effects and α-blocking effects may cause symptoms but these are usually secondary and not fatal

Sx: Anticholinergic symptoms—dry mouth, dry skin, confusion, palpitations

Si: Tachycardia, altered mental status, hypotension, seizures, coma

Crs: When these problems occur, they do so rapidly—altered mental status (J Toxicol Clin Toxicol 1992:161), cardiac conduction defects, arrhythmias, and seizures are poor prognostic indicators

TOXICOLOGY

(Am J Emerg Med 1986:496). Hypotension due to cardiogenic shock has high mortality

Cmplc: ARDS (Chest 1989:852; Ann Pharmacother 1993:572), pancreatitis (J Toxicol Clin Toxicol 1994:425)

Diff Dx: Consider other similar toxic overdoses (wide QRS with seizures) such as cocaine, lithium, phenothiazines, antihistamines, carbamazepine, quinidine, quinine, propoxyphene, propranolol, phenothiazines, bupivacaine, and lidocaine

Lab: EKG looking for right axis deviation (Ann Emerg Med 1989:348), wide QRS, or prolonged QT (Am J Cardiol 1986:1154); glucoscan; CBC with diff; metabolic profile; ABG; ETOH level; acetaminophen level; salicylate level; urine toxic drug screen

ED Rx:

- Airway, O_2
- IV access, consider naloxone and thiamine 100 mg IV as overdose/coma protocol
- Gastric lavage if within 2 hours of presentation, followed by activated charcoal (AC) 1 mg/kg—AC is the most important tool (J Emerg Med 1995:203); be prepared to protect the airway if necessary since sudden deterioration is a possibility
- $NaHCO_3$ 1–2 mg/kg IV bolus, followed by 2-cc/kg/hour drip of 1 L of D_5W with 2 amps of $NaHCO_3$ added. Use $NaHCO_3$ if wide QRS (>0.1 seconds), refractory hypotension, or cardiac arrhythmias noted. Goal of Rx is pH 7.50–7.55
- Lidocaine is second-line drug for arrhythmias, and would specifically avoid disopyramide, imipramine, procainamide, quinidine, flecainide, propafenone, β-blockers, and calcium channel blockers
- Role of phenytoin to be elucidated for cardiac arrhythmias (Ann Emerg Med 1981:270)
- Benzodiazepines for seizures, followed by phenobarbital
- Hypotension refractory to fluids and $NaHCO_3$ should be Rx'ed with norepinephrine (Levophed) 2–80 µg/min, avoid dopamine (Am J Emerg Med 1988:566)
- Perhaps Fab or single chain Fv fragment (sFv) fragments for desipramine overdose (Toxicol Lett 1995:801)
- Consider extracorporeal circulation if not responding to usual methods (Am J Emerg Med 1994:456)
- Admission for continuous cardiac monitoring for 24 hours if not toxic (Jama 1985:1772)

25.3 ASPIRIN

Drug Saf 1992:292

Cause: Ingestion of >10 g of ASA in adult; topical treatment absorption (Cutis 1992:307)

Epidem: Common in all ages, and many times unintentional

Pathophys: Oxidative metabolism uncoupling, with early stimulation of respiratory centers as well; CNS stimulant; gastric irritant

Sx: Nonspecific; dizziness, abdominal pain, nausea

Si: Fever and hypermetabolic state; confusion; seizures; hematemesis or melena

Crs: Variable with mild cases requiring IV fluid for dehydration and alkalosis, severe cases as seen under **Complications**

Cmplc: CNS ischemia secondary to decrease in CNS ATP and cerebral edema; pulmonary edema; altered glycemic control, with hypoglycemia common in peds; cardiac arrhythmias; and rarely renal failure. Nomogram not accurate in enteric-coated formulations, for dosages spread out over time such as acute ingestion on top of chronic therapy (Ann Emerg Med 1989:1186); some salicylate assays cross-react with diflunisal (J Emerg Med 1987:499)

Diff Dx: Cocaine, ethylene glycol, isoniazid, methanol, iron, cyanide poisoning. NSAIDs (Drug Saf 1990:252) usually not as severe as salicylates, with major problem if co-ingested with anticoagulants —the antiplatelet effect increases risk of bleeding. GI (ulcers) and renal (interstitial nephritis, metabolic acidosis, failure) side effects are most common with overdose, with less likely pulmonary (bronchospasm), hepatic (hepatitis), anaphylaxis, and CNS (aseptic meningitis). Rx is supportive

Lab:
- Salicylate level at admission and 6 hours postingestion (see Figure 25.2); ABG (respiratory alkalosis followed by metabolic alkalosis); acetaminophen level; ETOH level; CBC with diff; PT/PTT; metabolic profile; U/A; urine toxic drug screen; EKG
- X-ray: abdominal flat plate to look for salicylates in GI tract

ED Rx:
- IV access
- Activated charcoal 1 g/kg po, most effective when repeated q 4 hours × 3 (Ann Emerg Med 1988:34); with cathartic such as

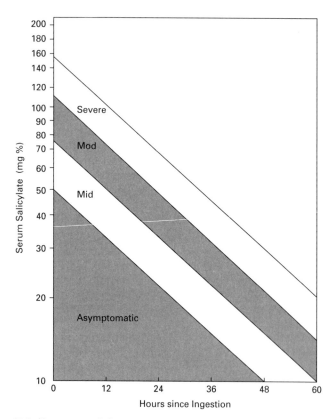

Figure 25.2. Nomogram relating serum salicylate concentration and expected severity of intoxication at varying intervals following the ingestion of a single dose of salicylate. (Reproduced with permission from Done AK, Salicylate intoxication: Significance of measurements of salicylate in blood in cases of acute ingestion. Pediatrics 1960;26:805.)

sorbitol (Ann Emerg Med 1990:654) or $MgSO_4$ (Arch Intern Med 1984:48)

- Vitamin K for prolonged protime (controversial if no clinical effects of prolonged PT)
- Intravenous glucose for ASA-induced hypoglycemia
- Metabolic acidosis treated with IV $NaHCO_3$, 2–3 amps in liter of D_5W at 100 cc/hr, and follow serum/urine pH. Consider dialysis if

severe, correct lytes—still treat with alkalinization if going to dialysis (Clin Nephrol 1998:178)

- Consider hemodialysis for initial level >120 mg% or 6-hour level >100 mg%; or if renal failure, pulmonary edema, or persistent CNS problems

25.4 BENZODIAZEPINES

Curr Opin Pediatr 1996:243; Drug Saf 1997:181

Cause: Ingestion or parenteral use of benzodiazepines; mixed overdoses common (J Forensic Sci 1997:155)

Epidem: Common intentional overdose, occasionally miscalculated medicine dosing

Pathophys: CNS receptors activated, inducing anxiolysis and sedation

Sx/Si: Nonspecific; sleepiness

Crs: Most recover from pure ingestions; the elderly may present as being delirious

Cmplc: Co-ingestions usually cause most problems with coma, respiratory depression, or hypotension; withdrawal from benzodiazepines may precipitate seizures—avoid this if at all possible

Lab: Search for co-ingestions with ETOH level; acetaminophen level; salicylate level; CBC with diff; metabolic profile; urine toxic drug screen; EKG

ED Rx:

- IV access, fluid if hypotensive
- Airway support if necessary
- Activated charcoal 1 g/kg po
- Do not reverse with flumazenil (Romazicon) (Crit Care Med 1992:1733; Am J Emerg Med 1992:184) unless adverse side effect of parenteral sedation in ED or hospital in patient who is not ETOH or benzodiazepine dependent. Otherwise, may precipitate seizure. Dose of flumazenil is 1 mg over 3 minutes q 1 hour prn

25.5 CARBON MONOXIDE

Ann Emerg Med 1994:242

Cause: CO inhalation, from combustible sources

Epidem: Common sources are car exhaust, cigarette or any fire smoke, gas appliances with closed space inhalation

Pathophys: CO has a 200× affinity for Hgb than O_2, with a slow dissociation rate (Circulation 1981:253A). It shifts the Hgb dissociation curve to the left, which means that it also decreases O_2 dissociation

Sx: Cherry red skin; headache; dizziness; altered mental status (Arch Surg 1973:851)—30–40 mg% CO; coma—>40 mg% CO

Si: Cherry red skin; retinal hemorrhages

Crs: Recovery may take months

Cmplc: Ischemic heart and CNS disease

Lab: Serum CO level (look for level >10 mg%); ABG; CBC with diff for significant exposures to assess for anemia; screen for co-ingestions (see 25.4) if possible suicide attempt

ED Rx:

- High-flow O_2, with non-rebreather mask and 15 lpm flow rate; treat longer if pregnant (Science 1977:680)
- Use of hyperbaric O_2 is controversial, but would use if available (J Emerg Med 1985:443; Undersea Hyperb Med 1996:215); more efficacious if metabolic acidosis (J Accid Emerg Med 1999:96)
- Exchange transfusion is controversial

25.6 CYANIDE

J Emerg Med 2000:441; Occup Med (Lond) 1998:427

Cause: Ingestion, inhalation, or transdermal absorption of cyanide (CN); past use of Laetrile (Ann Emerg Med 1983:449)

Epidem: Common inhalation toxin from house fires, yet overall serious toxicity from all sources is uncommon

Pathophys: Cytochrome oxidase poisoning, which renders cells unable to use O_2 (J Toxicol Clin Toxicol 1987:121)

Sx: Nonspecific, but may include headache and dyspnea; rarely history of "almond smell"

Si: Cyanosis if respiratory arrest; mental status change with coma possible

Crs: Inhalation exposures usually recover rapidly with removal of patient from toxic environment

Cmplc: Arrhythmias; metabolic acidosis; diabetes insipidus; seizures; respiratory arrest

Diff Dx: Cocaine, ethylene glycol, isoniazid, methanol, salicylates, iron poisoning

Lab: Serum CN level (look for level >40 µM/L); CO level; ABG—look for lactic acidosis (Bmj 1996:26); ETOH; methanol level; ethylene glycol level; salicylate level; acetaminophen level; metabolic profile; CBC with diff; urine toxic drug screen; EKG

ED Rx:

Consider calling for *Lilly Cyanide Antidote Kit*, which contains amyl nitrite, sodium thiosulfate, and sodium nitrite (Am J Emerg Med 1995:524)

- O_2
- IV access
- Amyl nitrite for inhalation, exact mechanism of action unknown although proposed activity through formation of methemoglobin; potentially dangerous in the setting of cotoxicity with CO
- Sodium thiosulfate ($Na_2S_2O_3$) to form SCN which can then be excreted 12.5 g IV in adult
- Sodium nitrite ($NaNO_2$) 0.2 cc/kg of 3% solution to a maximum of 10 cc IV
- Perhaps hydroxocobalamin (vitamin B_{12}) to complex CN for acute treatment, or preventative role in those receiving nitroprusside (Crit Care Med 1993:465)
- Dicobalt edetate (Kelocyanor) and 4-dimethylaminophenol (DMAP) used in Europe, no proven efficacy over the Lilly kit. Previous cobalt experiments without benefit (Proc Soc Exp Biol Med 1965:780)
- Research active using stroma-free methemoglobin solution (SFMS) (Am J Emerg Med 1985:519)
- If resuscitating patients with a cyanide overdose, it is possible to have significant exposure (J Forensic Sci 1989:1280)

25.7 DIGITALIS

Prog Cardiovasc Dis 1984:21; J Card Surg 1987:453

Cause: Ingestion or parenteral use of digitalis (digoxin)

Epidem: Common accidental overdose

Pathophys: The primary clinical action of digitalis as an Na/K pump inhibitor is the same action that causes its lethality, with consequent heart blocks and arrhythmias. More common in people with renal disease since digoxin has renal elimination (Ger Med Mon 1966:316)

Sx/Si: Weakness, fatigue, yellow halos, other nonspecific findings

Crs: Variable, with acute toxicity more likely to have GI symptoms and hyperkalemia, and chronic toxicity with more nonspecific findings

Cmplc: Co-ingestion with β-blockers, Ca-channel blockers, and quinidine may increase toxicity

Diff Dx: Rarely seen from toad venom bite in U.S.

Lab: Serum digoxin level; metabolic profile including calcium and magnesium (hypomagnesemia) (Am Heart J 1970:57); EKG, with a myriad of arrhythmias, PVCs most common (Geriatrics 1965:1006); cardiac markers if EKG changes

ED Rx:
- IV access, and cardiac monitor
- Activated charcoal 1 g/kg po for acute poisoning
- Digoxin antibody or Fab fragments (Digibind) (Conn Med 1986:835) for ventricular arrhythmias or bradyarrhythmias not responding to standard therapy (see below). May also be used for hyperkalemia (Am J Emerg Med 1986:364). Dose is 40 mg of Fab (1 vial) / 0.6 mg of digoxin (actual) (Clin Pharmacokinet 1995:483), and number of vials = serum digoxin level × weight (kg) / 100 (good estimate)
- Bradyarrhythmias—atropine 0.5–1 mg IV, consider MgSO$_4$ 2 g IV, and cardiac pacing. Co-ingestion of β-blockers and Ca-channel blockers may make it difficult to use standard therapy. Perhaps try glucagon 1 mg IV if β-blockers co-ingestion. *Do not use CaCl$_2$ or other calcium compounds in digitalis overdose*—it may worsen cardiac effects of digitalis
- Hyperkalemia—may use NaHCO$_3$, glucose, insulin, and Kayexalate, but avoid CaCl$_2$ since may worsen cardiac effects of digitalis

- Ventricular arrhythmias—consider lidocaine, or phenytoin (Dilantin) (Dis Chest 1968:263) or fosphenytoin; phenytoin/fosphenytoin bolus is the same as for seizures at 15 mg/kg. If no effect, consider MgSO$_4$ 2 g IV. Quinidine, procainamide, and amiodarone should not be used since they depress AV node conduction

25.8 ETHYLENE GLYCOL

Med Toxicol 1986:309; J Toxicol Clin Toxicol 1999:537; Crit Rev Toxicol 1999:331

Cause: Usually inadvertent ingestion of antifreeze

Epidem: Unsure, since we do not screen every intoxicated patient for ethylene glycol ingestion, and they probably have no clinical problems if the ingestion of ethylene glycol is minimal and they are intoxicated with ethanol

Pathophys: Alcohol dehydrogenase (ADH) converts ethylene glycol to glycolic acid which is metabolized to oxalate; this process gives a metabolic acidosis with a high osmolar gap (Vet Hum Toxicol 1980:255). Glycolic acid is a physiologic marker which correlates with severity of disease (Toxicol Sci 1999:117). Other metabolites include lactate and glycolate (Am J Clin Pathol 1966:46)

Sx/Si: Intoxication, with CNS effects of seizures and coma in severe cases

Crs: Variable degrees of end-organ damage to the heart, lungs, and kidneys may occur if this overdose goes unchecked

Cmplc: Respiratory, cardiac, and kidney failure may be the result of this end-organ damage

Diff Dx: ETOH, cocaine, salicylates, methanol, iron, isoniazid, cyanide poisoning

Lab: ETOH level; ethylene glycol (look for level >20 mg/dL), methanol, and isopropyl alcohol levels; ABG—metabolic acidosis may be lacking if coincident ingestion, such as lithium (Am J Kidney Dis 1994:313); metabolic profile including calcium and magnesium; salicylate level; acetaminophen level; CBC with diff; EKG; U/A; urine toxic drug screen

TOXICOLOGY

ED Rx:
- IV access
- Thiamine 100 mg IV and pyridoxine 100 mg IV (J Nutr 1977:458)
- Correct Ca and Mg deficiencies if necessary
- IV ETOH is 10% ETOH in D$_5$W—bolus 10 cc/kg, then 1.6 cc/kg/hr infusion. An oral loading dose of 20–50% ETOH solution with maintenance of 20% solution po gives just as good if not better results (N Engl J Med 1981:21)
- 4-Methylpyrazole (Fomepizole) may substitute for ETOH as first-line Rx (J Toxicol Clin Toxicol 1986:463; Toxicol Lett 1987:307)—15 mg/kg load, then 10 mg/kg every 12 hours IV for a total of 4 doses
- Hemodialysis for those with CNS dysfunction, visual complaints, or methanol level >50 mg/dL (Acta Med Scand 1984:409). Do not withhold ETOH Rx pending dialysis

25.9 IRON

Cause: Ingestion of either form—ferric or ferrous—in dose >20 mg/kg

Epidem: Common, and many prove to be accidental

Pathophys: Direct corrosive effect on GI mucosa; iron salts are hepatotoxic; subsequent release of iron and ferritin leads to vasodilatory effect and shock (Adv Exp Med Biol 1994:239)

Sx: Nausea, abdominal pain, seizures; then 2–3-hour respite, then protracted/fatal seizures

Si: Hematemesis; melena/hematochezia

Crs: Systemic toxicity occurs in 4–40 hours postingestion

Cmplc: Possible late complications include GI strictures, obstruction, and perforation

Diff Dx: Cocaine, ethylene glycol, isoniazid, methanol, salicylates, cyanide poisoning

Lab:
- Serum iron level (look for level >300 μgm%)—deferoxamine can interfere with this measurement and radioimmunoassays are unreliable here; TIBC (Ann Emerg Med 1999:73), and transferrin and ferritin (Ann Emerg Med 1991:532) are unreliable predictors; salicylate level; acetaminophen level; CBC with diff; metabolic profile including Ca and Mg; U/A; urine toxic drug screen; urine for

deferoxamine challenge test, with rose-colored change if serum-free iron is present, is not a reliable indicator. Leukocytosis and hyperglycemia not indicative of severity in adults (Am J Emerg Med 1996:454)

- X-ray: single view flat plate abdomen to look for iron tablets, low sensitivity and specificity

ED Rx:

- IV access
- Gastric lavage if <2 hours, otherwise just activated charcoal 1 g/kg
- Chelate with L1 (Br J Haematol 1994:851), which also complexes aluminum
- Deferoxamine 1-g IV bolus, then 15 mg/kg/hour continuous infusion; this is safe in pregnancy (Am J Hematol 1999:24); start this immediately if patient is symptomatic
- Perhaps magnesium hydroxide 4.5 g po per g elemental iron if <1 hour postingestion (Acad Emerg Med 1998:961)
- Consider L1,1,2-dimethyl-3-hydroxypyris-4-one (Deferiprone) (Toxicol Lett 1995:1)
- Hemodialysis if renal failure

25.10 ISONIAZID

Cause: Ingestion of isoniazid (INH)

Epidem: Uncommon

Pathophys: INH inhibits glutamic acid decarboxylase, which leads to decreased GABA levels. This decarboxylase enzyme is pyridoxine dependent

Sx: GI symptoms

Si: Change in mental status including seizures or coma

Crs: Seizures predispose to a metabolic acidosis

Cmplc: Protracted seizures (South Med J 1976:294)

Diff Dx: Cocaine, ethylene glycol, methanol, salicylates, iron, cyanide poisoning

Lab: Serum INH level (look for >2 mg/L); ETOH level; methanol level; ethylene glycol level; salicylate level; acetaminophen level; ABG—profound acidosis (Am J Emerg Med 1987:165); CBC with diff; metabolic profile with Ca and Mg; urine toxic drug screen; EKG

ED Rx:
- IV access
- Activated charcoal 1 g/kg, but less helpful if >1 hour postingestion (Hum Toxicol 1986:285)
- Pyridoxine gm/gm of INH ingested, give 5 g IV if unknown (Ann Emerg Med 1983:303). This is first-line treatment for seizures in these cases as well (Jama 1981:1102)
- Benzodiazepines for protracted seizures—diazepam or lorazepam
- Hemodialysis rarely needed

25.11 LEAD

N Engl J Med 1973:1289; 1973:1229

Cause: An acquired porphyria from lead (Pb) ingestion; found in paint, battery fumes, pottery glazes, smeltering, indoor firing ranges, radiator repair shops, moonshine; tetraethyl lead from gas only results in encephalopathy, not porphyria or blood changes

Epidem: Unknown incidence in adults and usually via work exposure, common in children (pica)

Pathophys: Pb chelates sulfhydryl groups of ALA dehydrogenase, ferrochelatase, and ALA synthetase. Induces gout and gouty nephropathy in adults—gouty nephropathy commonly associated with Pb intoxication

Sx: Abdominal pain, better with palpation; associated family pet illness

Si: Gingival margin lead line (Am J Hematol 1981:99), peripheral motor neuropathy (e.g., wrist drop), neuroses, psychoses (Am J Psychiatry 1984:1423)

Crs: Chelation helps avoid seizures, not other neurologic complications

Cmplc: Hypothyroidism; gout; gouty nephropathy (N Engl J Med 1981:520); encephalopathy (50% mortality without Rx, 3% with); mental and neurologic disabilities; HTN (Environ Health Perspect 1988:57) (look for creatinine >1.5 mg%)

Diff Dx: Other causes of encephalopathy (CNS lesion, drugs, metabolic, infectious, CO) or psychiatric disorders

Lab:
- CBC with diff, look for RBC stippling; serum lead level (Arch Intern Med 1987:697), all other tests for lead not as accurate; metabolic profile and U/A if suspect renal involvement; consider TSH

- X-ray: Acute ingestions may show lead pills in bowel; children with lead lines at metaphyseal calcification areas

ED Rx:

All Patients
- IV, O_2 if encephalopathy
- For seizures, see 13.11
- If lead pills noted in bowel, polyethylene glycol solution (Golytely)

Level of 10–25 µg %
- Find source, oral Fe to decrease Pb absorption, mandatory follow-up

Level of 25–45 µg %
- Find source, oral Fe, consider chelation

Level of 45 µg % or higher
- Chelation

Chelation Rx
J Pediatr 1968:1
- EDTA (ethylenediaminetetraacetic acid) 1500 mg/m^2 IV for 24 hours 4 hrs after BAL, 1000 mg/m^2 in children who are not encephalopathic (J Pharmacol Exp Ther 1987:804)
- BAL IM (2,3-dimercaptopropanol) 75 mg/m^2 in adults, 50 mg/m^2 in children who are not encephalopathic
- DMSA (2,3-dimercaptosuccinic acid) (Clin Pharmacol Ther 1985:431), 10 mg/kg po q 8 hours × 5 days, and then q 12 hours × 14 days
- CDTA (cyclohexanediaminetetraacetic acid) (Arch Environ Contam Toxicol 1990:185)
- Succimer (dimercaptosuccinate) po
- Perhaps zinc supplementation (Toxicology 1990:129)

25.12 THEOPHYLLINE

J Emerg Med 1993:415

Cause: Usually iatrogenic (Ann Intern Med 1991:748), with aminophylline or oral theophylline used for chronic lung disease; this chemical has a narrow therapeutic window, has many interactions with other medications, and is influenced by thyroid function (Clin Pharm 1988:620)

Epidem: Becoming more uncommon as use of theophylline is waning; increased risk if >60 years of age, increased levels secondary to drug interactions (e.g., some antibiotics, estrogens, allopurinol, cimetidine), and lower levels cause more toxicity in chronic users (Ann Intern Med 1993:1161)

Pathophys: Unknown, but many hypotheses with theophylline interaction with phosphodiesterase-2 (PDE-2), cAMP, prostaglandins, release/synergism with catecholamines, and adenosine antagonism. These interactions may occur at some level, but not known which are predominant at the levels that we use (usually <20 µg/mL). Reaction to theophylline also appears to be idiosyncratic and avoiding toxicity is only reliably done via serum levels (Jama 1976:1983)

Sx: Headache, irritability, GI upset, agitation (as with other methylxanthines such as caffeine); seizures

Si: Tachycardia, hypotension, seizures, coma

Crs: Dependent on level and chronicity

Cmplc: Status epilepticus, ventricular arrhythmias (rare), rhabdomyolysis (rare)

Lab: CBC with diff looking for leukocytosis; metabolic profile looking for metabolic acidosis, hypokalemia, hypophosphatemia, and hypomagnesemia; theophylline level; EKG looking for ectopic beats, sustained arrhythmias rare (Chest 1990:672) and perhaps T wave inversion corresponding to severe toxicity (Chest 1989:429)

ED Rx:
- Activated charcoal 1 g/kg po (Crit Care Med 1984:113), with sorbitol
- Airway control if seizing, for status epilepticus refer to 13.11, may need to move quickly to pentobarbital
- Arrhythmias should follow standard protocols for atrial and ventricular arrhythmias; adenosine may precipitate bronchospasm; consider labetalol or esmolol (Ann Emerg Med 1990:671) if β-blockade considered—caution in those with bronchospastic disease
- Hemoperfusion/hemodialysis/plasmapheresis (Crit Care Med 1991:288) for acute toxicity and level >100 µg/mL, or chronic toxicity and level >60 µg/mL (Am J Med 1990:567)

26 Trauma

26.1 BURNS

Cause: Thermal (majority of burn unit admissions), chemical (3–16% of burn unit admissions), or electrical (3–4% of burn unit admissions) (Clin Plast Surg 2000:133) injury with subsequent tissue damage

Epidem: Annually, a minority of patients with massive (>75% of total body surface area) burns, ~3% in children (Jama 2000:69). Major burns with worse outcomes in infants and the elderly (Burns 2000:49). Scald burns of the perineum and lower extremities are common and preventable injuries in infants and the elderly (Burns 2000:251)

Pathophys: Tissue (skin) damage from the three above mentioned causes is inherent in their physical properties—heat, acidic or alkaline extremes, or electrical destruction. Thermal burns can cause acute or subacute ocular and airway damage that is linked to the initial insult or steam generation with consequent inhalation. Steam injury to the lungs can be quickly overwhelming (Burns 1996:313). Chemical burns have a predisposition for ocular and oropharyngeal damage. Chemical burns to the lungs can occur from a hydrocarbon source as seen in huffing, if linked with smoking (Burns 1996:566). For associated electrical injury problems, see 5.2

- Major burns are those involving >20% TBSA or any fourth-degree burns; or those with associated airway, fracture, or other secondary injury problems. Burns in infants or the elderly are at higher risk for secondary complications; as well as burns that involve the hands, feet, and perineum, cross major joints, or are circumferential
- Moderate burns are those involving 10–20% TBSA, with none of the aforementioned concerns of hands, feet, or perineum, crossing a major joint, or circumferential locations. Moderate burns may be

1999:203) if unable to interpret, or CT or MRI if specific abnormality noted on neurologic exam or plain films—if no abnormality, then 5-view C-spine (A/P, lateral, odontoid, obliques) if >16 years of age with CT/MRI if these are abnormal. Specific classifications are referrable to excellent work by Harris et al (Orthop Clin North Am 1986:15)

May advocate in those with high to moderate risk for C-spine fracture a lateral plain film with helical CT (J Trauma 1999:896, discussion, 902; Radiology 1999:117) or MRI (J Neurosurg 1999:54) initially, and perhaps any of the following risk factors and >16 years of age: 1) high-speed MVA >35 mph (56 kmph); 2) crash with death at scene; 3) fall from height >10 ft (3 m); 4) significant closed head injury or ICH on CT; 5) C-spine symptoms or abnormal neurologic exam; or 6) pelvic or multiple extremity fractures (AJR Am J Roentgenol 2000:713)

Flexion/extension plain films (Am J Emerg Med 1999:504) or MRI may be helpful if suspect ligamentous instability—this is rare (Am Surg 2000:326, discussion, 330). Patient must be alert and cooperative to have 5-view or flexion/extension studies completed, although evaluation in the obtund/comatose patient is active research area (Pediatr Neurosurg 1999:169)

ED Rx:

- Prehospital care should begin with long board, collar, and head immobilization. Infants require an item 3–4 cm in thickness posterior to the scapula when supine to maintain neutral head position (about the thickness of an adult hand)
- Maintain airway, with intubation facilitated by gum elastic bougie or fiberoptic instrumentation (J Neurosurg Anesthesiol 1999:11). Cricothyrotomy if airway needed and cannot intubate; remember in-line stabilization, not traction
- In moving patient from the board, control spinal alignment and move patient as a unit
- High-dose methylprednisolone at 30 mg/kg IV is controversial but is used for spinal cord injury (see 13.12)
- Neurosurgery consult for abnormal neurologic exam or radiographic abnormalities

26.3 COMPARTMENT SYNDROME

Hand Clin 1998:335

Cause: Increased pressure in a tissue (muscle) compartment that is contained by fascial and bony planes such that intercompartment muscle, nerve, and blood vessel viability is threatened or impaired. Various etiologies include fractures, blunt trauma, revascularization of ischemic extremity, venous occlusion, circumferential burns, chronic and repetitive exertion (Med Sci Sports Exerc 2000:S4), external compression by medical antishock trousers (pneumatic trousers) (J Trauma 1989:549), and prolonged limb compression from drug overdose (Clin Orthop 1975:81)

Epidem: Common

Pathophys: A function of the nonelastic properties of bone and fascia, with the critical mass found in medium-sized compartments in the forearm and leg being most vulnerable, but possible at any site; thigh has been reported and is uncommon (Orthop Rev 1990:421; J Trauma 1998:395). Hypotension is a risk factor, since the diastolic pressure has to exceed the pressure in the compartment for flow to occur through that compartment

Sx: Pain, swelling

Si: Tense edema, pallor, distal hypesthesia or anesthesia, lack of distal pulses, distal paralysis, pain with distal passive range of motion testing

Crs: Dependent on whether isolated injury or part of multisystem trauma; fasciotomy wounds associated with high infection rate

Cmplc: Ischemic (Volkmann's) contracture; renal failure, rhabdomyolysis, metabolic acidosis, hyperkalemia, multiorgan failure

Diff Dx: Muscle contusion; DVT; rarely de novo compartment syndrome secondary to neoplasm (J Surg Oncol 1994:198, discussion, 200) or ruptured aneurysm (J Vasc Surg 1993:295)

Lab:
- CBC with diff; metabolic profile; total CK; U/A and urine for myoglobin
- X-ray: to look for associated fracture
- Compartment pressure >30 mm Hg at a minimum for fasciotomy (ortho consult for procedure)—exact threshold number is controversial and depends on clinical exam (Clin Orthop 1975:43)

- EMG may be useful if diagnosis uncertain (Acta Belg Med Phys 1990:195)

ED Rx:
- IV access with fluid resuscitation if hypotensive
- IV narcotics
- If rhabdomyolysis, urinary catheter and 2–3 amps of NaHCO$_3$ (88–132 mEq) in 1 L of D$_5$W to keep urine pH > 6.5 (J Biol Chem 1998:31731); mannitol of no proven value (Ren Fail 1997:283)
- General or orthopedic surgery consult

26.4 PRESSURE INJECTION INJURIES

Am Surg 1989:714

Cause: Usually from industrial sources; high-velocity liquids such as grease, paint, or other material are injected into the body from accident with "gun"

Epidem: Most commonly involves hand

Pathophys: Mechanical obstruction of distal nerves, arteries, and veins is possible from pressure effects. Liquefaction necrosis if grease gun injury

Sx: Pain, swelling

Si: Erythema, tenderness, range of motion deficits, abnormal distal neurovascular exam

Crs: Ischemia, relieved with surgical debridement

Cmplc: Ischemia leading to necrosis if not recognized

Lab: None

ED Rx:
- IV access, parenteral pain control—**do not do a digital or local block**
- Tetanus update if needed
- Surgical consult for debridement and open wound treatment (J Hand Surg [Am] 1993:125); early amputation may be unavoidable (J Hand Surg [Br] 1998:479); early treatment desirable before complications develop

27 Urology

27.1 EPIDIDYMITIS

Sex Transm Dis 1984:173

Cause: Not always infectious, but infectious agents age dependent
- *<40 years of age*: chlamydia, occasionally gonorrhea or ureaplasma
- *>40 years of age*: gram-negative bacteria

Rarely from intravesical BCG instillation (Aust N Z J Surg 1993:70) or amiodarone (Can J Cardiol 1993:833)

Epidem: Rare under 18 years of age; peak incidence at 32 years of age. Perhaps increased risk with intact foreskin (J Urol 1998:1842)

Pathophys: Considered an STD in young adults, reflux of infected urine if gram-negative bacteria implicated; testes are spared. Considered a malfunction of the genitourinary tract in the 18 and under age group

Sx: Gradual pain onset, with the possibility of first symptom coincident with minor trauma; nausea; dysfunctional voiding characteristics

Si: Swollen and tender epididymis with normal testicle; Prehn's sign is negative (relief with elevation of testicle)

Crs: May last 7–10 days with Rx

Cmplc: Chronic epididymitis—consider noninfectious etiology (chemical inflammation from urine reflux); consider prostatitis or urethral obstruction of some degree in those >40 years of age; orchitis; abscess; rarely infarction (Acad Emerg Med 1998:1128)

Diff Dx: Testicular torsion; appendix testes torsion; symptomatic varicocele (Prehn's sign is positive—elevate the testicle and symptomatic relief); neoplasm

Lab: U/A; urine C + S; do penile swab first for GC/chlamydia if STD suspected

ED Rx:

Drugs 1999:743
- Scrotal support

- NSAID—ibuprofen 600 mg q 6 hours for 4–5 days; oral narcotics if needed; antiemetics if needed

<19 Years of Age
J Urol 1995:762
- Tm/S if pyuria, or consider for prophylaxis
- Refer to urology outpatient for imaging/urodynamic studies

20–40 Years of Age
- Ceftriaxone 250 mg IM × 1; or ciprofloxacin 500 mg po × 1; or ofloxacin 400 mg po × 1—along with doxycycline 100 mg po × 10 days, or azithromycin 1 g po × 1
- Condom use reviewed, and suggest partner testing
- Counseling/testing for syphilis and HIV
- 2-week follow-up with primary physician

>40 Years of Age
- Tm/S (Bactrim DS) 1 tab po bid for 2 weeks, increase to 4 weeks if prostatitis present; may use ciprofloxacin 250–500 mg po bid instead for same length of time
- 2–4-week follow-up with primary physician

27.2 PRIAPISM

J Urol 1969:576; Acad Emerg Med 1996:810

Cause: Medications (e.g., iatrogenic injection for impotence or abuse of cocaine (J Urol 1999:1817) or use of phenothiazines/trazodone), sickle cell disease, high spinal cord lesion, idiopathic, rarely leukemic infiltration

Epidem: Uncommon from all causes

Pathophys: Both corpora cavernosa engorged with blood

Sx: Pain if not a neurologic lesion

Si: Tense corpora cavernosa, the glans and corpus spongiosum may not be tense

Crs: Some are irreversible, such as some medications, spinal cord lesions, or if truly idiopathic

Cmplc: Infection, impotence

Lab: Dependent on cause—CBC with diff and O_2 sat in those with SSD or leukemia; trauma evaluation if new CNS lesion; urine toxicologic screen if considering cocaine use

ED Rx:

All causes
- Terbutaline 0.25–0.5 mg IM (deltoid)
- Urology consult; oncology consult if leukemic infiltration

SSD
- Transfuse RBCs
- Dilute epinephrine 1:1,000,000 (1 cc of epinephrine 1:1000 in 1 L of NS) irrigation of corpora cavernosa with 10 cc of solution (Blood 2000:78)
- Hyperbaric O_2

Other Causes Except SSD and Leukemic Infiltration
- Aspiration of engorged corpora cavernosa
- Instillation of 10 mg neosynephrine
- Perhaps unfractionated heparin instillation

27.3 TESTICULAR TORSION

Pediatrics 1998:73

Cause: May be seen in trauma or spontaneously

Epidem: Those <18 years of age appear to present later to ED and thus are at higher risk for orchiectomy (J Urol 1989:746)

Pathophys: Testicle is usually anchored inferiorly by the gubernaculum. Rotation causing torsion is usually an inward (medial) rotation in reference to the anterior part of the testes, and the rotation may be half a rotation or multiple rotations

Sx: Acute pain onset, either abdominal or scrotal; nausea

Si: Prehn's sign usually negative (pain relief with elevation of testes); high-riding testicle; loss of affected side cremasteric reflex (Pediatrics 1998:73)

Crs: Operate within 4–5 hours to save 70%, 15% saved if operative intervention within 10 hours

Cmplc: Infarcted testicle; sterility

Diff Dx: Torsion of appendiceal testes—a vestigial remnant on the superior/anterior aspect of the testis (look here for a blue dot = infarction), it is pedunculated and may infarct, conservative (pain meds, ice, support) and surgical treatment both appropriate; appendicitis; epididymitis

Lab:
- U/A; CBC with diff
- X-ray (Clin Radiol 1999:343): duplex U/S (Urology 1984:41) vs. testicular (radionucleotide) scan (Br J Urol 1995:628) may be helpful if symptoms >24 hours, but do not do this in pts with acute presentations in lieu of surgical consult (J Urol 1995:1508)

ED Rx:
- Once suspected, urologic/surgical consult (J Urol 1997:1196)
- IV access, pain control
- May attempt manual detorsion using conscious sedation protocols (midazolam, morphine) with gentle lateral/outward rotation; stop/reverse course if seems to worsen; endpoint is pain relief and this does not obviate the need for surgical exploration

27.4 URETHRITIS (MALES)

Jama 1981:381; Sex Transm Infect 1999:S9

Cause: *Chlamydia trachomatis*, *Neisseria gonorrhea*, less commonly *Ureaplasma urealyticum*; and many other less common pathogens (Sex Transm Dis 1991:76)

Epidem: Exact numbers difficult—1/3 of males with chlamydia and 2/3 of males with GC have no symptoms

Pathophys: An STD; GC septicemia more common in those strains with fewer genitourinary symptoms

Sx: Penile discharge or dysuria

Si: Tenderness over shaft or glans of penis; attempt to milk urethra for discharge; check for inguinal adenopathy

Crs: GC with ~7-day latent period; some may go onto chronic urethritis that is probably due to some degree of prostatitis, although antibiotic compliance, noninfectious inflammation, unusual organism, or resistant organism are also possibilities (J Infect Dis 1988:1098)

Cmplc: Epididymitis; sterility; GC may lead to rash, polyarthralgias with negative joint tap (immune complex disease), endocarditis, septicemia

Diff Dx: Reiter's syndrome

Lab: Gram's stain of penile discharge will show >4 polys/HPF—if no gram-negative diplococci, presumptive chlamydia; U/A may show white cells; these screening tests have poor sensitivity and specificity for disease (as well as the clinical sign of discharge) (Sex Transm Dis 1995:244). Do GC/chlamydia probe on all before obtaining U/A; consider culture if treatment failure—100% specific, 75% sensitive. Consider syphilis (RPR, VDRL) and HIV testing

ED Rx: All partners should be tested, barrier methods for birth control, report to State Public Health Office if appropriate, and the specific following treatments:

GC

- Ceftriaxone 125–250 mg IM × 1, treats syphilis, and both pharyngeal and resistant GC, or
- Cefixime 400 mg po × 1, or
- Cefpodoxime 200 mg po × 1, or
- Ciprofloxacin 500 mg po × 1, although not effective against syphilis and resistance appearing, or
- Ofloxacin 400 mg po × 1, or
- Second-line Rx with spectinomycin 2 g IM × 1—good if PCN allergy, but not effective against syphilis or vs. GC pharyngitis, resistance developing in Army where used as first-line drug in Korea
- If complications with septicemia or arthritis, hospitalize, and tap joint—irrigate joint if clinically worsens. Give 10 million U aqueous PCN until afebrile × 3 days, then 7 days of cefoxitin 1 g qid IV, or spectinomycin 2 g bid IM

Chlamydia

- Tetracycline 500 mg po qid × 7 days, 250 mg po qid × 14–21 days; or doxycycline 100 mg po bid × 7 days; or azithromycin (Zithromax) 1 g po × 1; or ciprofloxacin 500 mg po bid or ofloxacin 200 mg po bid × 7 days (Sex Transm Dis 1989:7); or minocycline 100 mg po qhs × 7 days

Index

Abdominal wall hernia, 90
Acalculous cholecystitis, 71
ACE inhibitors
  in acute coronary syndromes,
    12
  in CHF, 20
Acetaminophen overdose, 303
Acetazolamide
  in altitude illness, 54
  in pseudotumor cerebri, 178
Acetylcysteine, 305
ACLS guidelines, 300
Acquired angioedema, 2
ACTH, 231
Acute angle closure glaucoma,
  208
Acute coronary syndromes, 7
Acute leukemia, 113
Acute mountain sickness, 53
Acute renal failure, 159
Acute serotonin syndrome, 168
Acute tubular necrosis, 159
Addison's disease, 43
Adenosine, in PSVT, 31
Adrenal insufficiency, 43
Adrenoleukodystrophy, 44
Airway management, 270
Albuterol
  in asthma, 286
  in bronchiolitis, 251
  in COPD, 290
Allergic conjunctivitis, 209
Allopurinol, 231
Altitude illness, 52

Aminophylline
  in anaphylaxis, 2
  in asthma, 286
  in CHF, 20
  in COPD, 290
  in heart block, 22
Amiodarone in atrial fibrillation, 16
  in Vfib, 38
  in Vtach, 37
Amrinone in CHF, 19
Anaphylaxis, 1
Aneurysm
  abdominal aorta, 87
  in acute coronary syndrome, 9
  thoracic aorta, 33
Angioedema, 2
Angioneurotic edema, 5
Ankle dislocation , 217
Ankle fracture, 223
Antacids in PUD, 84
Anterior spinal cord syndrome, 194
Antibiotics
  in acute OM, 241
  in acute rheumatic fever, 296
  in asthma, 287
  in bites, 263
  in CAP, 289
  in cat scratch disease, 253
  in chronic OM, 242
  in complicated UTI, 167
  in COPD, 290
  in dental infection, 39
  in diarrhea, 78
  in epididymitis, 328

Antibiotics (*cont.*)
  in epiglottitis, 235
  in febrile neutropenia, 118
  in Fournier gangrene, 128
  in gallbladder disease, 71
  in gastroenteritis, 70
  in infectious endocarditis, 26
  in lyme disease, 135
  in meningitis, 138
  in parotitis, 243
  in periorbital cellulitis, 140
  in peritonsillar abscess, 244
  in pharyngitis, 246
  in PID, 103
  in retropharyngeal abscess, 247
  in serous OM, 242
  in sinusitis, 248
  in STDs, 108
  in syphilis, 147
  in tetanus, 148
  in uncomplicated UTI, 166
  in urethritis, 331
  in vaginitis, 111
Anticoagulation, in Afib, 17
Antidepressants, overdose, 305
Antidiarrheals, 78
Antifungals, in vaginitis, 112
Antihistamines, in urticaria, 6
Antiphospholipid antibodies, 124
Antivirals
  in Bell's palsy, 176
  in encephalitis, 181
  in urticaria, 6
Anusol HC, in hemorrhoids, 97
Apgar score, 300, 301
Appendicitis, 88
Aspirated foreign body, 284
Aspirin
  in acute coronary syndromes, 12
  in CVA, 173
Asthma, 285
Atherosclerosis, 7
Atrial fibrillation/flutter, 15
Atropine in heart block, 22

Automatic external defibrillators, 37
Avulsed tooth, 41

Babesiosis, 135
Bacillary angiomatosis, 253
Barotrauma, 233
Bartholin cyst abscess, 99
Behçet's syndrome, 297
Bejel, 146
Bell's palsy, 176
Benign paroxysmal positional vertigo,
    249
Benzodiazepines
  in acute serotonin syndrome, 169
  overdose, 309
  in vertigo, 250
Benzyl alcohol, in local anesthesia, 264
Beta blockers
  in acute coronary syndromes, 12
  in atrial fibrillation, 16
  in CHF, 20
  in thyroid storm, 50
Bipap, in CHF, 19
Bites, 262
Blindness
  atraumatic, 214
  traumatic, 214
Boerhaave syndrome, 66
Bowel obstruction, 89
Breech delivery, 203
Bromocriptine, in NMS, 190
Bronchiolitis, 250
Brown-Sequard syndrome, 194
Brugada syndrome, 36
Bupivicaine, in local anesthesia, 264
Burns, 319
Bursitis, 215
Button battery ingestion, 65

CABG, 13
Calcium channel blockers
  in atrial fibrillation, 16
  in CHF, 20
Canalith repositioning procedure, 250

Candidiasis, vaginal, 110
Carbon monoxide overdose, 310
Cardiac angioplasty, 13
Cardiac markers, 10
Cardiac stress test, 7
Cardiac tamponade, 28, 29
Cardiomyopathy, 26
Carotid sinus massage, 17
Carpal bones fracture, 227
Carvedilol, in CHF, 20
Cat scratch disease, 252
Catamenial pneumothorax, 292
Cauda equina syndrome, 115
CD4 cell lymphopenia syndrome, 131
Central apnea in CHF, 18
Central cord syndrome, 194
Cerebrovascular accident, 169
Cervical adenitis, 252
Cervical spine injury, 322
Chancroid, 105
Child abuse, 253
Chlamydia, 102, 105
Cholecystitis, 70
Cholelithiasis, 70
Cholinergic urticaria, 5
Cicatrizing conjunctivitis, 209
Ciguatera, 69
Cimetidine in anaphylaxis, 2
Clavicle fracture, 226
CNS/spinal cord neoplasms, 114
Cocaine
    in acute coronary syndromes, 7
    intoxication, 281
Colchicine, 231
Cold urticaria, 5
Community acquired pneumonia, 287
Compartment syndrome, 325
Concussion, 183
Congestive heart failure, 18
Conjunctivitis, 209
Conscious sedation, 274
Constrictive pericarditis, 29
Conus medullaris syndrome, 115
COPD, 289

Corneal abrasion, 210
Corneal foreign body, 210
Corticosporin otic suspension, 234
Corticosteroids
    in acute rheumatic fever, 296
    in adrenal insufficiency, 44
    in altitude illness, 54
    in anaphylaxis, 2
    in asthma, 286
    in Behçet's syndrome, 298
    in Bell's palsy, 176
    in bronchiolitis, 252
    for CNS mass effects, 115
    in COPD, 290
    in croup, 255
    in encephalitis, 181
    in envenomations, 4
    in epiglottitis, 235
    in increased ICP, 178
    in meningitis, 138
    in migraine headache, 189
    in pericarditis, 29
    in pharyngitis, 246
    in spinal cord injury, 195
    in temporal arteritis, 299
    in vertigo, 250
Craniopharyngioma, 115
Cricothyrotomy, 273
Croup, 254
Cryoprecipitate, 123
Cyanide overdose, 310
Cyclobenzaprine, 305
Cyproheptadine, in acute serotonin
        syndrome, 169
Cyproheptadine, in urticaria, 6

Dantrolene, in NMS, 190
Defibrillation
    in Vfib, 38
    in Vfib, biphasic, 38
    in Vtach, 37
    in Vtach, biphasic, 37
Dehydration, 46
Delirium, 279

Dental block, 267
Dental infection, 39
Dental trauma, 41
Dermatan sulfate in DIC, 117
Dermatographia, 5
Desmopressin in DI, 47
Diabetes insipidus, 46
Diabetic ketoacidosis, 44
Dialysis complications, 160
Diarrhea, 76
Diastolic dysfunction, in CHF, 18
Digit dislocation, 217
Digital blocks, 265
Digital intubation, 271
Digitalis overdose, 312
Digoxin
  in atrial fibrillation, 16
  in CHF, 20
Dihydroergotamine, in migraine
      headache, 188
Dimenhydrinate, in vertigo, 250
Diphenhydramine
  in anaphylaxis, 2
  in envenomations, 4
  in local anesthesia, 264
Dislocations, 216-219
Disseminated intravascular
      coagulation, 116
Diuretics, in CHF, 20
Diverticulitis, 64
Dobutamine
  in CHF, 19
  in Shock, 32
Dofetilide
  in atrial fib, 16
  in CHF, 20
Dopamine
  in CHF, 20
  in Shock, 32
Dressler syndrome, 9
Duodenal ulcer, 82

EACA, 175
Echocardiogram, 11

Eclampsia (toxemia), 206
Ectopic pregnancy, 197
Ehrlichiosis, 135
EKG, in acute coronary syndrome, 11
Elbow dislocation, 217
Elbow fracture, 226
Electrical cardioversion
  in atrial fibrillation, 17
  in PSVT, 31
  in stable Vtach, 38
Electrical injury, 55
  and cardiac arrhythmias, 55
Embolic CVA, 170
EMLA in local anesthesia, 265
Encephalitis, 178
  tick-borne, 178
Encopresis, 256
Envenomations, 3
Epididymitis, 327
Epidural abscess, 181
Epiglottitis, 234
Epinephrine
  in anaphylaxis, 2
  in local anesthesia, 264
  in shock, 32
  in Vfib, 38
Epistaxis
  anterior, 236
  posterior, 237
  thrombocytopenia, 237
Erythema multiforme, 6
Esophageal detector devices, 273
Esophageal foreign body, 65
Esophageal rupture, 66
Esophageal varices, 67
Ethanol intoxication, 281
Ethylene glycol overdose, 313

Facial bones fracture, 228
Factor replacement, in hemophilia,
      119
Febrile neutropenia, 117
Febrile seizures, 192
Femur fracture, 224

Fiberoptic airway devices, 274
Fibula fracture, 224
Filiforms and followers, 164
Flumazenil, 309
Foot fracture, 223
Foreign body
    aural, 238
    nasal, 237
    pharyngeal, 238
Fournier Gangrene, 127
Fractures, 219–229
    Salter classification, 220
Franklin's disease, 3
Fresh frozen plasma, 122
Friderichsen-Waterhouse syndrome, 43
Frostbite, 56

G IIb/IIIa agents, in acute coronary
        syndromes, 12
Gamow bag, 54
Gardenerella, 110
Gastric ulcer, 82
Gastroenteritis, 68
Glasgow coma scale, 301, 302
Glioma, 115
Glucagon, in esophageal foreign body,
        66
Gonorrhea, 102, 105
Gout, 229
Graves disease, 50
Green goddess, 84
Guillain-Barre, 142
Gum elastic bougie, 272

H2 blockers, in PUD, 84
Hand digits fracture, 228
Hashimoto thyroiditis, 49
Head trauma, 182
Heart block, 21
Heat exhaustion, 57
Heat stroke, 58
Heat urticaria, 5
Heat-related illness, 57
Helicobacter pylori, 83

Heliox
    in asthma, 286
    in croup, 255
HELLP syndrome, 207
Hemolytic-uremic syndrome, 69
Hemophilia, 118
Hemoptysis, massive, 291
Hemorrhagic conjunctivitis, 209
Hemorrhagic CVA, 170
Heparin
    in acute coronary syndromes, 12
    in CVA, 173
    in DIC, 117
    in DVT, 126
    in pulmonary embolus, 294
Hepatitis, 72–76
Hepatitis B exposure, 76
Herpes simplex virus, 105
Herpetic keratitis, 211
High altitude cerebral edema (HACE),
        53
High altitude pulmonary edema
        (HAPE), 53
Hip dislocation, 217
Hirschsprung's disease, 255
HIV, 128
    complications, 130
    testing, 132
    treatments, 132, 133
HTLV infection, 131
Human papilloma virus, 105
Humerus fracture, 226
Hydrocortisone
    in adrenal insufficiency, 44
    in shock, 32
    in thyroid storm, 51
Hydroxyzine in urticaria, 6
Hypercalcemia, 150
Hyperkalemia, 155
Hypermagnesemia, 152
Hypernatremia, 158
Hyperosmolar states, 46
Hyperphosphatemia, 154
Hypertension, 22

Hypocalcemia, 150
Hypoglycemia, 47
  glucagon, 48
  glucose, 48
  thiamine, 48
Hypokalemia, 154
Hypomagnesemia, 152
Hyponatremia, 156
Hypophosphatemia, 153
Hyporeninemic hypoaldosteronism, 44
Hypothermia, 59
Hysterical seizures, 192

Ibutilide, 16
Immunoglobulin, in Kawasaki disease,
      259
Incision and drainage, dental, 40
Increased intracerebral pressure, 177
Indomethacin, 231
Infectious conjunctivitis, 209
Infectious endocarditis, 25
Inferior wall MI, 13
Insulin
  in acute coronary syndromes, 13
  in diabetic ketoacidosis, 45
Intoxication, 280
Intraosseus technique, 276
Intussusception, 257
Ipratropium
  in asthma, 286
  in COPD, 290
Iritis, 212
Iron overdose, 314
Ischemic bowel, 92
Isoniazid overdose, 315
Isopropranolol intoxication, 281
Isoproterenol
  in CHF, 20
  in Shock, 32

Kawasaki disease, 258
Ketorolac in renal colic, 162
Kleihauer-Betke, 196
Knee dislocation, 217

Knee fracture, 224
Kussmaul sign
  in pericarditis, 28
  in right ventricular infarct, 13

Labetalol
  in hypertension, 24
  in increased ICP, 178
Laryngeal mask airway, 270
Lead overdose, 316
LET, in local anesthesia, 265
Lidocaine
  in local anesthesia, 264
  in migraine headache, 189
  in stable Vtach, 38
  in TCA overdose, 306
  in Vfib, 37
  in Vtach, 37
  viscous, in local anesthesia, 265
Light/solar urticaria, 5
Lightning injuries, 61
Lilly cyanide antidote kit, 311
Limb presentation deliveries, 204
Lithium, in thyroid storm, 51
Liver markers, in hepatitis, 74
Low back pain, 185
Lower GI bleed, 78
Lown-Ganong-Levine syndrome, 30
Lugol's solution, in thyroid storm, 51
LVH, in hypertension, 23
Lyme disease, 134

Magnesium sulfate
  in acute coronary syndromes, 13
  in asthma, 286
  in COPD, 290
  in Vtach, 37
Malignant bowel obstruction, 90
Malignant hypertension, 23
Mallory-Weiss tear, 86
Mandibular fracture, 228
Mannitol, in increased ICP, 178
Meckel's diverticulum, 82
Meclizine in vertigo, 250

Medical screening exam, 282
Medulloblastoma, 115
Meniere's disease, 250
Meningiomas, 115
Meningitis, 136
    aseptic, 137
    CSF, 138
    pathogens, 136
Metabolic acidosis, 149
Metacarpals fracture, 227
Methanol intoxication, 281
Metoclopramide, in migraine
        headache, 188
Midazolam, in envenomations, 4
Migraine headache, 187
Moxonidine, in CHF, 20
Multifocal atrial tachycardia, 15
Mycobacterium marinum, 232
Myocarditis, 26
Myoglobinuria, 191
Myxedema coma, 49

Narcotic intoxication, 282
Nasal pharyngeal airway, 270
Nasotracheal intubation, 271
Near drowning, 62
Necrotizing gingivitis, 39
Nephrogenic DI, treatment, 47
Nephrolithiasis, 161
Nerve blocks, 265
Neuroleptic malignant syndrome, 189
Neurosyphilis, 145
Nitroglycerin
    in acute coronary syndrome, 13
    in CHF, 19
    in esophageal FB, 65
    in esophageal varices, 67
Nitroprusside
    in CHF, 19
    in hypertension, 24
    in increased ICP, 178
    in thoracic aortic dissections, 34
Nitrous oxide, in migraine headache,
    189

Non-Q-wave MI, 14
Nonketotic hyperosmolar coma, 47
Norepinephrine, in shock, 32
NSAIDs, 307

Octreotide
    in esophageal varices, 67
    in upper GI bleed, 86
Oral lacerations, 40
Oral pharyngeal airway, 270
Orotracheal intubation, 271
Otitis externa, 238
Otitis media, 240
Ovarian cyst rupture, 100
Ovarian torsion, 101

Pacing in heart block, 22
Packed red cell transfusion, 123
Pancreatitis, 79
Paradoxical pulse, 28
Parkland formula, burns, 321
Parotid duct stone, 242
Parotitis, 242
Patella dislocation, 218
Pathogens
    in diarrhea, 77
    in gastroenteritis, 68
Pediatric bladder catheterization, 276
Peliosis hepatitis, 253
Pelvic inflammatory disease, 102
Pelvis fracture, 224
Peptic ulcer disease/gastritis, 82
Perforated viscus, 93
Pericarditis, 28
Perimortem delivery, 199
Periodontal abscess, 39
Periorbital cellulitis, 139
Perirectal abscess, 95
Peritonitis, 140
Peritonsillar abscess, 243
Peritonsillar cellulitis, 244
Pharyngitis, 245
Phenylephrine, in shock, 32
Pilonidal cyst abscess, 96

Placenta previa, 200
Placental abruption, 200
Platelet transfusion, 123
Pneumothorax, 292
Postobstructive diuresis, 164
Postphlebitic syndrome, 125
Precipitous delivery, 201
Precordial thump, 37
Preeclampsia, 206
Premature ventricular contractions, 35
Pressure injection injuries, 326
Priapism, 328
Probenecid, 231
Procainamide
  in stable Vtach, 38
  in Vfib, 38
  in Vtach, 37
Prochlorperazine, in migraine headache, 188
Proctitis, 85
Prolapsed cord, obstetrics, 204
Propafenone, in atrial fibrillation, 16
Protein C deficiency, 124
Protein S deficiency, 124
Proton-pump inhibitor, in PUD, 84
Pseudo-angioedema, 2
Pseudogout, 229
Pseudomonas pseudomallei (melioidosis), 45
Pseudotumor cerebri, 177
PTU, in thyroid storm, 51
Pulmonary embolus, 293
Pulseless electrical activity, 21, 37
Puncture wounds, 268
Pyelonephritis, 165
Pyloric stenosis, 259

Rabies, 142
Racemic epinephrine
  in bronchiolitis, 251
  in croup, 255
Radius/ulna fracture, 227
Ramsay-Hunt syndrome, 176

Ranson criteria, in pancreatitis, 80, 81
Rapid sequence intubation, 272
Renal-ocular syndrome, 213
Respiratory syncytial virus, 251
Restraint, chemical and physical, 278
Retrograde intubation, 273
Retropharyngeal abscess, 246
Reversible ischemic neurologic deficit, 172
Rewarming, in hypothermia, 60
Rhabdomyolysis, 326
Rheumatic fever, acute, 296
Rhinitis, 248
Rib fracture, 225
Right ventricular infarct, 13
Ruptured globe, 213

Salicylates
  in acute rheumatic fever, 296
  in Behçet's syndrome, 298
  in Kawasaki disease, 259
  overdose, 307
Saterinone, in CHF, 19
Scapula fracture, 226
SCIWORA, 322
Sclerosing peritonitis, 141
Scombroid, 69
Scorpion stings, 4
Seizures, 191
  outpatient treatment, 193
Sengstaaken-Blakemore tube, 68, 86
Sepsis, 143
Septic arthritis, 231
Septic shock, 143
Sexual assault, 103
  exam, 104
  lab evaluation, 104
  post-exam treatment, 104
Sexually transmitted disease, 105
Shaken baby syndrome, 182
Shock, 31
Shoulder dislocation, 218

Shoulder dystocia, 205
  and McRobert's maneuver, 205
  and Woods screw maneuver, 205
  and Zavenelli maneuver, 206
Shoulder fracture, 226
Sick sinus syndrome, 16
Sickle cell crisis, 121
Sickle cell disease, 120
Silver slider, 84
Sinusitis, 248
Slow ventricular tachycardia, 36
Snake bites, 4
Sodium bicarbonate
  in diabetic ketoacidosis, 45
  in local anesthesia, 264
  in TCA overdose, 306
Somatostatin
  in esophageal varices, 67
  in upper GI bleed, 86
Sotalol, in Vtach, 37
Spider bites, 4
Spinal cord injury, 194
Spinal shock, 194
St. John's wort, 305
Stanford classification of thoracic
    aorta, 34
Status epilepticus, 191
  treatment, 193
Stiff man syndrome, 148
Stress test, in acute coronary
    syndrome, 11
Stress urticaria, 5
Subluxed tooth, 41
Sudden death, 36
Sudden infant death syndrome, 260
Sulfinpyrazone, 231
Sumatriptan, in migraine headache,
    189
Superficial phlebitis, 125
Supraventricular tachycardia, 30
SVT, with aberrancy, 36
Syphilis, 144
Systemic inflammatory response, 143
Systolic dysfunction, in CHF, 18

Tabes dorsalis, 145
TAC, in local anesthesia, 265
Temporal arteritis, 298
Tendonitis, 215
Tension pneumothorax, 293
Testicular torsion, 329
Tetanus, 147
Tetralogy of Fallot, 256
Theophylline overdose, 317
Thiamine, in CHF, 20
Thoracic aortic dissection, 34
Thrombolytics
  in acute coronary syndrome, 12
  in CVA, 173
  in pulmonary embolus, 295
Thrombosed rectal hemorrhoids, 97
Thrombotic CVA, 169
Thyroid replacement, 49
Thyroid storm, 50
Tibia fracture, 224
Tobacco use, 8
Toe digits fracture, 223
Torsades de Pointes, 38
Transfusion guidelines, 122
Transient ischemic attack, 172
Transient synovitis, 232
Translaryngeal insufflation, 273
Transvaginal ultrasound, 198
Trichomonas, 110
Trimethaphan, in aortic dissection,
    34
Tympanic membrane perforation, 233

Universal precautions (hepatitis), 76
Unstable angina, 14
Upper extremity DVT, 125
Upper GI hemorrhage, 85
Uremic pericarditis, 29
Urethritis, 330
Urinary retention, 163
Urinary tract infection, 164
  and indwelling catheter, 166
Urticaria, 5
Uterine rupture, 196

Vaginitis, 110
Vasopressin
  in shock, 32
  Vfib, 38
Venous thrombosis, 124
Ventricular fibrillation, 35
Ventricular shunt management, 276
Ventricular tachycardia, 35
Vertebral body fractures, 225

Vertigo, 249
Vitamin A, in encephalitis, 179

Wandering atrial pacemaker, 15
Water deficit calculation, 47
Wolff-Parkinson-White syndrome, 15
Word catheter, 99
Wound management, 267
Wound repair, 268

Yaws, 146